MARY ADELAIDE NUTTING

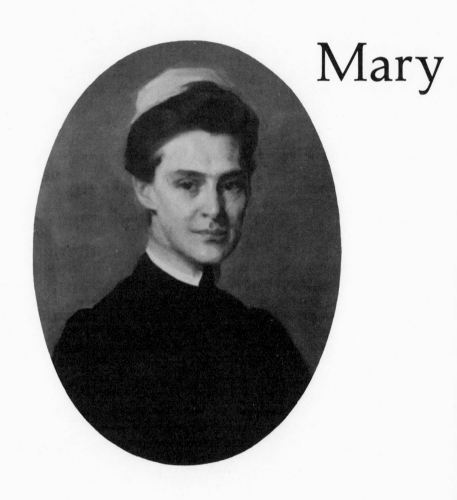

Mary

Adelaide Nutting

PIONEER OF MODERN NURSING

HELEN E. MARSHALL

THE JOHNS HOPKINS UNIVERSITY PRESS
BALTIMORE AND LONDON

Frontispiece: Portrait of Adelaide Nutting by
Cecelia Beaux, 1906, courtesy of the author.

The Johns Hopkins University Press, Baltimore, Maryland 21218
The Johns Hopkins University Press Ltd., London

Library of Congress Catalog Card Number 72-174557
ISBN 0-8018-1365-4

Contents

Foreword

In a letter to a former student, Adelaide Nutting wrote that she "could hardly wish her anything more satisfying than the discovery of the heroisms, the devoted labors and superb achievements of those nurses whom our beloved calling has built up."[1] Miss Nutting's own life was one of dedication and achievement. She was a woman of rare charm and dignity, with a gift for friendship. She had intelligence, vision, an insatiable desire for knowledge, determination, and ideals, as well as ideas and a remarkable sense of timing, and was ready when opportunities to advance nursing arose.

For years after Miss Nutting retired, friends urged her to write her memoirs and tell of her work in behalf of nursing and nursing education, but she always brushed aside the suggestion, saying there was more immediate work to be done. Like Florence Nightingale, Miss Nutting had a penchant for consistently saving materials of historical import: first her notebooks as a student, later her own lecture notes, various drafts of articles that she wrote and speeches that she made, committee reports, clippings and scrapbooks, travel itineraries, programs of meetings, carefully annotated quotations that impressed her, and great files of correspondence with nursing leaders, friends, former students, and members of her family. At the insistence of Isabel Stewart, she wrote a few pages of pertinent facts about her family and childhood that might later be helpful in writing the story of her life. Later on a weekend holiday in Atlantic City, Miss Stewart jotted down answers Miss Nutting gave to questions about her education and choice of nursing as a career.

After Miss Nutting's death a group of women, led by Isabel Stewart and Mary Roberts, who were cognizant of her role in building nursing into a profession and who realized the significance of her

[1] Adelaide Nutting (New York) to Amy Miller (Baltimore, Maryland). 1930, MAN Papers.

papers, set about to conserve them and to add other pertinent letters and reminiscences in the hope that a biography of the great nursing leader might be written. Virginia Dunbar, dean emeritus of the New York–Cornell University School of Nursing and a graduate of The Johns Hopkins Hospital School of Nursing, was a graduate student at Teachers College, Columbia University, and became acquainted with Miss Nutting in her emeritus years; she meticulously collated the correspondence between Miss Stewart and Miss Nutting and indexed and typed the Nutting family papers. The work of these "Friends of Adelaide Nutting" facilitated the writing of this biography, which was supported in whole by the U.S. Public Health Service, under grant NU 0017–01. Research was conducted in the New York City Public Library; The Johns Hopkins University Library, The Johns Hopkins Medical Library, the Library of The Johns Hopkins Hospital School of Nursing, and the Enoch Pratt Free Library, Baltimore; The National Archives, the Library of Congress, and the National Red Cross Library, Washington, D.C.; the National Medical Library (formerly the Surgeon General's Medical Library), Bethesda, Maryland; Butler Library and Teachers College Library, Columbia University, New York; and the Public Library, Waterloo, Quebec, Canada.

I am grateful to all who have assisted in any way in the preparation of this biography. Special acknowledgments are due Dr. Robert G. Bone, president of Illinois State University, and Dr. Arthur H. Larsen, dean, who made possible my two-year leave from the Department of History; Dr. Eleanor Lambertsen, director of the Division of Nursing Education, Teachers College, Columbia University, who provided office space and unrestricted access to departmental records; Mrs. Mary S. Price, director of The Johns Hopkins Hospital School of Nursing, for the hospitality of Hampton House and access to school records; Mrs. Anne Cohen, Nurses' Library, The Johns Hopkins School of Nursing; Mrs. Dorothea S. Robertson, executive secretary, The Johns Hopkins Nurses Alumnae Association; Mrs. Lois Miller, librarian, American Journal of Nursing Company; Inez Haynes, director of the National League of Nursing; Dr. Faye Abdellah, assistant surgeon general, U.S. Public Health Service, for her interest and encouragement; Mrs. Alice J. Buckland, Waterloo, Quebec; and Mrs. Duncan Campbell, Mangrove Bay, Bermuda.

Effie Taylor, Anna Wolf, Stella Goostray, Mrs. Rachel Louise Metcalf McManus, Lillian A. Hudson, and Mrs. Jessie Black McVicar have shared with me memories of their association with Miss Nutting as colleagues and former students. Isabel Stewart bequeathed notes that have been invaluable.

Virginia Dunbar has read the entire manuscript and given valuable assistance relative to sources, content, and the history of nursing and nursing education. Anne Austin, who collaborated with Isabel Stewart in the last revision of the Nutting and Dock *History of Nursing* contributed important side-lights on the friendships of Miss Nutting, Isabel Stewart, Lavinia Dock, Annie Goodrich, and other leaders in nursing. Dr. Isabella Harris has made helpful suggestions as to style.

Adelaide Nutting was a proud and devoted nurse, a farsighted and inspiring teacher, and a leader in her profession. This study seeks to bring to subsequent generations a sense of commitment and kinship with one of America's most useful women.

HELEN E. MARSHALL

MARY ADELAIDE NUTTING

I

Frost Village, 1858–1881

Winter had come early to the Eastern Townships of Canada. Vespasion Nutting turned the logs in the fireplace and as the flames leaped high, a warm glow fell across the room where his ashen-faced wife lay with a tiny new-born baby close to her side. This baby was small and frail, like her first baby, Ella Frances, who had died eleven years before. Harriet Nutting loved her sturdy sons, Charles now nearly nine, four-year-old Arthur, and Jim barely two, and she prayed this daughter might be spared.

Vespasion led his sons in to see their sister. Harriet smiled wanly as the boys clustered at her bedside and looked in wonderment at the pink and wrinkled face. Vespasion lifted Jim so that he might more easily see the sleeping baby. For several minutes they stood there in silence; then Arthur, awed and uncertain, looked up to his older brother. Charles bent over and kissed his mother, then Arthur kissed her, and Jim leaned over as if to touch the baby. By nightfall there was not a household in Frost Village that had not heard of the Nuttings' new baby.[1]

Slowly the child's cheeks began to fill out and the voice grew stronger, more persistent. With the first thaw of spring, Harriet decided that her daughter should be baptized, and she reminded her husband that the names of the other children had not yet been inscribed on the church rolls. Vespasion did not agree with the Reverend David Lindsay, rector of the Frost Village church, on matters of religion, but he concurred in his wife's decision. On March 8, 1859, Harriet Nutting took the four children to the small, gray stone church with the white spire, and in the presence of the rector's wife, had Mary Adelaide and her three brothers baptized and their names writ-

[1] *Advertiser and Eastern Townships Sentinel* (Waterloo, Canada East), November 11, 1858, p. 4 (hereinafter cited as *Waterloo Advertiser*).

1

ten in the Register of Marriages, Baptisms, Births, and Burials of the local parish.[2]

The families of Vespasion Nutting and Harriet Peasley were United Empire Loyalists. The Nuttings came from Groton, Massachusetts, where the family plied the trade of shoemaking. Vespasion Nutting was the son of George Veraines Nutting, and the grandson of Loyalist Captain David Nutting, who settled near Mansonville, Quebec. George Veraines Nutting was married to Elizabeth Blanchard in nearby Potton in 1793; there Vespasion, one of their six children, was born November 3, 1816.[3]

Harriet Sophia Peasley was the daughter of Moses Peasley and his second wife, Polly Ayers, and the granddaughter of Jonathan Peasley, who moved to Canada from Ware, New Hampshire, in 1801. Moses Peasley and Polly Ayers were married on October 16, 1806, and were the parents of eight children. Their sixth child, Harriet Sophia, was born July 3, 1824, in Bolton, Quebec.[4]

When Vespasion Nutting was sixteen, he went to Lowell, Massachusetts, to perfect his skill in shoemaking. After serving an apprenticeship he set up a shop of his own. On June 25, 1845, he married Harriet Sophia Peasley. He was twenty-nine; she was twenty-one.

Harriet Peasley was a beautiful woman with a fine carriage and an alert mind, and she was clever with her hands. In addition to the housewifely arts of cooking, sewing, carding, spinning, and knitting, her mother had trained her in the woods and garden remedies to be used in sickness: mandrake for gargle; syrup of spikenard for coughs and colds; catnip, tansy, and hop teas for stomach ache and indigestion. Harriet loved beauty, in nature, in fabrics, in style and line, music and poetry. Books were her great delight. As a mother she was devoted and ambitious.

Vespasion Nutting was a religious man, skilled in his trade, but easygoing. On a fine day in spring he set out with his fishing rod, in

[2] "Charles Albert, born August 7, 1849; Arthur Knowlton, born February 23, 1854; James Peasley, born August 1, 1856; Mary Adelaide, born November 1, 1858. Children of Vespasion Nutting and his wife, Harriet Sophia Peasley, baptized by David Lindsay, Rector. Parents were sponsors, witnesses: Sophia Lindsay and H. S. Peasley [Nutting]." Certified copy, Register of Marriages, Births, and Burials, Parish Church of St. Luke's County of Shefford, Quebec, Canada, 1859, fol. 10, Mary Adelaide Nutting Papers (hereinafter cited as MAN Papers).

[3] John Keep Nutting, *Nutting Genealogy: A Record of the Descendants of John Nutting of Groton, Massachusetts* (Syracuse, N.Y.: C. W. Borden, 1908), pp. 70 and 104; F. H. Parkin (Mansonville, Quebec) to Charles A. Nutting (Waterloo, Quebec), March 20, 1908, MAN Papers.

[4] Adelaide Nutting, "The Peasley Family Record," MAN Papers.

fall with his gun.[5] He had a good voice, and between stints of shoe-making, repairing, and gardening he conducted singing schools. Although he was a careful workman, he was scarcely able to provide the barest necessities for his wife and children. Seeking a more advantageous location, he moved his family in 1854 to Frost Village, about twenty miles from the community in which he grew up.[6]

The Nuttings lived in Frost Village for seven years, but their financial situation failed to improve, and in order to provide more for the children, Harriet Nutting began to sew and do millinery work for her more affluent neighbors.

As the town of Waterloo, three miles away on the Yamaska River, began to develop and expand after the advent of two railroads there, families began to leave Frost Village. In 1861 R. W. Laing moved his academy to Waterloo. Gone too was the Mechanics Institute and Library Association, which had given a certain tone to Frost Village through its books and occasional lecturers. Because the children had to go to school, Harriet Nutting decided the family would have to move to Waterloo.

Harriet Nutting appealed to Seth Huntington, an influential man in the Eastern Townships for help. He had established himself in Waterloo in 1856 and founded the town's first newspaper, *The Advertiser and Eastern Townships Sentinel.*[7] In addition to politics, he was interested in railroads and milling. Was there not some job he could find for Vespasion in Waterloo? People were buying factory-made shoes, and Vespasion, once proud of his craft, was now little more than a cobbler. Huntington, who admired and respected Mrs. Nutting, agreed to do whatever he could to help her husband.

Vespasion lost no time preparing to move his family to Waterloo. He bought a narrow and inexpensive lot near the eastern end of the town's principal street.[8] In the rear it sloped gently to the river. Across the river was a grove of trees and in the distance were the Shefford Mountains. Close to the street he built a modest brick house. By late

[5] Adelaide Nutting, "Notes for Story of Life," *ibid.*; Isabel M. Stewart, "Reminiscences of Mary Adelaide Nutting, Atlantic City, New Jersey, April 17, 1940," Nutting–Stewart Correspondence (hereinafter cited as MAN–IMS Correspondence); Isabel M. Stewart, "I Remember," Isabel Maitland Stewart Papers (hereinafter cited as IMS Papers).

[6] Obituary, "Vespasion Nutting, Esq.," *Waterloo Advertiser*, February 19, 1904; clipping, MAN Papers.

[7] George C. Foster and John P. Noyes, *Sketches of Some Early Shefford Pioneers* (Waterloo, Quebec: Public Library, 1905), p. 7; *Sherbrooke Daily Record* (Sherbrooke, Quebec), November 2, 1962.

[8] This part of the principal street was known as Main Street, but in 1964 it was changed to Foster, long the name of the western part of the thoroughfare.

summer, 1861, the family was settled in the new home, and on November 6, Harriet gave birth to a strong, healthy daughter, Harriette Armine.[9]

On December 19, a government appointment as clerk of the circuit court came through for Vespasion,[10] but it was not very remunerative and Harriet was compelled to engage in dressmaking and millinery on a more extensive scale, hiring help for the household chores and an assistant for the sewing.[11]

The Nutting boys were promptly enrolled in the local school. Because Charles was especially studious, his mother developed great ambitions for him. Arthur learned easily but soon became impatient and restive. It was too early to predict about Jim. Adelaide ("Addie") was the first to catch the usual childhood diseases and the last to recover, always requiring extra care and protection. She delighted in singing the songs her father taught her, and almost immediately assumed responsibility for her baby sister. Her mother thought she made "a perfect little mother," and hoped both of her daughters would "marry well and not always have to live under the shadow of debt and drink."

After an argument with the Reverend Lindsay over some obscure doctrine, Vespasion moved his church affiliation to the Methodist congregation, where his services as choir director were greatly appreciated, and for years he was superintendent of the Methodist Sunday School.[12] There was no argument over religion in the Nutting home. For many years Vespasion conducted daily family prayers. The children attended the Anglican church with their mother and returned home to Sunday dinner and a Methodist blessing by their father.

On Sunday afternoons the children took long walks in the woods with their father and the dog, "Mr. Pip." The boys called Minnie, robust, athletic, and impulsive, "the tomboy," and Addie, frail and delicate, "the weakling." Vespasion had a clear, observant eye. In the spring he always spied the first jack-in-the-pulpit and the places where the blue violets were bluest and the white violets thickest. He could identify the tracks of rabbits, fox, and deer, and of the smaller animals that lived in the Canadian underbrush. He knew the trees—

[9] Harriette Armine Nutting ("Minnie") named for her mother, but the spelling of the name was that preferred by her father. Armine Nutting married William Gilbert Gosling in Halifax, Nova Scotia, on January 2, 1888. She died in Bermuda on December 15, 1942.

[10] Document, MAN Papers.

[11] Mrs. Nutting's accounts with local customers and Montreal wholesale firms are among the family records, *ibid.*

[12] Adelaide Nutting, "Notes on Family History" (n.d.), *ibid.*

beech, birch, fir, pine, elm, and maple—by leaf, bark, and smell. He knew the names of birds and could identify them by song when they were hidden from sight. He taught the boys the skills and lore of the forest and stream. In the spring he and the children were likely to take a basket on their jaunts and return with mushrooms. In the summer it was blueberries, in the fall wild grapes, but always there was enough for a pie or a pot of marmalade.[13]

Each spring Vespasion Nutting planted a garden, a few acres that stretched from the woodpile back of the house to the tangled clump of alder and wild roses near the river's edge. He grew neat rows of peas and beans, potatoes, onions, marrow, beets, squash, and turnips, hearty vegetables that were good for summer eating and stored well for winter. He also planted tomatoes, corn, and cucumbers, and a few flowers for Harriet. Plump and tasty vegetables, fish, squirrel and rabbit, pheasant and partridge, wild duck and goose were Vespasion's contributions to the family larder.

Harriet dried peas, beans, and corn for winter use and carefully saved the down and soft feathers from the geese and ducks for extra pillows or comforters. Shoe-repairing and harness-mending were sometimes bartered for apples and for the maple sugar the children enjoyed so much on hot cakes and porridge. Years later Adelaide wrote, "We were poor but we were never hungry."[14]

The duties of the clerk of the court were such that Vespasion was able to handle short stints at the harness and shoe-making trades. He trained an apprentice from time to time and once managed a local hotel. With five children in school and heavy debts, he needed to earn every cent possible. Harriet was determined that Charles go to McGill University in Montreal when he finished at the local academy. Only on Sunday did she lay aside her needle and thimble. When her fingers and back ached and the fabric slipped from her hands, she would pick up a book and lose herself in the world of Shakespeare, Byron, or Carlyle. The girls would have elocution, music and drawing, and the graces suited to the society in which she herself had longed to move.

In 1872 Harriet Nutting realized one dream when Charles graduated in law from McGill University with honors. He was dignified and handsome with his fine complexion, thick black hair, and heavy moustache, and looked very much like his father before he grew a beard. Harriet visualized her son as a brilliant barrister, "Queen's Counselor," established in a fine office in Montreal, Ottawa, Quebec,

[13] Adelaide Nutting. "Notes: Conversation with Charlie while Visiting in Waterloo, August, 1929," *ibid.*
[14] Adelaide Nutting, "Notes for Family History, 1929," *ibid.*

or Toronto. He might even be elected to Parliament. She could not avoid some misgivings, therefore, when he returned to open a law office in Waterloo, where there were already twelve practicing lawyers. She suspected that red-haired Lizzie Haskell was responsible for the decision.

It was not that Harriet disliked Lizzie. Maria Elizabeth Haskell was a kindly, forthright young woman, a faithful worker in her church, and an active participant in the Temperance movement. Harriet would bide her time; she had four other children to think about.

As the younger children grew up, they became increasingly aware of the family's poverty. Arthur and Jim tried to find odd jobs around town. Charlie wanted to save his money in order to marry Lizzie Haskell. Arthur, who had no desire to be a lawyer or a doctor, was indolent in school and was allowed to leave early. His mother secured him a position with Thomas May and Company, Montreal, a firm from which she bought dressmaking and millinery supplies, hoping that he would prove to be a reliable employee.[15] Jim applied himself to his studies at Shefford Academy, but he, too, looked forward to the time when he could strike out on his own. He loved sports and fun, but was more stable than Arthur.

When Addie and Minnie passed Asa Foster's mansion, with its eight imported marble fireplaces, and the homes of Waterloo's other prosperous citizens, they were sharply conscious of the austerity and shabbiness of their own home and its hodge-podge surroundings. The simple brick house had been built near the end of a tree-shaded street. Soon, however, hotels, stores, butcher shops, and livery stables crowded in. Then, almost directly across the street, a market was built. On the first floor were meat and general food stalls; in the basement was a jail, seldom occupied. Above the market, and reached by a long, wide, outside stairway, was the spacious town hall, in which entertainment of various kinds was held. In back of the stores were piles of barrels and packing boxes, weeds, unsightly privies, and feeding troughs for farmers' horses and mules.

The wagons and buggies hitched along the street by farmers added to the dust and flies in summer and to the muddy ruts in other seasons. To the girls, Waterloo seemed very different from the Lowell their parents talked about, and the beautiful Ottawa and gay Montreal of Jim's and Charlie's letters.

At Shefford Academy the meagerness of the Nutting girls' ward-

[15] *Ibid.*

robes was in strong contrast to the expensive and beautiful garments that their mother made for their classmates.

The girls were conscientious in school. Good marks were a way of expressing appreciation for their mother's sacrifices and of maintaining self-esteem in the community, where they imagined their family was relegated to a very humble place. Learning did not always come easily for Adelaide, but she was intelligent and persistent.[16] The girls attended school parties, Sunday School picnics, toboggan parties, and sugar-offs, and despite their self-consciousness made friends among the young people of the town. Adelaide was especially devoted to Russell Huntington.[17]

When Adelaide was fifteen, she spent a year studying French and music at the convent in a nearby town. Later, for a short time, she attended a private school in Montreal, Bute House. It was typical of private schools of that day, devoting much attention to social accomplishments, French, drawing, music, and literature. Adelaide remembered with particular affection her music teacher, Monsieur Ducharme, who encouraged her to continue with voice and piano lessons.[18] The following year she spent the winter with Uncle Daniel and Aunt Helen Peasley Hamblett and their daughters, Edna Adelaide, Viola, and Alice, in Lowell, where she studied design at an art school and took private music lessons.[19]

Meanwhile, Armine continued her studies, preparing to be a teacher. After returning from Lowell, Adelaide spent the next three years helping her mother with sewing and devoting her spare time to music and drawing. A girl was hired to do household chores. All the so-called better families in Waterloo employed daughters of the French farmers to perform the menial tasks of laundering, cleaning, and stoking the fires. Mrs. Nutting reasoned that it was better to release Adelaide from exhausting household tasks and direct her limited energy into the more remunerative tasks.

In 1877, through the influence of Seth Huntington, then postmaster general of Canada, Jim Nutting secured a low-paying position in the Postal Department in Ottawa. Charlie was sufficiently established in

---

[16] Mary Manning, a niece of Lizzie Haskell Nutting, quoted Charles Nutting as saying his sister Adelaide was not brilliant in school (Mary Manning [Montreal, Canada] to Isabel M. Stewart, n.d., IMS Papers).

[17] Russell Huntington studied law at McGill University and joined the staff of the *Montreal Herald*. He died of typhoid fever in November, 1878.

[18] Adelaide Nutting, "Notes for Story of Life," MAN Papers.

[19] William H. Way (Lowell, Mass.) to Adelaide Nutting (Waterloo), June 24, 1878, *ibid*.

his law practice to support a wife modestly, and on September 5, 1878, he and Lizzie Haskell were married. They moved into a two-story house on a high rise of ground at the apex of the triangle formed by Patrick and Court streets and the Canadian Pacific tracks, and directly across from Shefford Academy.

After a year or more with Thomas May Company, Arthur lost interest in his work and returned home. His mother helped him secure a deputy clerkship under his father, but he soon gave it up, and with the opening of land in western Canada he headed for Calgary.[20]

The family's debts now amounted to something over $700, a formidable sum in those days.[21] Harriet Nutting's health was such that she could not sew as much as she had formerly, and many of her customers now shopped for materials in Montreal, so her profits were less. She did not want to ask Charlie for money; Arthur seldom kept his promise to return a loan or to help out; and Jim's salary was barely enough for himself.

The thing that troubled Harriet Nutting most was that Addie and Min were unhappy and longed for things Waterloo did not afford. Secretly she shared their feelings and sometimes felt snubbed by her more affluent neighbors.[22] After long talks with her husband and Charlie, she wrote to Jim. She proposed to rent the house in Waterloo, ship the furniture to Ottawa, rent a flat there, and keep house for him. Perhaps Addie could give music lessons and Minnie could teach elocution. By careful economy, they could all live together. She reminded her husband that Addie was twenty-three and Min twenty, and that they had had few opportunities to meet desirable young men. When old enough, most of Waterloo's promising youth left for careers in Ottawa, Montreal, Quebec, or Toronto.[23]

Vespasion, however, was loath to leave Waterloo, his clerkship, his cronies, and the Methodist choir. Charlie and Lizzie offered him an upstairs room that he could furnish.

"Perhaps you will change your mind," the girls said as they helped their mother with the packing.

Vespasion patted his dog on the head. "No," he said, "Mr. Pip and I will stay here."

[20] Adelaide Nutting, "Notes on Family History," ibid.

[21] Vespasion Nutting (Waterloo) to Adelaide Nutting (Ottawa), January 9, 1885, ibid.

[22] Harriet P. Nutting (Ottawa) to Armine Nutting (St. John's, Newfoundland) January, 1882, ibid.

[23] Harriet P. Nutting (Waterloo) to Addie and Minnie Nutting (St. John's), April 3, 1883, ibid.

II

Ottawa, 1881-1882

It was the first time in the thirty-six years that Harriet and Vespasion Nutting had been married that they had been apart for any length of time. Whatever misgivings they might have had about the breakup of their home, each was determined to make the best of the situation. Despite his weaknesses, Harriet deeply loved her husband, and letters were exchanged frequently. Jim seemed happy to have a home where he could bring his friends. Harriet was careful to let her husband know that he was welcome to join the family at any time. "Minnie," she wrote, "is quite charmed with Ottawa and so is Addie."[1]

Vespasion made no attempt to hide his loneliness. He spent most of his time in his office, except when he was doing chores for Charlie in exchange for his room and board. At the office, unless someone dropped in to chat, Vespasion read the Montreal *Witness*, *Vox*, *Truth*, and various religious papers and tracts or wrote long letters in his strong, legible hand to his wife and children. Arthur and Jim seldom answered, but he could always expect a reply from Harriet and his daughters. He tried to inject a cheerful note by relating to them the small doings about the town, the weather, Lizzie's precarious health, his own well-being, and that of "Mr. Pip." In summer he wrote of his garden and of his hunting and fishing.[2]

At the church in Ottawa, Addie's fine mezzo-soprano voice stood out well in the congregational singing. She practiced diligently, while Armine continued her studies to prepare for teaching. Neither of the girls obtained pupils, but they never regretted the move.

[1] Harriet P. Nutting (Ottawa), to Vespasion Nutting (Waterloo, Quebec), June 28, 1881, MAN Papers.

[2] Vespasion Nutting (Waterloo) to Minnie and Addie Nutting (St. John's, Newfoundland) December 12, 1882; and Harriet P. Nutting (Ottawa) to Vespasion Nutting (Waterloo), June 28, 1881; *ibid.*

Ottawa was a beautiful city with tree-lined streets bordered by rows of stone mansions or more modest homes of red brick, and its skyline was accented here and there by the spires of churches and the standpipes of factories. Especially imposing were the cream-colored Parliament buildings, with their red sandstone arches and Ohio free-stone trim, high above Wellington Street. The two-hundred-foot tower of the central building was visible from most parts of the city.

At the first opportunity Jim took his mother and sisters on a tour of Parliament Hill. He pointed out the special features of the chambers. On important nights Commons was crowded with politicians and ladies. The ceremonies of opening and closing Parliament took place in the Senate. The throne was occupied by Her Majesty's representative, the governor general, at that time the marquis of Lorne. The opening was a great event that the girls would enjoy, with the gay military uniforms, the rich dress of the ministers, the scarlet gowns of the judges of the Supreme Court, and the varied and beautiful dresses worn by the ladies. Afterward anyone who had a ticket and wore evening clothes might attend the "drawing room" and meet the representatives. Jim was quite sure he could get tickets through one of his friends. They walked past the Parliament library at the rear of the Senate to the summerhouse at the edge of the cliff, where there was a manificent view of the Ottawa River.

Down in the city the streets were crowded with delivery wagons, hansom cabs, phaetons for the rich, and horsecars for the poor, and there was the clatter of hooves and wheels on stone pavements and the clanging of bells. The store windows glistened with their displays of imported fabrics, furs, and jewels, and, though Addie and Min could not purchase, they enjoyed looking and getting ideas for working over old garments.

The girls read in the papers about the theaters and balls, so different from the Quadrille Club in Waterloo.[3] There were libraries, too, where books could be borrowed. Minnie often read aloud while Addie and Mother Nutting sewed or knitted. Sometimes they paused to discuss the possible outcome of a romance, the author's style, or to repeat a sentence or phrase that appealed to them.

When friends called, Mrs. Nutting served biscuits and tea with great éclat, as though her worn silver and china compared with the finest on Sherbrooke Street. Because living in Ottawa required the strictest economy, guests were usually invited only for tea.

Early that winter Minnie was asked to take charge of a Church of

[3] Harriet P. Nutting (Waterloo) to Adelaide Nutting (St. John's), December, 1882, *ibid.*

England School for Girls, in St. John's, Newfoundland, and despite the great distance she decided to accept the offer.[4]

In 1882, St. John's was far from being an attractive city. When Minnie, tired from the long journey, first saw her new home, her heart sank. The streets were badly laid out, and the stores and houses, dingy and drab against the winter snow and ice, looked as though they were made from packing boxes. Church steeples seemed to be the only redeeming pieces of architecture in the sordid town spread out before her.

Minnie was seven hundred miles from home, and there was no turning back, for she did not have the price of a return ticket. Suddenly she realized how much she depended on her sister.[5]

Minnie had not even arrived in St. John's when Mother Nutting began a letter: "Darling Minnie, after you left everything wore such a funeral aspect that I could do nothing but weep." The neighbors "came in to cheer us up and so the dreary hours wore on until bedtime and blessed sleep brought forgetfulness." Addie had been invited to the Russells for tea to meet their guest, a young Scotsman, and was disappointed to find him ugly, freckle-faced and red-haired. Jim had been invited to two parties, but Addie had not been asked to either. Mother Nutting wondered whether Addie's tongue had made her a great many enemies who might just as well have been friends. "Down to Sunday night," she wrote Minnie, "not a being of the male persuasion has poked his nose inside the door since you left." By Tuesday, however, things were looking up. That afternoon the Russells and the young Scotsman had called with a "pair of blacks and a nice sleigh and had taken Addie for a drive." In the evening Addie would sing "Loch of Narledean" at the Temperance festival at St. Andrews Church, accompanied by Duncan Scott at the organ.[6]

As the winter wore on and spring approached, Addie's social horizon looked brighter and Minnie's letters became more cheerful. At Mrs. Coens' boarding house Minnie had met a pale, quiet youth, Gilbert Gosling, who seemed far older than his eighteen years. He shared her interest in books and current affairs. He had come from Bermuda the previous June to work for Messrs. Harvey and Company, one of the largest business concerns in Newfoundland. Minnie was beginning to like St. John's.[7]

---

[4] Armine Nutting Gosling, *William Gilbert Gosling: A Tribute* (New York: Guild Press, 1935), p. 17.

[5] *Ibid.*, p. 18.

[6] Harriet P. Nutting (Ottawa) to Armine Nutting (St. John's), January 15, 16, 17, 1882, MAN Papers.

[7] Gosling, *William Gilbert Gosling*, pp. 11, 18.

Only from Waterloo did discouraging news come. Charlie and his father wrote anxious letters about Lizzie's declining health. No longer was she even able to direct Mary Ann, the hired girl, in the household tasks. Because the doctor seemed unable to help her, Charlie appealed to his mother, and she returned to Waterloo in April, leaving Addie to keep house for Jim.

Mother Nutting seemed to be just the tonic Lizzie needed. By late summer Lizzie was able to accompany Mrs. Nutting on a visit to the summer home of her niece, Addie Puffer, near Salem, Massachusetts.[8] While they were enjoying the cool sea breezes, Addie came from Ottawa to be with her father and Charlie.

Minnie continued to write enthusiastic letters about her school. When she proposed that Addie join her in the fall, teach music in the school, and take private pupils, a solution seemed to be found for the family's ever-present problem of funds. Lizzie was not yet able to take over the management of the Waterloo home. It was decided that Jim should rent the Ottawa flat and take lodgings until the family could be reunited. Mother Nutting was happy to be able to do something for Charlie. It would be easier in many ways; there would be no laundry to do, and she got along very well with Mary Ann.

Addie borrowed money from Charlie and in October joined Minnie in St. John's. Adelaide and Armine, as the girls were now trying to remember to call each other, were delighted to be together again. Music in the school was an exciting adventure, and they hoped many parents would want private lessons for their children.

Mother Nutting grieved for her daughters so far away. "Addie, dear," she wrote:

> I do not forget that Wednesday next is your birthday and I can not remember you as I wish on that day but I will do one little thing for you. On that day I will, D. V., pay Mrs. Fay the two dollars due from you to her and that will relieve your mind of so much and you must consider that an equivalent for a present, and as for Minnie, the dear child who remembered my birthday so magnificently I can not do a thing for her. I wonder if it will always be so with me and I shall never have anything of my own to give. My blessing and my prayers are all that I have for my poor darlings.[9]

Of life in St. John's, Minnie wrote a long letter in late November:

> Addie and I derive much amusement on Sundays from sitting in the window, watching the people pass to and from the different churches.

[8] Harriet P. Nutting (Salem, Mass.) to Adelaide Nutting (Waterloo), August 4, 1882, MAN Papers.
[9] Harriet P. Nutting [Waterloo] to Adelaide Nutting (St. John's), [late October, 1882], *ibid.*

Some we know, but the majority, of course, are strangers to us. The cut of the male garments here is so extremely antiquated, and I am sure Noah would, if resurrected, recognize certain fashions adopted by the feminine portion of this community. . . . All the men wear tall silk hats . . . tweed suits are a thing unknown.

Minnie complained of the lack of newspapers and information about what was going on in "civilized society" and of the expense of food. Her school was growing slowly but surely and had already won a reputation. Music in the curriculum was an added attraction. She ended her letter, "Kiss Pip for me."[10]

In reply, Vespasion, lonely for his daughters, assumed they were homesick too.

My dear little girls, I suppose you would like to see the old place again but in patience possess ye your souls, and I trust you will do so, in time I hope to see you again in Shefford. . . . We think of you every hour. . . . Little Pip is beside me. He is just as nice as ever and when we call Minnie or Addie he starts and goes around the house to see if he can find you.[11]

When Adelaide wrote that she was thinking about buying a piano, her mother hastened to advise her.

Don't Addie dear, not just yet at any rate. I should feel you were a fixture for life in Newfoundland if you went sixty pounds in debt and I can not bear to think of it . . . something may turn up so that you can come back next summer if you do not go into debt.[12]

For Mother Nutting the winter in Charlie's home had its boring overtones. Snow and ice and strong blasts of freezing wind kept the family in and the callers out. She deplored the "devices to which they resorted to keep from stagnation." The "one nice cheering thought" that she could write her girls was that "all my boys are temperate. . . . a subject for devout thanks. You can hardly imagine what a burden it was off my mind."[13]

Mother Nutting became apprehensive when neither Minnie nor Addie alluded to private music pupils. As Lizzie's health improved,

[10] Armine Nutting (St. John's) to Vespasion Nutting (Waterloo), November 26, 1882, ibid.

[11] Vespasion Nutting (Waterloo) to Armine and Adelaide Nutting (St. John's), December 12, 1882, ibid.

[12] Harriet P. Nutting (Waterloo) to Adelaide Nutting (St. John's), January 18, 1883, ibid.

[13] Harriet P. Nutting (Waterloo) to Adelaide Nutting (St. John's), January 21, 1883, ibid.

Harriet began to worry about Jim being alone in Ottawa and to consider the possibility of reopening the house there. She wrote her daughters: "I have been accumulating the greatest amount of odds and ends with which we will make some lovely things when we get together. I sometimes compare myself to an old magpie who is always picking up things to carry away to its nest."[14]

The girls kept their parents informed of the school, social gatherings, tea at the rectory, and made reference to the young men they had met, those who walked them home from church, and those who called. Mother Nutting was especially interested in the latter and offered sage advice.[15]

When Adelaide failed to secure private music pupils and the financial burden of music in the school fell on Minnie, they decided Adelaide should return home when the school year was out.

Since February Mrs. Nutting had been making plans to return to Ottawa. She had embroidered table covers and charted ways in which, by careful economy, she and her children could live together again. When Minnie wrote in April that it was quite probable that she would stay in St. John's another year, Harriet Nutting was crushed. "Dear little Min," she wrote.

> I could not keep the tears from coming and my heart cried out, "How can I bear it," or how can you, and I bowed myself upon the bed and said "Oh, Thou who seest the end from the beginning, give what is best, we commit ourselves to Thy care and guidance and in meek submission say, "Thy will be done," and so in trust and in confidence that whatever you decide to do will be for the best, I await your next letter.[16]

Although Minnie could ill afford a vacation, she decided to make the long journey home with Addie. When Jim came to visit Charlie in June, Mother Nutting decided to return with him to Ottawa, bidding "adieu to poor old Waterloo with scarce a feeling of regret."[17]

[14] Harriet P. Nutting [Waterloo] to Adelaide and Armine Nutting (St. John's), March 8, 9, 1883, *ibid.*

[15] Harriet P. Nutting (Waterloo) to Armine Nutting (St. John's), February 28, 1883, *ibid.*

[16] Harriet P. Nutting (Waterloo) to Armine and Adelaide Nutting (St. John's), April 21, 1883, *ibid.*

[17] Harriet P. Nutting (Waterloo) to Armine Nutting (St. John's), May 28, 1883, *ibid.*

III

Return to Ottawa, 1883

By the first of July, Mother Nutting had the Ottawa flat in order. Tuesday, July 3, would be her fifty-ninth birthday. "I can hardly fancy myself almost sixty years old," she wrote her husband. "It seems as though I have just hurried through life with never a moment to rest by the way." She hoped Vespasion would come up and see the girls before Min went back to St. John's in August.[1] She refused to let Charlie and his father pay the fares for the three women to come to Waterloo because of the added expense this would entail. As Min's stay would be short, Mother Nutting and Addie would be busy sewing and getting Min's clothes ready for the next year. Addie was already heavily in debt to Charlie, so Min would come down from Montreal alone.[2]

The days with Minnie passed all too swiftly. "Addie sat day after day and stitched away on Minnie's clothes till she was wearied out," Mrs. Nutting wrote her husband. As for Minnie, "I think she felt very badly at leaving us all again and as for myself . . . so many partings and changes have left a weight upon my heart never to be lifted in this world." She wrote that she was glad her husband's garden had done so well. "It is awfully good of you to send us a box now and then." Everything in Ottawa was expensive, especially meat and berries. Seldom could meat be bought for less than fifteen cents a pound.

> I did have a little of these things when Minnie was with us because they have hardly any fruit in Newfoundland and have to practice greater economy in consequence this month. . . . every indulgence we have, is greater self-denial afterwards. . . . We ought to be thankful that she has

[1] Harriet P. Nutting (Ottawa) to Vespasion Nutting (Waterloo, Quebec), July 1, 1883, MAN Papers.
[2] Harriet P. Nutting (Ottawa) to Vespasion Nutting (Waterloo), [mid-July], 1883, *ibid.*

got such a good place and can earn six hundred dollars a year, and be treated as well as she is there. I do not mean to worry about her as I used to do for I think she is very capable of taking care of herself.[3]

It was late October before Addie finally completed the sewing for Min and had the box ready to be shipped to Newfoundland. Her mother explained the delay:

> Addie's eyes have been very bad and pained her so she could not work by lamp light a good deal of the time. . . . You ought to like your evening dress for Ad spent more than a week over it and exhausted all her ingenuity in trying to make it uncommonly pretty. I do not believe she would have taken as much trouble for herself. I embroidered the lace that is on it which was no trifling task but I am glad I did it for it improved the dress wonderfully. . . .[4]

Addie would soon be twenty-five years old. At that age Harriet Nutting had been married five years and was the mother of two. Minnie seemed to be "very well set up" with her school and a sound matrimonial prospect.[5]

It looked, though, as if the family finances would never straighten out. Arthur had come for a visit in early December and the wake of unpaid bills he left behind necessitated a curtailment of expenditures at Christmas—no presents, no cards, and only the simplest dinner.[6]

The new year, 1884, however, began with bright prospects. Arthur wrote that he had been appointed sheriff of Calgary and the territory for forty miles around, a position which paid around $1,500 a year. He would sell his claim and invest in mining stocks. In Ottawa a vacancy had occurred in the Finance Department, and, although fourteen clerks went up for the examination, Jim was the successful one. His transfer to the Finance Department carried with it the almost certain prospect of promotion and a salary of $1,100 a year. Addie, who had been having a "rather dolorous time" and was rarely invited to the parties Jim attended, received some money from her father which would be spent on new clothes for the social season ahead.[7]

[3] Harriet P. Nutting (Ottawa) to Vespasion Nutting (Waterloo), September 1, 1883, ibid.

[4] Harriet P. Nutting (Ottawa) to Armine Nutting (St. John's, Newfoundland), October 30, 1883, ibid.

[5] Harriet P. Nutting (Ottawa) to Vespasion Nutting (Waterloo), November 2, 1883, ibid.

[6] Harriet P. Nutting (Ottawa) to Armine Nutting (St. John's), December 7, 1883, ibid.

[7] Harriet P. Nutting (Ottawa) to Armine Nutting (St. John's), January 9, 1884; and Harriet P. Nutting (Ottawa) to Vespasion Nutting (Waterloo), January 27, 1884; ibid.

In fact, the situation looked so bright that the family decided to have a party. Afterward Mother Nutting wrote Min about the affair:

Our party was voted a success, and so it ought, considering the trouble and expense it gave us. It was rather over doing the thing for a small affair, I thought. We had the Chesleys, Andrews, Phinneys, Mc-Lymonts, Huntons, Mr. Duggan, Jim's chief on the Hansard, Mr. Cunningham, Mr. Jack Christie, Mr. P. Taylor, Miss Corson, and Miss Wood of the Ladies College. All I can say I am glad it is over and we might as well have had a dozen more as we had plenty of good things to eat for refreshments. We had lots of jellies, oyster patties, charlotte russe, cakes and oranges, grapes, etc., and coffee, claret cup (which was most delicious) and all *ad libitum*.[8]

Through his position in the Finance Department and as a calligrapher for the House of Commons, Jim was able to obtain tickets for the Speakers Gallery and invitations to various social affairs at Rideau Hall, as the official residence of the governor general was then called.

Government House, two miles from the city, could be reached by carriage, hackney coach, carry-all, or sleigh, depending on the season. In the 1880s Rideau Hall was a piecemeal agglomeration of buildings of incongruous brick, plaster, and stone situated on a ninety-acre plot of gardens, grass, and forest. Famous for its balls, banquets, and receptions, Government House also had facilities for such winter sports as skating, curling, and toboganning.

The toboggans were two feet wide and six or eight feet long, with the front curled up and held taut by thongs of deer sinew. The sides were built up slightly to accommodate cushions and the tucking in of buffalo robes or blankets. Two or three persons could ride a toboggan. The women wore red, blue, or white blanket coats, with white scarves wound about their heads, thick woolen stockings, mittens, and moosehide boots. After the women were tucked in, the steerer jumped on. A push—and off they rushed at twenty miles an hour down the steep slope and through the cold, crisp air.

When Lord Lorne came as governor general in 1878, he introduced tobogganing by torchlight. Hundreds of Chinese lanterns were hung in the trees or in festoons about the pavilion. The toboggan course was outlined by master torches and there was a great bonfire. In the nearby shelter, hot mulled cider and coffee were served to the tobogganers and skaters.[9]

When the invitation for four February "At Homes" arrived, Mother Nutting was elated, and promptly sent the card to her husband. She

[8] *Ibid.*
[9] George Monro Grant, *Picturesque Canada* (Toronto: Belden Bros., 1882).

was proud to have people in Waterloo know that the Nuttings were being entertained by His Excellency, the governor general and marquis of Lansdowne, and told him not to lose the card, for she "liked to keep such things."[10]

The money Vespasion sent Addie for Christmas provided her with a new tobogganing outfit, moccasins, and a pair of long gloves and left two dollars for a dress. Addie bought the nicest white Hudson blanket that she could find and made it into a coat, which she wore with a blue toque and matching mittens. Mother Nutting was very pleased with her daughter's appearance when Addie and Jim set out for the first "At Home" at Rideau Hall. The following day she wrote a long letter to Minnie. Addie and Jim "had a grand good time, as Ad expressed it, for which I am truly thankful for she has been to hardly anything this winter." Mr. Cunningham, one of Jim's friends, had gone with them. "Mr. Fisher was there and took Ad for a couple of slides on the toboggan, and several others did the same so that she did not have to stand and see the others go by."[11]

As it was not considered proper in Ottawa for a young unmarried woman to go about evenings without a chaperone, Mrs. Nutting felt obliged to accompany Addie to the House of Commons. She wrote Minnie that she had gone to the House twice one week. On Friday night they sat in the front row of the Speakers Gallery. She "thought Ad enjoyed it because Mr. McMaster spied her there, and managed to meet us and speak to her afterward." This was "private gossip" to which Min must not allude. She also wrote that at last Addie had a music pupil, Mrs. Brewer's younger sister.[12] Later, writing to her husband for some money, she explained:

> We sit in the Speakers Gallery and most of the ladies, especially the younger ones go in full dress which makes it a little hard on us. I begin to realize Addie is twenty-five years old and if we ever expect to see her respectably settled in life we must not put her in the kitchen and make her do the work of a servant and dress her like one, as we have been doing of late. I have resolved not to permit it any longer and so I have commenced going with her to the House and elsewhere, when it is any place I can wear my cloak as that is the only respectable thing I have.
>
> You spoke of sending me some money, if I needed it. I need it, no

[10] Harriet P. Nutting [Ottawa] to Vespasion Nutting (Waterloo), January 25, 1884, MAN Papers.

[11] Harriet P. Nutting (Ottawa) to Armine Nutting (St. John's), February 3, 1884; and Harriet P. Nutting (Ottawa) to Vespasion Nutting (Waterloo), February 22, 1884; ibid.

[12] Harriet P. Nutting (Ottawa) to Armine Nutting (St. John's), February 12, 1884, ibid.

mistake, but can you spare it, that is the question. It might bring you back four-fold sometime and I want to give Addie one more chance to get settled in life. Ten dollars would be most helpful.[13]

On February 16, Mrs. Nutting accompanied Jim and Addie to Rideau Hall. She sat near a window where she had a good view of the people going down the slide and those skating on the lake. She seemed to enjoy her role as chaperone. At sessions of the House, arguments between the members were exciting and she enjoyed meeting Addie's and Jim's friends. As she wrote to Min: "We stayed until twelve last night and Mr. McMaster walked home with us. By the same token he is down in the drawing-room now, having just called to see Ad and I have gathered up my writing material and beat a retreat to my room because I must write this letter tonight and I *might* be one too many."[14]

The next week's letter told of another Saturday afternoon which the three Nuttings had spent at Rideau.

> Mr. Cunningham, one of Jim's chums asked the pleasure of our company and took us down, and also Addie, and myself as chaperone to the opera in the evening. . . . Mr. Fisher and Dr. Rogers were at Rideau yesterday. The member from Brome took Ad down the slide once, and the doctor took her in for a cup of coffee, and altogether she had a very good time, Mr. Cunningham being in attendance when there was no one else.[15]

Lady Lansdowne's final skating and toboganning party on March first was a gala affair, "with bonfires, Chinese lanterns, and a grand supper, and all the rest of it. About eleven hundred invitations were given, and I am sure every one of them was there. . . . Mr. Cunningham, a very bashful youth by the way, hovered about Addie like a shadow."[16]

Mrs. Nutting lamented that, with Lent coming on, the only diversions would be tobogganing, going to the House of Commons, listening to the debates, and looking at the dresses. "Nearly all the ladies who sit in the Speakers Gallery wear full dress, and our tickets admit us to the charmed circle." At her insistence Addie had taken her mother's black Spanish lace and made it into a very pretty evening

[13] Harriet P. Nutting (Ottawa) to Vespasion Nutting (Waterloo), February 22, 1884, *ibid.*
[14] Harriet P. Nutting (Ottawa) to Armine Nutting (St. John's), February 24, 1884, *ibid.*
[15] *Ibid.*
[16] Harriet P. Nutting (Ottawa) to Armine Nutting (St. John's), March 3, 1884, *ibid.*

dress, and Mrs. Nutting was no longer ashamed of her when they went to the House in the evening.

> Addie also made the old black brocade into a sort of coat, and trimmed it with all the old black fur that was in the house and it looks very well but is worthless so far as wearing is concerned. It is like paper and you can [put] your finger through it anywhere, and she will wear it in fear and trembling for fear it should burst.
> . . . 10:30 o'clock. Ad has just returned with McMaster. I hope she won't make a mess of her affairs but the old proverb of "two stools" you know, is apt to land one on the floor. It is wisest to take what one can get than always striving for something out of reach. Do not on any account refer to anything I have written but I think Cunningham is, to use a slang expression, pretty badly smitten and he is oceans good for Ad, and is a thoroughly good fellow, goes with very good people and belongs to one of the old families, rather good looking, and though not quite so impressive as McMasters, I have no doubt is a thousand times better. . . .[17]

Mother Nutting vacillated in her preference for Addie's suitors. The next week as she was writing to Minnie the door bell rang. It was after nine o'clock. Mr. McMaster had just arrived in town and was calling on Addie before going to the House. "What do you think of it?" she wrote Min. "A man of his years and position ought not to be fooling. It would change the aspect of affairs materially . . . if he would marry Addie."[18]

[17] Harriet P. Nutting (Ottawa) to Armine Nutting (St. John's), March 6, 1884, *ibid.*

[18] Harriet P. Nutting (Ottawa) to Armine Nutting (St. John's), April 7, 1884, *ibid.*

IV

Mother Nutting, 1883–1884

And so the winter passed. The snows melted, Easter came, and the parliamentary sessions closed. Addie continued to teach her one music pupil and to copy records for one of the government offices at fifteen cents a page, hoping to pay Charlie the money she owed him. While she copied, her mother, with the occasional help of a girl, kept the house, cooked, knitted, and masterminded the family economy. Rent on their flat was sixteen dollars a month, but, investigating the possibility of cheaper quarters, she found that rents were increasing everywhere and she resolved to economize in some other way. She knitted all of her own stockings, Jim's, and some of Addie's, and even found time to make a winter's supply to send her husband. Vespasion had sent boxes of staples from his garden: potatoes, turnips, onions, and squash. The past summer he had even dried corn, following his wife's recipe. The bars of soap, so carefully wrapped and stuck in the box corners, had also been made according to her old and reliable method.[1]

When Vespasion sent ten dollars in April, Mother Nutting was especially cheered and grateful. "You can hardly imagine how much ten dollars can do when laid out judiciously. I hope in your case it will be like casting your bread upon the waters after many days, and I can not help thinking the outlook for her is brightening a little."[2] That spring she had an irresistible longing for Waterloo, Vespasion, Charlie and Lizzie, and her old friends. She wondered about Sophia Lindsay, her friend of so many years. She had admired the way Sophia could talk a confirmed drunkard into signing the pledge of abstinence! Un-

[1] Harriet P. Nutting (Ottawa) to Vespasion Nutting (Waterloo, Quebec), December 7, 1883, MAN Papers.
[2] Harriet P. Nutting (Ottawa) to Vespasion Nutting (Waterloo), April 21, 1884, *ibid.*

21

fortunately, Vespasion's contempt and dislike for the Lindsays had not abated with the years.

In mid-May, Mother Nutting left Addie to keep house for Jim and returned to Waterloo for the summer.[3] It was good to be back with Charlie and Lizzie and to see Vespasion looking so well. She wrote Addie how she and Lizzie read together every day and "discoursed" on literary subjects. There was such a number of magazines—*Harpers*, *Good Words*, *Century*, and several others—and no end of papers, that she had to ration her reading to protect her eyes.[4] She felt unusually strong, and, when Esther, the hired girl, became ill just as guests were arriving, she took to the kitchen.

It was a happy holiday for Mother Nutting. On warm afternoons she sat in the new hammock "hung in the same old place under those glorious pines" and wrote letters.[5] Because spring had been late, Vespasion's garden had been slow, but by the end of July the family was enjoying fresh peas, green beans, cucumbers, new potatoes, and tomatoes. Disciplined to strictest economy in Ottawa, Mother Nutting reveled in their abundance. Having no money to buy Jim a present for his birthday, she sent him a box containing several pints of raspberries and preserves and some of his favorite cookies.[6]

Mother Nutting went with Charlie and some of his friends to Brome to a political picnic sponsored by Wilfred Laurier and Edmund Blake, and there she renewed old acquaintances and had dinner with her nephew, Frank Williams, and his wife. Her sister Betsey was there, very proud of her newest grandchild. Blake's speech was quite as eloquent as any she had heard him make in the House the previous winter. It was such a pleasant outing that when Frank's wife invited her to return for a week's visit the last of July she hastened to accept. It would be nice to have a long visit with Betsey, and she would enjoy holding Frank's baby.[7]

Just as she was about to leave for the visit, however, she was taken ill with such pains in her back that she could not straighten out. After three days the pain shifted to her abdomen and she could not turn in

[3] *Ibid.*

[4] Harriet P. Nutting (Waterloo) to Adelaide Nutting (Ottawa), [May, 1884], *ibid.*

[5] Harriet P. Nutting (Waterloo) to Adelaide Nutting (Ottawa), June 5, 1884, *ibid.*

[6] Harriet P. Nutting (Waterloo) to Adelaide Nutting (Ottawa), July 23, 1884; and Harriet P. Nutting (Waterloo) to Armine Nutting (St. John's, Newfoundland), August 4, 1884; *ibid.*

[7] Harriet P. Nutting (Waterloo) to James P. Nutting (Ottawa), June 22, 1884; and Harriet P. Nutting (Waterloo) to Adelaide Nutting (Ottawa), June 22, 1884; *ibid.*

bed without agony. The frightened family sent for Dr. Phelan, who ordered flannels wrung out of boiling water and sprinkled with turpentine kept on her abdomen constantly until the pain subsided. When she was at her worst, the hired girl took sick with cholera morbus, Lizzie was in bed, and the nursing fell to Charlie and his father. "They were as kind as possible," she wrote Minnie, "only it is very hard for men to take proper care of a sick person."[8] Charlie sent for Addie, who was camping with Jim and some friends. She came at once and, although everyone was better by the time she arrived, it was decided that she should stay until her mother was ready to return to Ottawa.

As the pain subsided, Mother Nutting thought of the things for which she could be grateful. She was gaining strength, there were many good things in the garden, and Vespasion was "sober as a judge." Her letters to Minnie were longer and more cheerful. "Ad got a letter from the M. P. the day after she arrived."[9]

The first week in October, Addie and her mother returned to Ottawa. Although Mother Nutting insisted that she had recovered sufficiently to travel, the journey and the change of trains in Montreal were exhausting. The old pain returned, and she took to her bed. Hot turpentine compresses brought no relief, and an Ottawa physician was called.[10]

On October 23 Addie sent a frantic telegram to Minnie in Newfoundland, "Take first steamer home. Mother ill. Telegraph us how soon you can come."[11] A week later Minnie arrived and the two girls took turns keeping vigil at the bedside, with Jim helping when he could. When the doctor predicted that the end was near, the girls sent for their father, Charlie, and Aunt Betsey Williams. They were all there when Mother Nutting died, November 17, 1884.

Grief-stricken, the family decided to take her back to Charlie and Lizzie's home and to ask the Reverend Lindsay to read the last rites. Then they would lay her to rest in the little Protestant cemetery in the block below Charlie's house. When they took stock of their funds, however, they found that there was not enough money to buy mourn-

[8] Harriet P. Nutting (Waterloo) to Armine Nutting (St. John's) August 4, 1884, ibid.

[9] Harriet P. Nutting (Waterloo) to Armine Nutting (St. John's), August 28, 1884, ibid.

[10] Georgia Nevins, "My Friend, Mary Adelaide Nutting," The Johns Hopkins Nurses Alumnae Magazine, April, 1949, p. 52; Adelaide Nutting, "Notes for Story of Life," MAN Papers.

[11] Telegram (Anglo-American Telegraph Co. Ltd.), Adelaide Nutting, (Ottawa) to Armine Nutting (St. John's), October 23, 1884, MAN Papers.

ing garments for Addie and Minnie and pay their fares to Waterloo and back, so the girls remained in Ottawa and did not attend their mother's funeral.

To Addie and Minnie, the house seemed strangely still in the quiet that followed their mother's death. It was a world without her, yet so much of the house proclaimed her presence; the piano scarf, the bookcase drape, the table cover she had embroidered, the chairs she had upholstered, the books she had read, the pots and pans she had used.

Charlie and Aunt Betsey wrote the details of the funeral. In Montreal, Aunt Betsey had bought linen handkerchiefs for the pallbearers and the clergy. Reverend Lindsay was ill, so they were obliged to have the Reverend Magill conduct the service. The house was more than filled, and as they walked to the cemetery "the sun shone brightly as a last benediction to closing a useful life."[12]

When the black crepe and cloth which Aunt Betsey had purchased for them in Montreal arrived, Addie and Minnie began working over their wardrobes to conform to the amenities of mourning. Three weeks later, Min, dark-clothed and heavily veiled, set out for St. John's.

Back in Waterloo, Vespasion Nutting took long walks with his dog. It was difficult to reconcile himself to the fact that Harriet, who had been so much a part of his life for forty years, was gone. Charlie, looking out of his window toward the freshly made grave, searched for a way of paying tribute. "Jim," he wrote, "what do you say if you and I swore off rum in toto. Say yes. Will be best for us and we owe it to mother's memory and trials to be as good as we know how."[13]

[12] Charles A. Nutting (Waterloo) to Armine and Adelaide Nutting (Ottawa), [November 19, 1884]; and Betsey Williams (Knowlton, Quebec) to Adelaide Nutting (Ottawa), November 21, 1884; ibid.

[13] Charles A. Nutting (Waterloo) to James P. Nutting (Ottawa), December 1, 1884, ibid.

V

The Journey to Hopkins,
1884–1889

After her mother's death, Adelaide struggled with grief and the problem of her future. Charlie and Lizzie opened their home to her, Aunt Betsey Williams invited her to pay a long visit to Knowlton, and Cousin Addie Puffer asked her to spend the winter in Lowell. She declined their offers. For the present she believed her obligation to her mother's memory could best be met by staying in Ottawa and making a home for Jim. She would secure some copying and help reimburse Charlie, whose debts had been increased by their mother's illness and death.[1]

The monotony and loneliness of the household was broken in February by a visit from Cousin Addie Puffer, a joyous soul who was loving and reassuring. The two women had much in common besides their names and ancestors. Both enjoyed reading and music and fine needlework. Addie Puffer was quick to admit that, in all three, her Canadian cousin was the more skilled. Again she invited Adelaide to come to Lowell if any changes were made in the Ottawa living arrangements. Adelaide was hopeful that she might yet have some music pupils, although at twenty-six she had abandoned her youthful ambition of a professional music career.[2]

She continued to sing at church and club affairs. To the end of her life she cherished an engrossed scroll from the Ottawa Rowing Club after its moonlight excursion aboard the steamer *Peerless*. It was signed by James Cunningham, "Honorable Secretary" of the club, and it embodied a resolution passed at its meeting on June 9, 1885, ex-

[1] Adelaide Nutting (Ottawa) to Vespasion Nutting (Waterloo, Quebec), [March, 1885], MAN Papers.

[2] An English music teacher who accompanied the duke and duchess of Lorne when he assumed the governor generalship in 1878 had heard Adelaide sing. He thought she had professional possibilities and asked to teach her. Isabel M. Stewart, "Notes: Conversations with Adelaide Nutting, Atlantic City, New Jersey," *ibid.*

pressing appreciation of her kind and able assistance in contributing to the success of the vocal and instrumental portions of the program on a recent excursion.[3]

On September 16, 1885, Jim was married to Claire Lizzie Sinclair. After putting the house in order for the new bride, Adelaide went on a camping trip with friends; then she visited her cousins in Montreal and later went on to Waterloo.

The family was kind, but Adelaide felt she could not remain. Waterloo held too many unhappy memories: the family poverty, her mother working long hours to give her children some of the better things of life, her aging, lonely father who had failed so miserably as a provider and who now in his grief brought them embarrassment and humiliation in his drunken slovenliness.

Just as the future seemed darkest, an insistent letter came from Addie Puffer. She expected Adelaide to come to Lowell and would send money for her ticket. Furthermore, she was saving her sewing for her Canadian cousin so she would be able to pay for voice lessons from one of Lowell's best teachers. Adelaide decided to go for the winter at least.

It was good to be in Lowell again, with Addie and Stephen, Uncle Daniel, Aunt Helen Hamblett, and the other cousins, Alice and Viola.[4] They all lived comfortably and happily. Adelaide soon found herself entering into the gaiety of family parties, sleigh rides, and the social and cultural affairs the Hambletts and Puffers attended. The women read to each other and discussed books and magazines as they sewed or knitted. Sometimes a sonnet or a paragraph brought Adelaide vivid memories of her mother; she would have loved this consorting of minds. Occasionally Adelaide went to nearby Bradford to visit her father's sister, Aunt Jane Stickney.

In January, Minnie gave up her position in St. John's and returned to Montreal with the exciting news that she was engaged to be married to Gilbert Gosling. She would spend the next few months visiting relatives and friends and learning to cook and acquire skill in the other housewifely arts. Gilbert was not a wealthy man, and she expected to do her own work. She would assemble her trousseau and travel to Bermuda to visit Gilbert's family.[5]

In early spring, 1886, Jim wrote that Claire was ill, pregnant, and

[3] The scroll was found among her papers next to an engrossed citation from the government of Finland for her world-wide contribution to nursing. *Ibid.*

[4] Harriet P. Nutting's younger sister, Helen A. Peasley, was married to Daniel Hamblett in 1852.

[5] Armine Nutting Gosling, *William Gilbert Gosling: A Tribute* (New York: Guild Press, 1935), p. 20.

that he needed help. Adelaide returned to Ottawa, thinking that perhaps she could do some copying and pay her way while at Jim's. Aunt Betsey wrote, "Many times have I heard your mother say, 'How I would love to have a grandchild to love and care for—for I never had time to love and care for my own as I wanted to,'" and promised Adelaide that she would be a grandmother to Jim's baby.[6]

On August 20 a son was born to Claire and Jim. He was christened Harold Headley Sinclair Nutting. The new baby was a never-ending source of joy to Adelaide. She would never forget the thrill she felt the first time his tiny fingers clasped hers, the excitement of his first tooth, or his first step.[7]

Adelaide's social life now centered more on Claire's and Jim's friends and Cathedral Church than on the House of Commons and Rideau Hall. She entered into Min's plans for marriage and immediately took to her needle to hem linens, refurbish her sister's old dresses, and make a few new ones.

Adelaide had met Gilbert Gosling when she was with Armine in St. John's. She admired him as a man of purpose, high ideals, and an insatiable thirst for knowledge. He was gentle and kind. Min often read his letters aloud. "Not much is going on. My work is the chief thing. I think I shall take up the study of some language. I must have an outside interest—something that will sharpen my intellect." Another time he cautioned Armine: "You and I must not let ourselves get mentally slack. We should set aside a definite portion of our time for study and for reading good books, and if we don't do it systematically the chances are it will not be done at all."[8] Mother Nutting would have approved of Gilbert wholeheartedly.

Minnie spent the winter of 1886/87 with Gilbert's parents in Bermuda, and in January Gilbert came home for his first real vacation in six years. A year later Gilbert met Minnie in Halifax, and they were married there on January 2, 1888.[9]

After Minnie's marriage Adelaide felt strangely alone. Min's happiness made her own indecision stand out more clearly. Now approaching thirty, she realized that she should, as Aunt Betsey had advised, "give some thought for the morrow." She had had offers of marriage

[6] Betsey Williams (Knowlton, Quebec) to Adelaide Nutting (Ottawa), April 23, 1886, MAN Papers.

[7] Harold Headley Sinclair Nutting, son of Claire Lizzie Sinclair and James Peasley Nutting, was born in Ottawa on August 20, 1886. He married Bertha Oliver Waters in December, 1919. MAN Papers.

[8] Gilbert Gosling (St. John's, Newfoundland) to Armine Nutting (Ottawa), January, 1886, quoted in Gosling, William Gilbert Gosling, p. 21.

[9] Gosling, William Gilbert Gosling, p. 29.

and twice been engaged, once to a young curate at the church in Waterloo where she played the organ. He was devoted and persistent, but she did not feel she could be permanently happy with him. She wondered if she overidealized her childhood love for Russ Huntington, who years before had moved away, married another, and was now dead. Throughout her life she was to believe that he was the only man she could ever have loved enough to marry.[10]

While at Addie Puffer's in Lowell, Massachusetts, Adelaide had talked about taking up nursing. She had heard of trained nurses, but had never seen one. She could not forget how wholly unprepared she had been when her mother had become ill. Surely there were things she could have done to spare her mother pain if she had known. She thought of poor Lizzie, sick so often, and of Claire and the baby. "I am convinced," she told her cousin, "I must learn how to take care of my family."

As a young girl growing up in the British Empire, Adelaide had read fascinating stories of Florence Nightingale. The Lady of the Lamp, the heroine of Scutari, was a woman to be admired and reverenced. Adelaide had even written a paper about her for one of her classes. After reading another life of Florence Nightingale while at Addie Puffer's, Adelaide had sent for Miss Nightingale's *Notes on Nursing*. Long afterward she wrote: "Never can I forget the day it came into my hands quite accidentally. Then indeed I felt 'like some watcher of the skies when a new planet swims into his ken.' "[11]

On inquiring, she found that there were hospitals in the United States that offered training along the lines that Miss Nightingale prescribed. One was the Massachusetts General Hospital in Boston, and another, the Bellevue Hospital in New York City. She learned it was possible to attend a hospital training school and receive board, lodging, and a small stipend while studying and working in the wards. This would solve her financial problem. She simply could not ask Charlie for more money.

The more Adelaide thought about nursing, the more it seemed the thing she wanted to do. Just after she made application to Bellevue, the Montreal *Weekly Witness* carried an article about the new hospital and training school being established in connection with The Johns Hopkins University in Baltimore, Maryland. Its buildings and

[10] Russell Huntington (son of Seth Huntington, member of Parliament from Shefford), a graduate of McGill Law School, became a journalist on the *Montreal Herald*. He married Ellen Underwood, of Belmont, Mass., but died of typhoid fever in 1878. Obituary, *Waterloo Advertiser*, November 14, 1878.

[11] Adelaide Nutting, "Notes for Story of Life" MAN Papers.

equipment were to be the most modern and progressive of any hospital in America, and nurses were to be trained in the most approved techniques. Three Canadians had been appointed to the staff: Dr. William Osler, a graduate of McGill and now on the staff of Philadelphia General Hospital; Dr. Henri A. Lafleur; and Miss Isabel Hampton, as principal of the Training School for Nurses.

Adelaide wrote for a circular and read it carefully. Confident that she could pass the examination in reading, penmanship, simple arithmetic, and English dictation required at the end of the probationary month, she dispatched a letter to Miss Hampton.

> Waterloo, East, P. Q.
> Canada
> September 6, 1889

My dear Madam,

I have received the circular which you kindly sent me concerning your Training School for Nurses, and wish to apply for entrance. I submit the following information you ask for in regard to myself and hope you may find it satisfactory.

I was thirty years old on the first day of November last, am five feet five inches in height, weighing one hundred twenty-nine pounds. Though not remarkably strong, I have a good deal of endurance and have not had an illness of any importance since childhood. I have no diseases or physical defects that I am aware of. I have been educated almost entirely at home, and spent some time studying music, with the hope of going on with it elsewhere, which I was obliged to abandon for lack of means.

I am single and live with my brother who is married. My mother is dead, and my father, though elderly, is not an invalid. I have never been a nurse elsewhere, but I applied to Bellevue, New York, some days ago, from whence I have as yet received no reply. Hearing since then, that their replies are often delayed many weeks and sometimes months, I decided to apply to you, being anxious to avoid suspense, and also to begin my work at the earliest possible date. I enclose copies of letters from my clergyman and physician and should you wish for further information regarding me, beg to refer you to the Hon. G. G. Stevens of this place and to the Hon. Sir Hector L. Langevin, K. C., M. G., Minister of Public Works, Ottawa, Ontario.

Tho' aware that I am applying very late this year I earnestly hope that my application may be accepted and that I may be further fortunate in securing an early entrance.

> Believe me, dear Madam,
> Very truly yours,
> Mary Adelaide Nutting[12]

[12] Mary Adelaide Nutting (Waterloo) to Isabel Hampton (Baltimore), September 6, 1889, The Johns Hopkins Hospital School of Nursing Archives.

The forthrightness, sincerity, and apparent refinement of this fellow Canadian appealed to Isabel Hampton, who immediately accepted her. Relieved of suspense, Adelaide replied:

Waterloo East
September 15, 1889

Dear Madam,

I have just received your letter of the 9th telling me that my application has been accepted.

I shall make the preparations you require without delay, and you may rely upon my being in readiness to go, whenever you send for me.

Believe me,

Most sincerely yours,
Adelaide Nutting[13]

Adelaide was hardly prepared for Miss Hampton's wire that she should come at once, although the formal opening of the school was on October 9. Because Charlie and Lizzie were having guests and she could not leave, she asked for a postponement. Miss Hampton wired that her entrance would be deferred until November 1.[14]

Adelaide's announcement that she was entering nurse's training brought forth expressions varying from surprise and admiration to frank disapproval. A rejected suitor sought to change her mind, but she was adamant. If she would not change her plans, she would at least permit him to accompany her to Baltimore.

Late on the night of October 31 Adelaide and her suitor arrived in Baltimore. The moon and stars were shining brightly when they entered the hansom cab that was to drive them across the city to the great new red brick hospital at the top of the hill overlooking the business and residential district. The two miles from the station seemed almost as long as the trip from Waterloo. When at last the cab arrived in front of the administration building with its lighted dome, the driver drew the reins up sharply, shouted to his horses to stop, and alighted from his seat. Turning to the man beside her, Adelaide shook her head. "No, Jack." The long journey to Hopkins was over.[15]

[13] Adelaide Nutting (Waterloo) to Isabel Hampton (Baltimore), September 15, 1889, ibid.

[14] Isabel M. Stewart, "Notes: Conversations with M. A. Nutting, Hotel Gramatan, Bronxville, New York," August 24, [1940], MAN Papers.

[15] Isabel M. Stewart, "I Remember," IMS Papers.

VI

Student Nurse, 1889–1891

Adelaide waited inside the huge circular foyer while a porter went to call Miss Hampton. She looked about the room with its white marble floor and wide marble stairway facing the entrance, the ballustraded gallery above, and up into the softly lighted dome. Finding herself in front of the life-size portrait of Johns Hopkins, she studied his face with its deep strong lines, firm jaw, tightly closed lips, and compassionate dark eyes.

At that moment Isabel Hampton entered the room. She was tall, at least three inches taller than Adelaide, large of frame, and carried herself with a dignified, confident, almost regal air. Beautiful and apparently overflowing with energy, she was wearing her matron's uniform of soft black silk, with its short, tight basque, leg-of-mutton sleeves, high neck and stand-up collar, and narrow cuffs of fine white lawn. Her wavy light brown hair, loosely brushed back from her face and coiled into a knot on the top of her head, was covered with a white cap designed like that of a Roman cardinal. Her complexion was fair, fresh, and petal-like, and her eyes were pansy blue. She smiled and extended her hand in welcome.

After Miss Hampton had showed Adelaide to her room in the Nurses' Home, they returned to her suite, where the housekeeper brought in a tray of warm food. As the two women drank their tea in front of the lighted grate, Miss Hampton talked of the hospital's founder, Johns Hopkins, and of her own dreams for the Training School for Nurses.[1]

It was sixteen years since Johns Hopkins had died, leaving seven million dollars for the building of a university and a hospital which were to bear his name. Johns Hopkins had been a Quaker merchant. When he was twelve years old, his impoverished father, Samuel Hopkins, had sent him to Baltimore to live with his uncle, Gerard

[1] Adelaide Nutting, "Notes on Mrs. Isabel Hampton Robb," MAN Papers.

31

Hopkins, a prosperous merchant. As the boy grew, he developed an unusual talent for business and was given much responsibility. When he fell in love with his cousin Elizabeth, however, Gerard Hopkins refused to accept him as a son-in-law, marriage between cousins being contrary to Quaker belief. Elizabeth felt she could not go against her father's wishes, and Johns Hopkins broke with his uncle and went into business for himself. The cousins remained close friends, and neither married.[2]

Hopkins amassed a fortune from his investments and built a fine home overlooking the Patapsco River. His interest in hospitals may have arisen from the terrible cholera epidemic that struck Baltimore in 1832 and nearly took his life. Later he served on the governing boards of several hospitals. In 1867, while on the Board of the Maryland State Hospital for the Insane, he was appalled that the nurses did not have the methods, energy, or intelligence to discharge their duties, nor was there a sufficient number of nurses. That year he had two bills introduced into the Maryland General Assembly, one for the incorporation of The Johns Hopkins Hospital and the other for the incorporation of The Johns Hopkins University.

Although the hospital was not to open for twenty-two years, Hopkins immediately set up a board of trustees, with Francis T. King, a Haverford merchant and clerk of the Baltimore Yearly Meeting of Friends, as chairman, to begin studying and planning for the institution that would be built after he surrendered the control of his estate.[3] In March, 1873, Hopkins asked his lawyer to draft a letter to the Board of Trustees requesting that they establish in connection with the hospital a training school for female nurses. This, he believed, would secure the services of women competent to care for the sick in the hospital wards and would benefit the community with a supply of trained and experienced nurses.[4]

Years of planning, Miss Hampton explained, had gone into the building and organization of the hospital. The board was determined that The Johns Hopkins Hospital should be the most modern of hospitals and have the finest staff. Five of the most distinguished physicians in America were asked to prepare essays on the best methods

---

[2] Ethel Johns and Blanche Pfefferkorn, *The Johns Hopkins Hospital School of Nursing* (Baltimore: The Johns Hopkins Press, 1954), p. 6.

[3] Alan M. Chesney, *The Johns Hopkins Hospital and The Johns Hopkins School of Medicine: A Chronicle* (Baltimore: The Johns Hopkins Press, 1943), 1:7.

[4] Johns Hopkins to Francis King, March 10, 1873; and "Minutes of the Board of Trustees, The Johns Hopkins Hospital, March 11, 1873"; quoted in Johns and Pfefferkorn, *The Johns Hopkins Hospital School of Nursing*, p. 8.

of construction and organization of a hospital. Although the ideas of all of the consultants were utilized to some extent, the essay by Dr. John S. Billings, assistant surgeon, U.S. Army, led to his appointment in July, 1876, as consultant for the construction of the hospital.[5] Dr. Billings spent three months in Europe observing hospitals, among them St. Thomas Hospital in London.[6] Francis King was greatly interested in the nurses training school and he took his daughter, Elizabeth, to England in 1875 to discuss the possibilities of the school with Florence Nightingale and Florence Lees. Miss Lees sent copies of Miss Nightingale's *Notes on Nursing* to the trustees and offered suggestions relative to the Nurses' Home.[7]

Miss Hampton was pleased that Adelaide had such a conversant knowledge of Florence Nightingale. As she rose to bid Adelaide goodnight, she said, "Ours must be the best of training schools." Adelaide was told to come to breakfast in the simple blue washdress that had been made according to directions in Miss Hampton's letter. After breakfast all nurses and pupil nurses would assemble in the hall outside Miss Hampton's apartment for morning prayers, after which they would be given orders for the day and changes in ward assignments. Nurses went on duty at 7:00 A.M and worked until 7:00 P.M., with an hour off for lunch, rest, and study.[8] Twice a week, classes would be held from five until six in the evening. Lectures by the doctors would be given in the evening from eight until nine.

At breakfast the next morning Adelaide met most of the thirteen other probationers. They were friendly and offered to help her find her way around the hospital. Some of them had been there before the school formally opened on October 9.[9] The hospital had opened in May under the direction of three head nurses, Caroline Hampton, Annie McDowell, and Louisa Parsons, and the matron or housekeeper, Rachel Bonner, who was not a nurse.[10]

[5] Johns and Pferfferkorn, *The Johns Hopkins Hospital School of Nursing*, pp. 10–11.

[6] John S. Billings, "Plans and Purposes of Johns Hopkins Hospital" (Address given at the opening of the hospital, May 7, 1889), p. 15; on file in The Johns Hopkins Hospital School of Nursing Archives.

[7] Johns and Pfefferkorn, *The Johns Hopkins Hospital School of Nursing*, pp. 22–23.

[8] Circular of Information, The Johns Hopkins Hospital, Baltimore, Training School for Nurses (n.d., possibly the first issued), The Johns Hopkins Hospital School of Nursing Archives.

[9] *The Johns Hopkins Nurses Alumnae Magazine*, June, 1939, pp. 10–11.

[10] The head nurses received $30 a month and maintenance; Miss Bonner, the matron, was paid $800 a year; and Miss Hampton, principal of the training school and superintendent of nurses, earned $1,000 a year. Johns and Pfefferkorn, *The Johns Hopkins Hospital School of Nursing*, p. 30.

Miss Parsons, formerly a British army nurse in the Sudan, had been in charge until Isabel Hampton came, at which time she resigned to become superintendent of nurses at the University of Maryland Hospital. Caroline Hampton was a niece of General Wade Hampton of South Carolina. Her family had lost their money in the Civil War, and Caroline had gone north to study nursing. She had graduated from the New York Hospital Training School for Nurses, where the surgeon, Dr. William S. Halsted, always requested her presence in the operating room.

The students said everyone loved Miss McDowell, who was in charge of the private ward. She was from County Cork in Ireland and had trained in London Hospital. During the summer, when the work load had increased, four new nurses had been added. Miss M. A. Selby, who had trained in St. Thomas Hospital in London, was the night nurse in Ward C. She too had served in the Sudan campaign and was "all covered with medals."[11] Before Adelaide could hear anything about the doctors it was time for prayers, which began at exactly 6:50 A.M.

The service was brief. Miss Hampton read from the Scriptures and the English Book of Common Prayer, and then a hymn was sung. She gave out assignments and announced that the first of the medical lectures would be given the following evening by Dr. Alexander Abbott on "The Physical Properties of the Atmosphere, Air Currents Resulting from Alterations in Temperature and Barometric Pressure."[12] Students were expected to take notes. Miss Hampton then dismissed the group but asked Miss A. Nutting kindly to remain.

The nurses and pupils hurried away to their respective wards. It was exactly 7:00 A.M. Adelaide quickly sensed Miss Hampton's respect for the military tradition in nursing. Soon they started on a tour of the buildings, each of which was connected to the next by an outdoor corridor or bridge. Miss Hampton pointed to the tall, ornamental fence that surrounded the hospital grounds. Mr. Hopkins had specified in his will that there should always be a fence around the hospital. To the rear of the administration building and directly opposite was the apothecary, or pharmacy, building. At the other end of the long corridor, just beyond the bathhouse and almost a block from the Nurses' Home, was the kitchen. From this central kitchen, food was transported to the wards. The two three-story buildings that flanked

[11] *Ibid.*, pp. 33–36.

[12] "Schedule of Lectures, The Johns Hopkins Hospital Training School for Nurses, 1889–1891," photostat, Record of Emma Cleaver, The Johns Hopkins Hospital School of Nursing Archives.

the north and south sides of the administration building and formed the open court overlooking the circular drive past the main entrance housed Ward B for women and Ward C for men.

East of the kitchen and opening onto Monument Street was a large building containing the amphitheater and the dispensary. Some distance beyond were the stables, and at the far end of the block was the small building where Dr. Welch did his pathological work. The laundry was at the opposite corner on Jefferson and Wolfe streets. In a direct line with the male patients' private ward was another series of buildings known as D–E, F, G, H, and I. At the south end of all floors a screened porch overlooked an expanse of lawn facing Jefferson Street. These buildings were also connected by wooden bridges. Ward I, a one-story building and farthest away, was "Isolation," where patients suffering from contagious diseases were treated. The D–E building was divided into men's and women's surgical wards; F was the male medical ward; G was the female medical ward; and H was the gynecological ward. Later there would be a separate urological ward for men.[13]

On their tour of the hospital, Miss Hampton and Adelaide met Dr. Hurd, the superintendent, and Dr. Osler of the medical staff. Henry Mills Hurd had come from Michigan on August 1 to relieve President Daniel Coit Gilman, who confessed that managing a hospital was far more exacting than heading a university. Dr. Hurd was a thin, wiry man in his middle forties, with a sharp nose, pointed chin, thin grayish hair, a moustache, and side whiskers. Although he seemed anxious to get on his way, he stopped to greet the new probationer and wished her well. As Miss Hampton was about to tell Adelaide about Dr. Hurd's interest in the mentally ill, Dr. Osler appeared.[14]

William Osler was a man of medium height, olive complexion, and slender build. Forty years of age, he walked with a firm, jaunty step

---

[13] *Johns Hopkins Hospital, 1889–1939*, fiftieth anniversary souvenir (Baltimore: The Johns Hopkins Hospital, 1939).

[14] Henry Mills Hurd (1843–1927), was superintendent of The Johns Hopkins Hospital from 1889 to 1911. In 1886 he received an M.D. from the University of Michigan and became assistant physician at the Michigan State Asylum, Kalamazoo. Later he became superintendent, Eastern Michigan Asylum for the Insane, Pontiac, where he abolished restraints and introduced occupational therapy. The University of Michigan conferred the Doctorate of Laws on him in 1895. His most important publication was *Institutional Care of the Insane in the United States and Canada*, 4 vols. (Baltimore: The Johns Hopkins Press, 1916–17). For further details see Thomas Stephen Cullen, *Henry Mills Hurd: First Superintendent, The Johns Hopkins Hospital* (Baltimore: The Johns Hopkins Press, 1920).

and had sparkling eyes that conveyed sympathy and understanding as well as irresistible gaiety. Adelaide was attracted at once to this fellow Canadian. He had graduated from the medical school at McGill University the same year that her brother Charlie had taken his degree in law. Osler had gone abroad for further study in London and Vienna. After two years he had returned to join the faculty of McGill as professor of medicine. In 1884 he had become professor of clinical medicine at the University of Pennsylvania. Adelaide noted his careful diction, his almost poetic speech. In the years to follow, they would find they had more in common than being fellow countrymen.[15]

As the tour continued, Miss Hampton told Adelaide that shortly after Dr. Osler had gone to Philadelphia he had been offered a place on The Johns Hopkins staff. At present only graduate courses were taught by the medical staff. It was necessary to wait until the hospital was running smoothly before launching the medical school. The Hopkins staff insisted on ward teaching as well as lectures and laboratory work.

At the door of Ward H, women's gynecological, Miss Hampton paused. It was one of the less crowded wards, and to it she assigned Adelaide. The head nurse, looking very efficient and businesslike in her stiff white uniform and cap, came forward. "This is Miss Adelaide Nutting. I am sure you will find her gentle, serious, and attentive." With that introduction, Miss Hampton gave Adelaide's hand a reassuring squeeze and departed.

Adelaide walked with the nurse down the long white room with its rows of white beds and tables on either side. Her nostrils dilated as she caught the first whiff of medication and disinfectant. The nurse, aware that this was the first time the new probationer had ever been in a hospital ward, explained: "Carbolic acid, corrosive sublimate, and chlorine are used as disinfectants. All hospital wards have a distinctive odor."

"Today," she said, "you will listen, watch what others do, and do

[15] William Osler (1849–1919) attended Trinity College, Toronto, and in 1872 received an M.D. from McGill University, Montreal; he then studied in London and Vienna from 1872 to 1874 and returned to McGill as professor of medicine in 1874. In 1884 he became professor of clinical medicine, University of Pennsylvania. Osler served on the staff of The Johns Hopkins Hospital from 1889 to 1905; he began teaching in the Medical School in 1893. In 1873, Osler published research on blood platelets and wrote *Cerebral Palsies of Children*. He married Mrs. Grace Revere Gross in 1892. Their only son, Revere, died of battle wounds in August, 1917. Osler became Regius Professor, Oxford, in 1905. See *The Johns Hopkins Hospital Bulletin*, July, 1919, pp. 186–208; Elizabeth H. Thomson, *Harvey Cushing* (New York: Schuman, 1950), pp. 76–77.

what you are told. After that, when you see something that needs to be done, do not wait to be asked or told." They approached the last bed, temporarily screened off for privacy. The nurse looked at her watch. A pupil nurse (as the student nurse was then called) pushed back the screens, smiled at the patient, and, gathering up the linen, nodded to the head nurse and left the ward. "Everything is on schedule," the nurse commented to Adelaide. "It is important that every patient and the ward be in readiness when the doctor makes his rounds."

Just then Dr. Howard A. Kelly, the gynecologist and obstetrician, appeared. He conferred briefly with the nurse and then began visiting his patients.[16]

Throughout the morning Adelaide helped with the routine tasks of the ward as demonstrated by the head nurse and the other probationers. At noon she helped with the patients' trays. In the afternoon she folded bandages. Although not all the beds were occupied and the work had not been strenuous, Adelaide was tired when she sat down to dinner. She met more of the probationers and learned from them about the doctors and classes. She was assured that late entrance would not throw her too far behind, for Miss Hampton had been very busy and so far had held only three class meetings. Several of the young women offered her the use of notes they had taken. As yet, the school had no library, and there were few textbooks in the field of nursing. Each student was expected to buy or borrow her own copy of Gray's *Anatomy* and Martin's *Human Body*. Miss Hampton and some of the head nurses owned copies of Clara Weeks's *Textbook of Nursing*, the first book of its kind written by a nurse for nurses.[17] Excerpts from it were slowly dictated to the probationers, who took copious notes for future study.[18]

Adelaide liked the young women who sat around the table with her. Some of them would be her life-long friends. Marion Turner, Susan Read, Mary Gross, and Georgia Nevins had been educated in private schools. Emma Cleaver, whose handwriting resembled finest copperplate engraving, not only was a college graduate but held a

[16] Howard Atwood Kelly (1858–1943), gynecologist and obstetrician, and a member of the original Johns Hopkins Hospital staff in 1889, became a member of the faculty of the Medical School when it opened in 1893. He was one of the Big Four, invented numerous surgical tools, and collected Nightingaliana. Johns and Pfefferkorn, *The Johns Hopkins Hospital School of Nursing*, p. 56.

[17] *Ibid.*, pp. 60–61; Clara S. Weeks, *A Textbook of Nursing for the Use of Training Schools, Families and Private Students* (New York: D. Appleton, 1885).

[18] Adelaide Nutting, "Notes for Story of Life," MAN Papers.

master of arts degree from Ripon College as well. She had taken the classical course, which included three years in Greek, and had taught school for five years. Kate Emory had been a kindergarten and public school teacher. Anna Hudson, Anna Rutherford, and Tillie Spencer boasted only good, plain English educations. Norma Anthony, like Adelaide, had specialized in music. Gertrude Hammerill, who had an excellent German educational background, spoke only limited English and some French. Ida May had left school at fourteen. Evelyn Hartley was a Quaker who always said "thee" and "thou." The oldest of the group was Mary Emory, a thirty-five-year-old widow and mother of five children.[19] As they talked, Adelaide compared her own educational background with theirs and wondered if she could compete with women who had been to college or had taught school.

That night, although weary, Adelaide started a letter to Min. Entering the hospital was like coming into a new and different world. Already she noted sharply defined regions of authority and chains of responsibility, the insistence on obedience and the deference to authority, silence, and military precision in performing certain tasks as though they were orders from some all-powerful commander.[20]

The next morning Adelaide returned to duty in Ward H. She was inducted into bedmaking "the hospital way" and the careful folding of the sheets so that the patient could be easily and gently moved. She assisted in the bathing of patients and watched the nurse make routine checks of temperature and pulse. She was shown how to quietly and unobtrusively carry out vessels used by the patients, then rinse them and place them in a strong cleansing solution before scrubbing, scalding, drying, and placing them in the storage closets. She was taught how to "damp dust" by wringing a dustcloth out in soapy water.[21]

Student nurses quickly noted but accepted as a matter of practice that a head nurse never performed a menial task if a probationer was available. Airing and ventilating the wards was another of the student nurses' responsibilities. Fresh air was greatly stressed at Johns Hopkins; in planning the pavilions, Dr. Billings had provided for cross-ventilation and sunshine by affording each bed a window.

Adelaide was pleased when patients remembered her from the day before. When Dr. Howard A. Kelly, the gynecologist, and his assistant, Dr. Hunter Robb, made their rounds, she was careful to do as the

[19] Johns and Pfefferkorn, *The Johns Hopkins Hospital School of Nursing*, pp. 64–65; *The Johns Hopkins Nurses Alumnae Magazine*, June, 1939, pp. 10–11.
[20] Adelaide Nutting, "Notes for Story of Life," MAN Papers.
[21] Mary Dixon Cullen, "Memories of a Probationer, 1900," *The Johns Hopkins Nurses Alumnae Magazine*, April, 1950, p. 65.

nurse directed and to note procedures. The head nurse first had a conference with the doctors relative to the various patients, then preceded
the doctors to the respective beds, with the probationers not otherwise
occupied following close behind. Much valuable information could be
picked up on rounds, and Adelaide seldom lost an opportunity to
acquire more information about disease and its treatment. Dr. Kelly
had been a colleague of Dr. Osler at the University of Pennsylvania,
and, although only thirty-one years old, was widely recognized in the
field of gynecology. Hunter Robb had been one of Kelly's most promising students, and, after two years as a resident physician at the
Kensington Hospital for Women, he had been invited by Kelly to
come to Hopkins.[22]

At lunchtime Adelaide again helped arrange the trays. After a
morning of scrubbing, cleaning, bedmaking, and ministering to the
patients' wants, she was glad to have an hour off for rest and study
before returning to the ward. She would also have off one afternoon a
week and part of Sunday. Student nurses were expected to attend the
church of their choice on Sunday.

After supper, Adelaide and her fellow-probationers hurried to the
room where they were to hear the first lecture by a member of the
medical staff. The room was small and was equipped with the barest
essentials: chairs, tables, an improvised blackboard, a skeleton, and
some model bones. The air became stuffy and uncomfortable, and
Adelaide had to struggle to listen and take verbatim notes on the first
of Dr. Alexander Abbott's six lectures on "Ventilation." These she
later edited, compared with the notes taken by the other pupils, and
then copied in ink. Miss Hampton had emphasized that, because the
school had no library and there were so few nursing textbooks available, it behooved each student nurse to keep a careful notebook, which
would later be graded on neatness, accuracy, and completeness.

From her first month's stipend of eight dollars, Adelaide purchased
her own copy of Clara Weeks' *Textbook of Nursing.* She read it care-

[22] Hunter Robb (1863–1940) was born in Burlington, N.J., and received his
M.D. from the University of Pennsylvania Medical School in 1884. In 1888 and
1889 he was resident physician in gynecology, Kensington Hospital for Women,
Philadelphia. A gynecologist at The Johns Hopkins Hospital from 1889 to 1894,
he then moved to Lakeside Hospital, Cleveland, Ohio, where he remained for
twenty years. In World War I, Major Robb served in the Medical Department
of the army from 1918 to 1919.

Robb married Isabel A. Hampton (1860–1910) in London in 1894; their sons
were Hampton and Philip. He married twice after her death. He was the author
of several books published from 1894 to 1914.

See clippings from the *Philadelphia Evening Bulletin*, May 16, 1940, and the
New York Times, May 16, 1940, MAN Papers.

fully, marked passages that she wanted to remember, defined terms in the margin, and occasionally entered a questioning "Why?"[23]

During the first year the formal classes in nursing were taught by Miss Hampton as regularly as her duties as director of the nursing services of the hospital permitted. At 5:00 P.M. she rushed breathless from her office into the classroom, a few notes and Mrs. Weeks' textbook clutched in her hand. There she met a group of weary young women who had been up since 6:00 A.M. and who often had had less than an hour free during the day. Greeting them with a sympathetic smile, she began. Soon the flush of her own fatigue vanished, her eyes brightened, and her voice became lyrical as she dwelt upon the role of the nurse and the importance of learning everything it was possible to know about the human bodies and minds to which they would minister.

Sometimes the students became so entranced by Miss Hampton's enthusiasm that they failed to take notes. Later they reproached themselves and gathered in little huddles over their copies of Gray, Martin, and Weeks and tried to recall just what Miss Hampton had said. Years later, Adelaide Nutting wrote: "Lecture books were the bane of our existence. We came home too fatigued to write and fill in the gaps."[24]

In addition to Miss Hampton's classes the first year, there were sixty-six lectures by thirteen physicians between November 1 and June 26: six lectures on ventilation; six on anatomy and physiology; thirteen on aseptic and antiseptic surgery and the care of surgical patients; ten on materia medica, poisons, and antidotes; one on fever; three on nursing diseases of the throat and nose; five on gynecological nursing, including operating room techniques; four on the care of infants and children in health and in disease; three on the care of diseases of the skin; two on the application of electricity; and three on the care of the nervous and the insane. The last lecture of the year was on occupational therapy.[25]

Three probationers entered after Adelaide, and in February, 1890, a new class of nineteen was enrolled.[26] The capacity of the hospital the first year was 272 beds. By January 1, 1890, the number occupied was 169, and additional staff was added. Six hundred fifty-five per-

[23] Adelaide Nutting's copy of Clara S. Weeks, *Textbook of Nursing* (1889 ed.), Adelaide Nutting Historical Nursing Collections.

[24] Adelaide Nutting, "Notes," possibly for a lecture [*ca.* 1900], MAN Papers.

[25] "Schedule of Lectures, The Johns Hopkins Hospital Training School for Nurses, 1889–1891," photostat, Record of Emma Cleaver, The Johns Hopkins School of Nursing Archives.

[26] *The Johns Hopkins Nurses Alumnae Magazine*, January, 1939, pp. 10–11.

sons were treated in the hospital during the first seven and a half months that it was in operation.[27]

Miss Hampton was a firm believer in the importance of dietetics, and in April, 1890, arranged for a cooking school to be organized under the direction of Miss Mary A. Boland, a graduate of the Boston Cooking School. This was an innovation for nursing schools and may have been the first of its kind. Miss Hampton persuaded Dr. Hurd and the Board of Trustees that suitable space in the main building should be converted into a diet kitchen. The organization of the cooking school was similar to that of a ward, with the teacher corresponding to the head nurse, and two students working for a month at a time. The students spent the first hour and a half of their day in the private wards, where each took charge of preparations for breakfast—making the toast and arranging the trays in order to have everything ready when the food arrived from the kitchen at eight o'clock. After serving the trays they left the wards at nine, going directly to the diet kitchen. During the month's training the students were taught to prepare 150 items that might appear in a patient's diet. Each student was required to make these items at least three times without direct supervision. In the afternoon theoretical instruction was given. There were oral, written, and practical tests.[28]

As yet the hospital had no pediatric service, so Miss Hampton arranged that on June 15, 1890, the Training School would take over nursing for the summer at the Thomas Wilson Sanitarium, a country vacation home for infants and children in nearby Green Spring Valley. Some children were sent only for the day, but there were cottages where mothers could come with their children and stay for as long as two weeks. A big frame house served as an infirmary. Miss L. Miller was named head nurse and would direct a rotating staff of three student nurses. Each student nurse would work for three weeks, but the three would be replaced one at a time. This provided only superficial experience in dealing with children, but Miss Hampton thought that the project might be useful from an educational and administrative point of view; she made biweekly inspections all summer long. Regular teaching was suspended during the summer months, when

[27] Of the 655 patients treated during the first seven and a half months, 409 were men, 246 were women. Of the men, 66 were Negro; of the women, 67 were Negro. In 1894 separate wards for Negroes were opened. Henry M. Hurd, *First Report of the Superintendent of The Johns Hopkins Hospital, May 15, 1889, to January 31, 1890.* (Baltimore: The Johns Hopkins Press, 1890).

[28] Johns and Pfefferkorn, *The Johns Hopkins Hospital School of Nursing,* p. 72.

disease was rampant and the student nurses and regular staff were constantly on call.

Night nursing was always difficult. It was twelve-hour duty instead of nine. The nights were long and lonely, and one dared not fall asleep. In the early months only the night superintendent was on duty, and one nurse was in charge of two floors. Miss Hampton had sensed from the beginning both Adelaide's determination and her lack of strength. One morning she stopped beside the table where Adelaide was working on a patient's record and whispered: "You are to go on night duty tonight. I have kept you from it as long as I can."[29]

Not long after Adelaide arrived at Johns Hopkins, Miss Hampton invited her to go to the theater, "perhaps to size me up," Miss Nutting wrote years later. This was the beginning of a long friendship. Both delighted in the theater, music, good books, and the companionship of bright and intelligent people. To her apt pupil, Isabel Hampton confided her dreams for the training school and nursing in general.

In September, 1890, Adelaide took her first vacation. She spent it in Bradford, Massachusetts, with Aunt Jane and Uncle Nathaniel Stickney and their daughter, Jennie. Jennie had a fine new horse, a new double-seated carriage, and a new coachman. "With this very flourishing outfit," Adelaide wrote her father, "we take our drives abroad daily and have I think pretty thoroughly explored Haverhill and Bradford and their environments. I had not an idea how pretty the country about here is, and the Merrimac deserves all of Whittier's songs." She also went to Lowell for a three-day visit with Aunt Helen and Uncle Daniel Hamblett and Cousin Addie Puffer and her new baby. The Puffer home was "full of pretty things," and Adelaide concluded that Addie and Stephen must be quite prosperous. She had to be back at the hospital by September 24 and thought she might return by water. "The trip between Boston and Baltimore is [a] particularly pretty and pleasant one, for they stop a whole day at Norfolk and it gives one a chance of seeing a scrap of Virginia."[30]

Although the vacation was short, Adelaide was happy to be back at the hospital to start her second year's work. This time she did not feel she was entering a different world. She knew the nurses and most of the doctors and was beginning to be quite fond of some of them, especially Dr. Osler and Dr. Welch. She had even made some friends in Baltimore: Dr. Osler's niece Georgia, who kept house for him be-

29 Adelaide Nutting, "Notes for Story of Life," MAN Papers.
30 Adelaide Nutting (Bradford, Mass.) to Vespasion Nutting (Waterloo, Quebec), September 19, 1890, ibid.

fore his marriage, the Gilmans, and the Kings. It was good to greet fellow-nurses-in-training. She especially liked Georgia Nevins, a slender, gentle blonde who shared her enthusiasm for plays, concerts, books, and travel. Adelaide was beginning to feel more sure of herself. When the first preliminary examinations were given in September, she averaged 94 and stood fifth in her class.[31]

Soon after Adelaide's return to Hopkins a new class was enrolled, and, in November, Lavinia L. Dock, a graduate of Bellevue, began her work as assistant to Miss Hampton. "Very soon we learned an extraordinary mind was among us," Miss Nutting wrote, "a scholar, a student, a teacher of rare originality and ability. I recall with delight how she would come into the ward to follow us up and see how we were doing our work, how she illuminated a task, every step in a process was interesting and significant."[32] The students were divided into three groups; seniors, middle class, and juniors. Classes for seniors were held on Monday, for the middle class on Tuesday, and for juniors on Friday, now from 3:00 to 4:00 P.M. rather than from 5:00 to 6:00 P.M.[33] Lectures by the doctors continued to be given twice weekly in the evenings. Miss Dock took over the classes for the middle group and the juniors. Under Miss Hampton the seniors were given instruction on nursing in surgery, in medical cases, hygiene, gynecology, pediatrics, materia medica, dietetics, and urinalysis. Miss Hampton also gave instruction in ethics, ward management, and private and district nursing. Obstetrical nursing was emphasized because of the many calls for nurses to come to private homes for such services. During the two years that Adelaide Nutting was a student, only one baby was born in the hospital, and everyone wanted to take care of it.[34]

In their last year student nurses were sent into homes to do private duty nursing. This was very much against Miss Hampton's principles, however, and she fought against it at every opportunity. Home nursing paid from fifteen to twenty-five dollars a week and was duty around the clock with time off only at the convenience of the family. Provisions for sleep and for meals were usually inadequate, and there was greater danger of contagion for the nurse on private duty than for nurses in the wards. Instead, Miss Hampton advocated visiting or

[31] Johns and Pfefferkorn, *The Johns Hopkins Hospital School of Nursing,* p. 75.

[32] Adelaide Nutting, "Notes for Story of Life," MAN Papers.

[33] Johns and Pfefferkorn, *The Johns Hopkins Hospital School of Nursing,* p. 76.

[34] Edith Ware, interview with Isabel M. Stewart, New York, November 11, 1940, The Johns Hopkins Hospital School of Nursing Archives.

public health nursing, a program whereby second-year students might be sent out under the direction of a specially trained nurse. It was a proposal made far in advance of the times.

Adelaide was sent out on a private duty case in which a man, the breadwinner in a family of four, had been ill with typhoid fever for five weeks. He was delirious and had a temperature of 105°, and he had not had his clothes off the entire time. His tongue was covered with such a thick black crust that Adelaide had to use surgical tweezers to remove it. It was a harrowing experience, but she did not contract the disease, and after weeks of careful nursing the patient recovered.[35]

In November, 1890, the *Trained Nurse and Hospital Review* announced as a "new departure" the offer of special prizes "to be awarded for an essay giving full particulars with notes, as to temperature, dietary, etc., of a typhoid fever case, describing if possible the case from its commencement to its termination." Adelaide submitted an account of her experience. It was simply written and bore testimony to thorough and exact observations by a bedside nurse long before the case study technique became popular. Reporting that its office had been "flooded" with entries, the magazine awarded a first prize of ten dollars to Miss M. A. Nutting, The Johns Hopkins Hospital, Baltimore; the essay would be published in March, 1891.

The first issue of The Johns Hopkins Hospital *Bulletin* reported a meeting of the Hospital Journal Club at which various physicians reviewed articles they had read in British, German, French, and American medical journals. Dr. Hurd thought highly of the club meetings, and on January 28, 1891, Miss Hampton called together the Hopkins nursing staff and students in the training school for the purpose of organizing a Nurses' Journal Club. Its object, she said, would be to promote an *esprit de corps* among the members of the school, to keep in touch with what was being done in other schools and hospitals by means of reports and discussions drawn chiefly from British and American medical and nursing magazines, and to insure the reading of such papers by all. Attendance at the biweekly Monday meetings would be compulsory for students, but only the head nurses, senior students, superintendent, and assistant superintendent would be expected to prepare papers. Junior members might join in the discussions.[36]

[35] Mary Adelaide Nutting, "A Case of Typhoid," prize-winning essay, *Trained Nurse and Hospital Review*, March, 1891, p. 121.
[36] Adelaide Nutting, "The Hopkins Journal Club," MAN Papers.

The same evening that Miss Hampton launched the Nurses Journal Club and appointed its officers, she addressed the group on "The Scope and Aims of The Johns Hopkins Medical School," to be opened within the next two years.

Isabel Hampton and Lavinia Dock were aware of the paucity of basic nursing literature and were determined to do something about it. While night superintendent at Bellevue, Miss Dock had been disturbed by many doctors' ignorance of drugs, as revealed in discrepancies in dosages prescribed. She had done extensive research and had written a book, *Materia Medica*, for nurses, but when it appeared in 1893 its most avid readers were medical men. Miss Hampton resolved that as soon as she could find the time she would write a textbook on nursing, a text more scientific and comprehensive than Clara Weeks's work. She had already made some notes for *Nursing: Its Principles and Practices*. Inspired by Miss Dock and Miss Hampton, Mary Boland began to write a textbook in the field of dietetics; it was published in 1894 as *A Handbook of Invalid Cookery*. Osler, Welch, Halsted, Kelly, Hurd—everyone at Hopkins seemed to be writing.[37]

As Adelaide's studies drew to a close, she thought of the future. Should she look for a hospital of her own, or did she need more experience? Miss Hampton spoke so enthusiastically of her sojourn in St. Paul's House, Rome, where she had gone after graduation from Bellevue, and of the travel and unusual cultural opportunities it afforded that Adelaide thought of applying for a place there.

Under the aegis of the American Episcopalian Church, St. Paul's House provided a staff of British and American nurses to serve wealthy travelers who fell ill while in Italy. When Isabel Hampton went there in 1884, the staff was composed of the director and six nurses, three British and three American. Each nurse agreed to stay one and a half years and was paid fifteen dollars a month; when a nurse was called to care for a patient outside the hospital, St. Paul's collected fifteen dollars a week from her wages. American nurses went over for two winters' work, while British nurses came in the autumn and returned in the spring.[38]

St. Paul's House was a large, square villa with beautiful yellow roses climbing over the front wall. In summer the nurses could go to

[37] Lavinia L. Dock, *Materia Medica* (New York: G. P. Putnam, 1893); Isabel A. Hampton, *Nursing: Its Principles and Practices* (Philadelphia: W. B. Saunders, 1893); Mary A. Boland, *A Handbook of Invalid Cookery* (New York: Century, 1894).

[38] Alice Warren (New York) to Adelaide Nutting (New York), May 29, [1940], MAN Papers.

a residence in Lucerne when not on duty. After the slums of New York's East Side, Miss Hampton had thrilled to the soft beauty of the Italian landscape, the Medici Gardens where she gathered violets, the fountains in the plazas, the opera, and the art galleries.

Patients there were different from the derelicts she had so often nursed at Bellevue. There was the gay Lady Colin Campbell, who did not conform to Isabel's code of conduct but who was nevertheless an interesting person to be around, and there was Mrs. William Astor, wife of the American ambassador to England, who became fond of Isabel and asked her to social affairs. Sometimes Isabel accompanied patients to France or Germany, and in her free time she visited museums, historical places, studied French and German, and attended concerts. She learned how to converse with the cultured and urbane. The sojourn in Rome brought the realization of her capacity and self-confidence, and she recommended the experience to students who might profit from it. She especially urged Adelaide to consider it.[39]

In a letter to her father on May 3, 1891, Adelaide intimated her plans: "Dear knows when I shall see you all again for I don't expect to take a vacation this summer. . . . I realize however fully that this work is carrying me farther and farther away from my old life and those dear to me—and the prospects are that I shall find myself doing fever nursing in Rome before two years are over."

After five months in medical under Dr. Osler, Adelaide was transferred to new work in general surgery, which she did not expect to like so well. After a month or two in surgery, she would probably go to the operating room and dispensary. Then would come the necessary four months of private nursing, which she "hated the thought of."

May promised to be a busy month, with final examinations extending into early June. Adelaide felt so ill-prepared that her heart went down to her boots every time she thought of them. She had studied hard, but her competitors were "very formidable." Three of the class had been teachers, one had a college degree, and all of them were physically stronger. The best she expected was to come out sixth.[40]

Final examinations averaged two a week, and each lasted from one and a half to two hours. All of the students passed the required mark of 70 percent, although several did not go far above it. Mrs. Emory ranked first with an average of 96.7 percent; Mary Gross scored a

[39] Evelyn Pope and Ruth Williams, graduates of The Johns Hopkins Hospital Training School in 1891, later served on the staff of St. Paul's House. Johns and Pfefferkorn, *The Johns Hopkins Hospital School of Nursing*, pp. 44–46.

[40] Adelaide Nutting (Baltimore) to Vespasion Nutting (Waterloo), May 3, 1891, MAN Papers.

close second with 96.0 percent; Ruth Williams was third with 94.9 percent; and Adelaide Nutting surpassed her own estimate by coming out fourth with 94.0 percent.[41]

Graduating exercises were held in the rotunda of the administration building. Chairs were brought in for the visitors. A space to the right and to the left of the grand stairway was roped off for the speakers, the trustees, and the nursing staff. Potted palms and ferns lent an air of dignity. Among those on the platform were Francis T. King, Dr. Hurd, the Reverend Dr. Goucher, the Reverend Griffin, Dr. William Welch, Dr. Osler, and Mrs. Daniel Coit Gilman. The *Baltimore Sun* reported the exercises "most impressive."

Near the stage sat the head nurses in "pure white." Miss Dock and three student nurses "played a march on two pianos" as the seventeen graduates, dressed in their light blue uniforms with stiffly starched white collars, aprons, and caps, followed by the student nurses, descended the marble stairway. When the last step was reached, the procession stopped. The Reverend Griffin gave the invocation and then the graduates and students seated themselves on the stairs. As president of the Board of Trustees, Mr. King introduced Miss Hampton, who looked tall and especially beautiful in her black uniform. She sketched the brief history of the school and spoke of the function of the nurse and the importance of good public relations. She was proud of this first graduating class and once more told her students that they were always to bear in mind the sacredness of their calling and the trust imposed upon them.[42]

When Dr. Osler came forward to make the address of the day, "Doctor and Nurse," which would become a classic in nursing literature, he was greeted by smiles of approval. He was by far the most beloved of the hospital physicians. Adelaide gave Georgia Nevins' hand a gentle squeeze as she glanced from the speaker to the portrait of Johns Hopkins and recalled the night she had stood in front of it eighteen months before.

In his characteristic light and gentle way, Dr. Osler began by saying that doctors and nurses remind men of their frailties. There is no time when birth, life, death are not associated with that grizzly group, physicians and nurses.

A master painter in words, Osler in a few terse sentences traced the historic interplay of science, medicine, and nursing. Then he

---

[41] Johns and Pfefferkorn, *The Johns Hopkins Hospital School of Nursing*, p. 83.

[42] Clipping from the *Baltimore Sun*, June 16, 1891, The Johns Hopkins Hospital School of Nursing Archives.

brought his audience up sharply to the present: "We no longer mock the heart prostrate in the grief of loss, with the words, 'Whom the Lord loveth, he chastiseth' when we know the milk should have been sterilized."

Turning to the young women seated on the stairs, he said:

> You will be better women for the life that you have led here, better women in that the eyes of your souls have been opened, the range of your sympathies has been widened, and your characters have been molded by the events in which you have participated during the past two years.
>
> Practically there should be for each of you a busy, useful and happy life, more you can not expect, a greater blessing the world can not bestow. . . . Happy lives should be yours, because busy and useful; having been initiated into the great secret—that happiness lies in the absorption in some vocation which satisfies the soul; that we are to add when we can *to*, not to get what we can out of life.
>
> And finally remember what we are, useful supernumeraries in the battle, simply stage accessories in the drama, playing minor but essential parts at the exits and the entrances, or picking up, here and there, a strutter who may have tripped upon the stage. You have been much by the dark river, so near to us all—and have seen so many embark, that the dread of the old boatman has almost disappeared and
>
>> When the Angel of the darker Drink
>> At last shall find you by the river brink
>> And offering his cup, invite your soul
>> Forth to your lips to quaff, you shall not shrink.
>
> Your passport shall be the blessing of Him in whose footsteps you have trodden, unto whose sick you have ministered, and for whose children you have cared.[43]

Eighty years later a copy of this address would still be given as a souvenir to each graduating Hopkins nurse.

Dr. Hurd conferred the diplomas and presented a scroll to each graduate. Mrs. Gilman presented each with a bouquet of LaFrance roses from Dr. Osler. After the benediction and recessional, relatives and friends hurried to congratulate the graduates and to inspect the Nurses' Home, where that evening there would be a reception for five hundred. According to her rank in the graduating class, Adelaide would stand fourth from Miss Hampton in the receiving line.

It was almost midnight when the last guest departed, but it was not too late for a few lines to Min. It was all over—no more lectures, no more classes, only four months of private duty. In September Adelaide would be on her own.

---

[43] William Osler, "Doctor and Nurse" (Address before the first graduating class of The Johns Hopkins Hospital Training School for Nurses, June 5, 1891).

VII

Head Nurse, 1891–1893

September came at last, after a summer of private duty and wards crowded with typhoid patients. A vacation was never more welcome to Adelaide. She started at once for visits with Aunt Jane, Aunt Helen, and the Massachusetts cousins. She would have liked to go to see Min and Gilbert in St. John's. In July, Minnie's second baby had been born, a girl who was named Harriet Armine. Jim and Claire had recently lost Kenneth, their second son, and would have been cheered by a visit. But, out of her stipend of twelve dollars a month, Adelaide was barely able to pay for the trip to Massachusetts. Only once had she written Charlie for money, and then for only fifteen dollars.[1]

While in Bradford a letter inviting her to come back to Hopkins as a "head nurse" made it "unexpectedly advisable" for Adelaide to buy the necessary linen and begin making the white uniforms. Thus she had to borrow money for the return trip to Baltimore. She planned to pay Aunt Jane in monthly installments in October and November. If she stayed on at the hospital, her December 1 check would be for thirty dollars. At the Puffers, Adelaide had "flourished the flag of independence wildly" and frightened Addie away from offering her anything, but not from cramming a new nightgown into her handbag. "It is a fool's idea to travel without a margin," Adelaide wrote Min, "and your sister not being a fool will never attempt it again. I have been in positive terror for fear of turning up in some predicament penniless."[2]

In addition to making three linen uniforms, Adelaide made a new basque, the old one "having actually gone to pieces." It disconcerted

[1] Adelaide Nutting (Baltimore) to Vespasion Nutting (Waterloo, Quebec), May 8, 1891; and Adelaide Nutting (aboard the S.S. *Essex*, en route to Baltimore) to Armine N. Gosling (St. John's, Newfoundland), September 24, 1891; MAN Papers.
[2] Adelaide Nutting (aboard the S.S. *Essex*, en route to Baltimore) to Armine N. Gosling (St. John's), September 24, 1891, *ibid.*

her that her clothes were so shabby. "I look older now than I really am and dress abominably when you realize that a gray dress trimmed with fur is to be worn this year for the sixth winter."[3] After she got her first thirty dollars she hoped to buy a dress on sale. Oh, to be able to buy Christmas presents!

Adelaide returned to Baltimore by ship. Cousin Jennie accompanied her to Boston, where they learned to Adelaide's consternation that the sailing of the *Essex* had been delayed twenty-four hours. Jennie generously suggested that they stay overnight at the Adams House, browse in the shops and go to a play, and that for the sake of company she would gladly pay the bill.

Adelaide loved the sea. The first night on board the *Essex*, as she sat alone on deck looking at the stars and listening to the waves, she thought over the past two years and that first journey to Baltimore. After two months' duty she would be a full-fledged graduate nurse. She was suddenly engulfed in loneliness and confessed in a letter to Min: "I wished among other things I had not put an end to my friendship with dear old Jack. I miss him sorely and now I starve with nothing, were I surfeited with too much not so very long ago."[4]

Late Sunday night Adelaide arrived in Baltimore, sound and refreshed despite the fact that she "had not gained a pound of flesh where tons were expected." She was growing weary of comments about her thinness. She puffed out her hair a bit and patted her cheeks before going down to breakfast and to receive her new assignment. To her delight, Dr. Osler had chosen her to be his head nurse, and Miss Hampton had approved. The Men's Medical, being Dr. Osler's ward, was the pet ward of the hospital.

Adelaide reasoned that this was what Miss Hampton had had in mind when she told her to have white uniforms in readiness.[5] Adelaide's classmate Georgia Nevins would remain as head nurse in Ward B, and Evelyn Pope as head nurse in the dispensary.

Although it was not apparent to Adelaide at the time, as vacancies occurred Miss Hampton was deliberately replacing the original staff of head nurses with nurses of her own training, and thus was eliminating dissension among the head nurses who had diverse and unchangeable ideas about nursing procedures, ideas that in many instances baffled and confused the young women in training. Isabel Hampton believed in conformity. The Hopkins way would perforce be the Hampton way. By October, 1890, all of the night nurses except the

3 *Ibid.*
4 *Ibid.*
5 *Ibid.*

head nurse were students. Miss Hampton was determined to build a Hopkins *esprit de corps* as quickly as possible; however things went wrong, she was always loyal to her nurses and she inspired loyalty in them.[6] She was sensitive to relationships within the hospital hierarchy and to the authority which her position as superintendent of nursing services and principal of the training school conferred upon her. Occasionally she clashed with physicians if she found them trying to interfere with her assignment of nurses, and she would listen unmoved to their complaints when favored nurses had been transferred to other wards. Her wrath might be swift in its descent, but it was short-lived.

Miss Hampton and Miss Dock, both graduates of Bellevue, were in complete agreement about the relation of the training school to the nursing services. Both accepted the Nightingale military tradition. As Miss Dock wrote in her lecture notebook for a class in professional ethics:

> The nurse is a soldier, absolute and unquestioning obedience to a superior officer is the fundamental idea of the military system in order that responsibility may be rightly placed. . . . There is a necessity for drill in producing quickness, skill, and quiet. Criticisms are not accusations. Strictness and exactness produce better nurses.[7]

Adelaide's position as a graduate nurse brought her into a new and closer association with Miss Hampton and Miss Dock. When she became better acquainted with Lavinia Dock, she became more aware of her rare mind and her love of books and music. Sometimes they played piano duets, and sometimes Adelaide sang while "Dockie" played her accompaniment.

Dockie was an ardent feminist and a great admirer of Susan B. Anthony and Lucy Stone. Adelaide and Isabel were sympathetic but not militant supporters of the cause. Adelaide quoted her father, who had always contended that women had as much right to vote as men. The three often breakfasted together on Sunday mornings and discussed matters relating to nursing services and nursing education, as well as the activities of doctors Osler, Halsted, Kelly, and Welch, who, while waiting for the Medical School to open, were reading, researching, and writing.

The senior residents in medicine, surgery, gynecology, and pathology, all unmarried, had suites in the administration building, and

---

[6] Ethel Johns and Blanche Pfefferkorn, *The Johns Hopkins Hospital School of Nursing* (Baltimore: The Johns Hopkins Press, 1943), p. 87.
[7] *Ibid.*, p. 7.

when not on duty the graduate nurses saw much of them. There were games of tennis and croquet on the lawn, and tea and parties in the Nurses' Home. Dr. Hunter Robb, Dr. Kelly's resident in gynecology, was quite devoted to Miss Hampton, and through him they learned much about the Triumvirate, Welch, Kelly, and Osler, and their hobbies and idiosyncrasies. Welch, the pathologist, and an authority on hog cholera, was a connoisseur of fine food. Osler, writing his magnum opus, *Principles and Practices of Medicine,* had practically taken over the "Robin's study," as he called Dr. Robb's sitting room, where now and then he broke the monotony of writing by playing practical jokes.[8]

"At Hopkins, we try things," Halsted had said. Only the year before, a simple technique had been introduced in his operating room which would soon become standard practice in all hospitals. While Caroline Hampton was Halsted's head nurse, she had developed eczema of the hands from plunging them into strong disinfectants. Observing Dr. Welch's use of rubber gloves in the pathological laboratory, Dr. Halsted asked the Goodyear Rubber Company to make some thin, elbow-length rubber gloves that could be worn by a nurse. Dr. Joseph Bloodgood, noting that the gloves had not impaired the nurse's dexterity, then posed the question, "Why should not the surgeon as well as the nurse wear rubber gloves?"[9]

There was little time for luxuriating at breakfast on weekdays. Sometimes in the evening Adelaide, Isabel Hampton, and Lavinia Dock met in Miss Hampton's apartment to discuss plans, or as Miss Dock would say, "to map strategy." The hospital's services were expanding, and a demand for Hopkins graduates was growing. In March, 1892, Adelaide wrote her father:

> This is the dearest old hospital in the world and I offer up perpetual psalms of thanksgiving that I came here instead of elsewhere. The work never loses its interest, nor the place its charm and though it is undeniably hard it is not uncongenial. . . . Whenever you think of me, let it be as contented and happy in my lot.[10]

Baltimore had come to be something like home to Adelaide. She had become acquainted with several Baltimore families and thought if she had any leisure she might "go about a good bit." Georgina Osler,

[8] Harvey Cushing, *Sir William Osler,* 2 vols. (Oxford: Clarendon Press, 1925), 1:349, 358.

[9] W. G. MacCallum, *William Stewart Halsted, Surgeon* (Baltimore: The Johns Hopkins Press, 1930), quoted in Johns and Pfefferkorn, *The Johns Hopkins Hospital School of Nursing,* p. 33.

[10] Adelaide Nutting (Baltimore) to Vespasion Nutting (Waterloo), March 6, 1892, MAN Papers.

who kept house for her uncle, often invited Adelaide for Sunday dinner or Saturday night supper. Adelaide discussed books and public affairs with Dr. Osler, and sometimes he took the girls to concerts or "squired" them to balls. Georgina was engaged to Dr. Alexander Abbott, who had delivered the first medical lecture to Adelaide's class. Although it had not yet been announced, Dr. Osler would soon marry Grace Revere Gross of Philadelphia, the widow of his friend Dr. Samuel W. Gross.[11] In Mrs. Osler, Adelaide would find another friend, and in years to come when she was looking tired and exhausted the Oslers would take her in their carriage to their home, No. 1 West Franklin Street, for a weekend of rest.

Adelaide was not absolutely settled about going to Rome in November, but she felt certain she would go sooner or later. Miss Hampton invited her to go with her to the Berlitz School of Languages, as she thought it would be good for her to study a little Italian. Adelaide thoroughly enjoyed her studies, and a knowledge of the language renewed her interest in history and literature.[12]

What she really wanted to do was to spend two years nursing in Rome and on the Continent, and then come home and take over a training school and see what she could do with it.[13] Often she had wished she had her sister's training and ability to teach. She observed Miss Hampton and Miss Dock and the devices they used to make nursing concepts clear, to create a feeling for their calling and an awareness of the trust imposed. Miss Hampton was building a Hopkins tradition.

Before the second class of Hopkins nurses graduated in June, 1892, members of the first class were invited to return and assist in the organization of an alumnae association. At that time there were only two other nursing school alumnae associations in the United States: one at Bellevue, organized in 1889; and one at the Illinois Training School, established in 1891. On the afternoon of June 3, twenty-five members of the two classes met in the Nurses' Home. Helena Barnard, class of 1892, was elected president; Adelaide Nutting, class of 1891, was elected secretary and treasurer; and Susan C. Reid, class of 1891, was elected corresponding secretary. A few days later Isabel Hampton and Lavinia Dock were invited to become honorary members of the new association. A committee was set up to draft a constitution and

[11] Dr. William Osler and Mrs. Grace Revere Gross were married in Philadelphia, May 7, 1892. Georgina Osler and Dr. Alexander C. Abbott were married in Toronto, Canada, August 30, 1892. Cushing, *Sir William Osler*, 1:362, 366.

[12] Adelaide Nutting, "Notes on Mrs. Isabel Hampton Robb," MAN Papers.

[13] Adelaide Nutting (Baltimore) to Vespasion Nutting (Waterloo), March 6, 1892, MAN Papers.

bylaws and to incorporate the organization under the General Laws of the State of Maryland.

The purpose of the association was to promote unity and good feeling among the graduates and to advance interest in the profession of nursing. It also had the ambitious objective of a home for its members and provision for them when ill or disabled.[14] As an officer of the association and as a member of the hospital staff, Adelaide was close to the organization in its early years and became a dynamic influence twenty-five years later when it took on the responsibility of fundraising. She was proud of her Hopkins pin, a Maltese cross in blue and black enamel (The Johns Hopkins University colors) on a gold background with the letters "JHH" in the center. On the back was inscribed the date of her graduation, 1891, and the motto "Vigilando," a reiteration of the nurse's moral responsibility for abiding watchfulness.[15]

To everyone at Johns Hopkins, the delay in the opening of the Medical School was a matter of great concern. Despite an endowment of three and one-half million dollars, the trustees wisely used only accrued income in constructing the plant. Most of the Hopkins endowment consisted of Baltimore and Ohio Railroad stock, and, in 1887, when the company failed to pay dividends, the opening of the school had to be postponed. The enthusiastic and competent faculty that had been employed were now being called to other institutions. Dr. Hunter Robb resigned to go to Cleveland in January, 1892, and subsequently Dr. Alexander C. Abbott went to Philadelphia, Dr. F. J. Brockaway to Columbia University, and Dr. W. T. Councilman to Harvard. Harvard was angling for Dr. Welch, and McGill wanted Dr. Osler.[16]

The future of the Medical School was precarious, but the trustees were adamant that the school could not be opened with less than half a million dollars.

Learning of the dilemma through their families, Elizabeth T. King, daughter of the president of the Board of Trustees; Mary Garrett, daughter of the president of the Baltimore and Ohio Railroad; Mary Gwinn, daughter of Johns Hopkins' own attorney; Carey Thomas, daughter of a trustee; and their friend Julia Rogers determined to save the Medical School and retain its unusual faculty. They arranged for

---

[14] The Act of Incorporation provided for chartering the organization as "The Alumnae Association of the Johns Hopkins Training School for Nurses of Baltimore City. In 1933 this cumbersome official name was changed to "The Johns Hopkins Hospital Nurses Alumnae Association, Incorporated." Johns and Pfefferkorn, *The Johns Hopkins Hospital School of Nursing*, pp. 91, 362–65.

[15] *Ibid.*, p. 365.

[16] Cushing, *Sir William Osler*, 1:350, 351, 372, 379.

a meeting of public-spirited women at Miss King's home on May 2, 1890. Miss Hampton attended but took no part in the deliberations. A Women's Fund Committee was organized.

Dr. Carey Thomas, dean at Bryn Mawr and soon to be its president, had wanted to enter the Ph.D. program at The Johns Hopkins University but was permitted only to take some Greek courses under Professor Gildersleeve. She resented the attitude of the authorities toward women and after a year withdrew to complete her studies in Zurich. She and her friends were keenly interested in opening up more educational opportunities for women. They reasoned that, if they could raise a sufficient sum of money toward the endowment of the Medical School, the trustees might be compelled to accept the gift, despite the stipulation that women be admitted to the school on the same footing as men.

The women formed committees for propaganda, and in every city where one or two socially prominent volunteers could be secured, they launched a campaign for funds. Miss Garrett led off with a great reception, to which Baltimore's social and wealthy elite and distinguished outsiders were invited. Among those who came were Mrs. Benjamin Harrison, wife of the president of the United States, and Mr. and Mrs. Richard Watson Gilder, of Century Magazine. Mrs. Harrison allowed her name to be used as honorary chairman of the Washington committee. Subsequently, letters appeared in Century in behalf of the fund-raising women from such prominent persons as Dr. Mary Putnam Jacobi, Josephine Lowell, Dr. William Osler, and His Eminence, James Cardinal Gibbons, archbishop and head of the Roman Catholic hierarchy in America.[17] Miss Hampton, Miss Dock, and Miss Nutting did not take part in the fund-raising of the so-called embattled ladies, but they privately gave them their blessing.

Miss Garrett and Miss Thomas started the campaign by donating substantial sums and promising more if the trustees would raise a corresponding amount. After raising one hundred thousand dollars within eight months, the Women's Committee felt it was in a position to dictate terms. Miss Garrett came forward with the money needed to meet the committee's goal of half a million dollars, but in a letter of petition to the trustees she prescribed unequivocally the conditions of the gift, the standards for the school, and the position of women in it.[18]

[17] Alan M. Chesney, The Johns Hopkins Hospital and The Johns Hopkins University School of Medicine: A Chronicle, 3 vols. (Baltimore: The Johns Hopkins Press, 1943–63), 1:194–203.

[18] The Johns Hopkins Hospital Bulletin 3 (1892): 139; Cushing, Sir William Osler, 1:388.

President Gilman and Drs. Osler and Welch were somewhat startled by the high standards outlined by the women. No other medical school in America set such severe admission requirements. Later it was learned that Miss Garrett had gone to her lawyer, Charles J. M. Gwinn, also the attorney for the trustees, and he had given her a document which Welch had prepared when he came to Baltimore ten years before. The women had assumed that this was exactly what the medical faculty wanted. Neither Osler nor Welch signed the petition accompanying the letter to the trustees. Both were sympathetic toward women in nursing, where, as Dr. Hurd said, they were an extension of the physicians' hands, but they did not welcome women in the medical profession. Miss Garrett was adamant in her refusal to substitute "equal" for "same" in the terms of admission and training for women and men students; furthermore, according to the petition, the medical classroom building would be known as the Women's Memorial Building, and a lay committee of six women appointed by the trustees would supervise the extracurricular affairs of the women students.[19] Osler is said to have told Welch, "It is lucky that we got in as professors; we could never enter as students."[20] On December 22, 1892, two days after Miss Garrett's letter was sent to the trustees, a special meeting of the board was called and her offer was accepted.

Not only was the hospital staff agog at the opening of the Medical School, but breakfast, luncheon, and dinner conversations often centered on the World's Fair soon to open in Chicago. Dr. John Billings, who designed the hospital and who came over from Washington each week to lecture to graduate students on the history of medicine, was enthusiastic about the International Congress of Charities, Correction, and Philanthropy to be held under the auspices of the fair. He was chairman of the section dealing with hospitals, dispensaries, and nursing, and Dr. Hurd was its secretary; Miss Hampton was asked to serve as chairman of a subsection on nursing.

In the winter of 1892, before plans for the congress had fully crystallized, Mrs. Ethel Gordon Fenwick, dynamic leader of British nursing and editor of *Nursing Record*, an independent journal later known as the *British Journal of Nursing*, came to Chicago to arrange an exhibit of British nursing publications, techniques, and appliances. She quickly sensed the possibilities of the fair and suggested a con-

---

[19] The original committee consisted of Mrs. William Osler, Mrs. Henry Hurd, Mrs. Ira Remsen, Miss Carey Thomas, and Mrs. Mary Gwinn. *The Johns Hopkins Hospital Bulletin* 3 (1892):131.

[20] Cushing, *Sir William Osler*, 1:386.

gress on nursing to the lady managers, who referred the matter to Dr. Billings.

On her return to London, Mrs. Fenwick stopped over in Baltimore to visit America's most modern and highly publicized hospital and to confer with Miss Hampton and her associates. Adelaide was delighted to join Miss Hampton, Miss Dock, and Mrs. Fenwick at meals and to enter into the discussions on nurses' associations, registration, standards for nursing schools, professional journals, and the way in which the Chicago World's Fair could be used to advance the cause of nursing in the United States and Canada. As yet, neither country had a counterpart of the British Nurses' Association.[21]

Mrs. Fenwick would not attend the fair, but she assured Miss Hampton that British nurses would be in attendance and would represent her point of view and speak for standards and registration by examination.

In preparation for the subsection on nursing, Miss Hampton corresponded with directors of nursing schools and recruited a substantial number who could be depended upon to be present, give papers, or participate in discussions. Forewarned by Mrs. Fenwick that Sir Henry Burdett, editor of *The Hospital*, official organ of the British Hospital Association, which opposed nurses' organizations on the grounds that they were trade unions, would be present, and that Florence Nightingale herself did not favor registration, Miss Hampton arranged for strong papers that would support other points of view. She even wrote to Miss Nightingale, asking her to prepare an address to be read at the opening session.[22]

The nurses' congress assembled in the Hall of Columbus at the Chicago World's Fair on June 15, 1893, and continued for three days. At the opening meeting Miss Hampton presented Miss Nightingale's keynote address, "Sick Nursing and Health Nursing." "Training," she read, "is to teach the nurse to help the patient to live. Nursing the sick is an art; and an art requiring an organized practical and scientific training; for nursing is the skilled servant of medicine, surgery, and hygiene."[23]

Miss Hampton addressed the general session of the section on hospitals, dispensaries, and nursing on "Standards for Nurses." Miss Dock's paper before the nursing subsection was on "The Relation of

[21] Lavinia Dock [Fayetteville, Pa.] to Isabel M. Stewart (New York), n.d., IMS Papers.

[22] Isabel A. Hampton (Baltimore) to Florence Nightingale (London), January 31, 1893, photostat, The Johns Hopkins Hospital School of Nursing Archives.

[23] Mary Roberts, "Florence Nightingale as a Nurse Educator," *American Journal of Nursing*, July, 1937.

Training Schools to Hospitals." Isabel McIsaac, one of Miss Hampton's former students at the Illinois Training School for Nurses, spoke on the "Value of Alumnae Associations," of which at that time there were fewer than six. Louise Darche, an old Canadian friend of Miss Hampton, now of the New York Hospital School of Nursing, outlined a plan for the proper organization of training schools. Edith Draper presented a paper on "The Necessity of an American Nurses Association." Miss Hampton summarized: "We must in time evolve alumnae societies, an American Nurses Association, and Superintendents' Association. Our meeting here is the first step; before this Congress adjourns we should form a society of superintendents of training schools for nurses."

About twenty persons responded to the call for a meeting.[24] Mrs. K. L. Litt of St. Luke's Hospital, Chicago, invited some of the superintendents to her room to discuss the pros and cons of organization, and at the close of the next morning's session eight stayed to develop an organization. A constitution was prepared overnight and adopted before the meeting adjourned, and pro-tem officers were selected. These officers, along with Miss Hampton and Miss Irene Sutliffe, constituted an executive committee, which promptly called for a meeting in New York on January 10, 1894.[25] Miss Hampton and Miss Dock went home happy in the accomplishment of a preliminary organization of an association of superintendents of training schools.

Lavinia reported to Adelaide, who had stayed in Baltimore to run the hospital, that Sir Henry Burdett had been there but that "he did not get very far." Adelaide was glad to have Miss Dock and Miss Hampton home again. She had felt the strain of added responsibilities while Miss Hampton was gone, especially since the typhoid season was underway in Baltimore. The previous October Adelaide had transferred from Dr. Osler's ward to Dr. Halsted's surgical ward. Miss Hampton had advised that a nurse should not concentrate too much in

[24] American Society of Superintendents of Training Schools for Nurses, *First Annual Report* and *Second Annual Report* (Harrisburg, Pa.: Harrisburg Publishing Co., 1897); Blanche Pfefferkorn, "Nursing Organizations in the United States: Their Origin, Purpose, and Some of Their Results," *Modern Hospital*, February, 1917, p. 1; Mary M. Roberts, *American Nursing: History and Interpretation* (New York: Macmillan, 1954), pp. 21–25; Isabel M. Stewart and Anne L. Austin, *A History of Nursing from Ancient to Modern Times: A World View* (New York: G. P. Putnam's Sons, 1926), pp. 199–201.

[25] The personnel of the executive committee were Grace Alston, president pro tem; Mary S. P. Davis, University of Pennsylvania Hospital; Irene Sutliffe, New York Hospital; Louise Darche, City Hospital School of Nursing, New York; Lucy Drown, Boston City Hospital; Sophia Palmer, Massachusetts General Hospital; Isabel A. Hampton, The Johns Hopkins Hospital, Baltimore.

one area if she eventually planned to take over a hospital, and that it was important to become acquainted with the different personalities in physicians as in patients. Dr. Halsted was kindly, quiet, reserved, meticulous, and somewhat aloof.

As a young resident physician in New York, Halsted and two interns had experimented in partial anesthesia through the use of cocaine, and before he was aware of what was happening, Halsted had become addicted. Dr. Welch, who knew him well, supported him as he fought to overcome the habit. In a sense Halsted came to Johns Hopkins on trial, although he and Welch no longer mentioned the matter. Dr. Halsted was a hard worker, an omniverous reader of medical literature, and a skilled technician. As Adelaide worked with him, her respect for him grew.[26]

After four months with Dr. Halsted, Adelaide spent the summer in a private ward and served as acting superintendent while Miss Hampton was vacationing. Her own plans included a trip to Newfoundland to visit Minnie and Gilbert and the children. The previous summer she had vacationed with her father and Lizzie and Charlie in Waterloo, and with Claire and Jim in Ottawa. Because Vespasion Nutting was now seventy-eight years old, she had some compunctions about going to Min's home in St. John's rather than to Waterloo. She hoped her father would not feel neglected.

Adelaide found Minnie and Gilbert very happy and comfortable, but she regretted that there was so little real intellectual companionship for them in St. John's.

One bright spot had appeared on the Newfoundland horizon, however, and would reappear from time to time. In the summer of 1892 Dr. Wilfred Grenfell, a British medical missionary cruising in the hospital ship *Albert* along the east coast of Canada, holding religious services in various settlements and treating some 900 sick persons, put in at St. John's harbor. Gilbert met him and brought him to his home. "We have seen a great deal of him," Minnie wrote Adelaide, "and we both like and admire him immensely. He is quite young and

[26] William Stewart Halsted (1852–1922), who graduated from Yale in 1874, was first renowned as an athlete; he graduated from the College of Surgeons, New York, in 1877 and interned at Bellevue Hospital, where he was selected to reorganize New York Hospital. From 1878 to 1880 he studied in Europe, chiefly in Vienna. Halsted specialized in surgery and became visiting surgeon at several New York hospitals, where he developed unusual operating techniques. Dr. William H. Welch brought him to Johns Hopkins in 1889 as acting surgeon, then professor of surgery. Halsted was noted for his work in cancer of the breast, gall bladder, thyroid, and tuberculosis. On June 4, 1890, he married Caroline Hampton. *Dictionary of American Biography*, 8:165.

attractive, full of enthusiasm about his work and has a kind of personal magnetism that makes him very appealing."[27] Eventually Adelaide met Grenfell and they became life-long friends.

In late summer, 1893, Lavinia Dock left Hopkins to take over the Illinois Training School in Chicago, and Adelaide was given some teaching assignments and was asked to serve as assistant superintendent. Most of Adelaide's classmates who had remained as head nurses had now moved on to other positions. Georgia Nevins wrote that she had been very successful in private nursing, never having been without a patient for more than a day, and that she had earned around $1,200. Susan Read, the last of those who had stayed on as head nurses, was now leaving, and Adelaide expected it would be rather lonesome. She had no close friends among the subsequent classes, and those who stayed on as head nurses would not "dream" of dropping in for the evening as her old classmates had done.

Although she would miss those visits, she would have more time to herself, and, considering the work she had laid out, it would be advantageous to have no interruptions. She knew she would have to study long hours to make a success of teaching. After her first class in anatomy, she wrote her father, "It is no joke to take thirty very wide-awake young women, and try to teach them something of which I am only indifferently sure, but I shall be very severe and rigid, and they shall have good discipline if nothing else."[28]

Adelaide found teaching easier than nursing only in the sense that she did not have to walk or stand so many hours. She found it more satisfying because, while preparing her lessons, she was "steadily acquiring a great deal of useful knowledge." Three evenings a week from six until seven she took lessons in French because she thought it a good idea to maintain some interest outside her regular work. Rarely did she indulge in self-pity and loneliness, but one wintry Sunday night she confessed to her sister:

> If you had to live on black bread and scrub for a living, you would still be rich and to be envied the possessing of two such fine children. And I do envy you—there is no doubt about it but draw the line at the children, for I have sense enough to know that I should make a husband the most miserable being on earth four days out of seven.[29]

[27] Armine Nutting Gosling, *William Gilbert Gosling: A Tribute* (New York: Guild Press, 1935), p. 35.

[28] Adelaide Nutting (Baltimore) to Vespasion Nutting (Waterloo), October 6, 1893, MAN Papers.

[29] Adelaide Nutting (Baltimore) to Armine N. Gosling (St. John's), February 4, 1894, *ibid.*

At other times her letters sounded so enthusiastic that one might suspect she was "whistling in the dark."

During Easter week, 1894, Adelaide spent two pleasant days in Washington. Dr. Sara Hackett Stevenson, who had been visiting Miss Hampton, invited her to accompany her on a visit to her relatives, Vice-President and Mrs. Adlai Stevenson. The Stevensons were spending the winter in a hotel in Washington and Adelaide and Dr. Stevenson would be their guests. "They were extremely kind," Adelaide wrote her father:

> At dinner I sat next to the Vice-president who discoursed amiably upon many subjects and dispensed anecdotes with a liberal hand. He seems to me like a simple, sensible, shrewd, unpolished product of the country, and they say he is a hard-headed western lawyer. His wife is a very nice little Southern woman.[30]

Adelaide accompanied the Stevensons to the funeral services for Senator Colquitt of Georgia, but was not impressed with the way Americans managed matters of state and ceremony.

> The truth is they abolish ceremony to such an extent that when an occasion arises where it becomes necessary—they simply can't fall into line and traces of disorder and confusion are visible everywhere, giving one always the uncomfortable sensation that there is a hitch somewhere behind the scenes.[31]

She also "sat in the Vice-president's seats in the chamber just behind where Mrs. Cleveland's family sit." Afterward they went for a pleasant drive about the city and took the elevator to the top of the Washington monument. Reassuring her father, she concluded, "If I lived here fifty years, I should still be the warmest kind of a Canadian."[32]

It had been a busy year at the hospital. In September, 1893, the Medical School had opened with eighteen students, and, to the discomfiture of Dr. Osler and others, three were women. In January, 1894, the organization meeting for the American Society of Superintendents of Training Schools for Nurses was held at the Academy of Medicine in New York. A constitution was approved, and arrangements were made for annual meetings. Linda Richards, who had the distinction of having received the first diploma from an American school of nursing, was elected president. Adelaide did not attend, but

[30] Adelaide Nutting (Baltimore) to Vespasion Nutting (Waterloo), April 4, 1894, *ibid.*
[31] *Ibid.*
[32] *Ibid.*

Isabel Hampton had a prominent place on the program and in the discussions. Lavinia Dock came from Chicago, and the two women helped launch discussions on such significant matters as the three-year training program, non-payment of student nurses, alumnae associations, journal clubs, and sickness funds.

Meanwhile, The Johns Hopkins Hospital was expanding its services and reputation. Each year there were more patients and more foreign visitors. Adelaide and Miss Hampton talked at length about ways in which nursing services and the education of student nurses could be improved. Miss Hampton was especially concerned with the matter of ethics and planned to write a book on the subject when she found time to put her notes together.

Isabel Hampton insisted that Adelaide take part in the social affairs of Baltimore and hoped that, if asked, she would join the reorganized Women's Club. She was convinced it was important to the hospital and to the profession that nurses mingle with the best of society. Adelaide enjoyed the company of men and on the whole was well liked by them. She had been very happy to go about with Miss Hampton and Dr. Robb, Dr. Welch, Dr. Barker, Dr. Flexner, and other unmarried physicians, but at thirty-six she had begun to think of herself as beyond the "pale of matrimony" and more or less wedded to her profession. She assumed that Isabel Hampton, two years her junior, felt very much the same. In the spring of 1894, however, rumors began to circulate that Miss Hampton was engaged to marry Dr. Hunter Robb, now professor of gynecology at Western Reserve University in Cleveland. Although Adelaide knew they corresponded and were good friends, she had not anticipated that they would ever marry, for, as everyone noted, Miss Hampton was at least two, possibly three, inches taller than Dr. Robb.

The full impact of the situation did eventually fall on Adelaide. She and Isabel had a long talk. Isabel had made up her mind that her life would not be complete without a home, husband, and children. She had decided to submit her resignation and would recommend Adelaide as her successor. Adelaide was stunned at first, but then began to understand why she had been given new responsibilities, and why Isabel had talked so intimately of her ambitions for the Hopkins School of Nursing. There were things Isabel had not been able to carry out: lengthening the course to three years and shortening the daily hours for head nurses and students. In her affectionate, trusting way, she was bequeathing Adelaide unfinished business, but she had faith and confidence.

The trustees considered no other applicants, but, instead of immediately naming Adelaide Nutting Miss Hampton's successor, they designated her acting superintendent. Privately she was assured that her appointment would ultimately be confirmed. Adelaide was troubled about the matter of salary. Miss Hampton had received $1,200 and maintenance. The trustees offered Adelaide only $900. Dr. Hurd thought it enough for a beginner. Adelaide refused the offer on principle but agreed to stay until they could find someone else. Dr. Osler advised her to stay, and she did so conditionally.[33]

Isabel Hampton asked Adelaide to present the fourth graduating class to the trustees at commencement. Meanwhile Adelaide searched her soul. Did she have Isabel Hampton's organizing ability? Could she plan, direct, and control as Isabel had, and with that same appearance of ease and assurance? Did she have the gift of not losing sight of goals while immersed in the day-to-day details of administration?

In a flurry of dressmakers' appointments, parties, and gay farewells, Isabel Hampton prepared to leave for London, where she would marry Hunter Robb. As for the cause and profession of nursing, Isabel assured her successor she would never abandon that.

Another quick squeeze of the hand, a kiss on the cheek, and Isabel was off.

[33] Isabel M. Stewart, "Conversations with Adelaide Nutting, Chalfonte-Hadden Hall, Atlantic City, New Jersey, April, 1940," *ibid.*

VIII

Assistant Superintendent, 1894–1895

Adelaide Nutting moved into Miss Hampton's suite, but she was too busy really to enjoy its attractive spaciousness. She worked at her desk in her office after morning prayers until nearly midnight. The hospital now employed thirteen head nurses and had twenty-four senior student nurses, thirty-six junior student nurses, and a diet kitchen teacher. There were more than a thousand requests for the training school circular in 1894 and four hundred requests for application forms; the incoming class had to be selected from more than a hundred completed applications. The first year Adelaide had no secretarial assistance, and to answer all the letters as satisfactorily as she wished required from four to six hours a day.

Sometimes Adelaide questioned whether her inability to cope with the work might be due to a lack of executive capacity. Everyone was considerate. Miss Bonner, the matron, always seemed to know when to appear with a refreshing cup of tea or a glass of lemonade. Dr. Osler joked and smiled encouragingly, and Dr. Hurd dropped in obviously to see how things were going and remained to relate an oft-repeated anecdote about a man he "once know in Pontiac" or to inquire whether any news had come from Miss Hampton.[1]

It was Miss Hampton's plan to spend three weeks in England before the wedding. She had been accompanied to London by two Baltimore friends, Miss McLean and Miss Julia Rogers. They would do some sightseeing and shopping together. Isabel wanted to see Mrs. Fenwick, visit some hospitals and training schools, and, if possible, to call on Florence Nightingale. She wanted to tell Mrs. Fenwick first hand about the organization of the American Society of Superintendents of Training Schools for Nurses and about Miss Dock's work for

[1] Harvey Cushing, *Sir William Osler*, 2 vols. (Oxford: Clarendon Press, 1925), 1:316.

an association of alumnae societies. The next step would be a national association of nurses, and then state associations.

Mrs. Fenwick was delighted to see Miss Hampton. She did not regard Isabel's marriage a defection from the profession; she herself, no longer engaged directly in hospital work, had made her most significant contributions to nursing since her marriage to Dr. Bedford Fenwick. Freed of the responsibilities of institutional management which she had had at St. Bartholomew's Hospital, as editor of the British journal *Nursing Record* Mrs. Fenwick was in a position to shape the course of British nursing. She was now about to spearhead a movement for the registration of nurses in England. Before many years her fertile imagination would project an international organization of nurses.[2]

On the Sunday before the wedding, Miss Hampton visited Florence Nightingale. Isabel thanked her again for the message she had sent to the nurses' congress in Chicago. Miss Nightingale asked many questions about American hospitals and training schools, especially The Johns Hopkins Hospital. They talked of many things, and when Isabel left she felt renewed inspiration for the work she proposed to do in nursing when she returned to America.

The wedding took place in St. Margaret's Church, Westminster, on Wednesday, July 11. Dr. Robb's two brothers, Mrs. Bonham Carter, Sir Henry and Lady Burdett and their daughter, Miss Amy Hughes, who had attended the nurses' congress in Chicago, Miss McLean, Miss Rogers, Lady Colin Campbell, and a few other English and American friends were present. Elizabeth Birdseye Merritt, a friend from Bellevue and Illinois Training School days, came down from Scotland with her husband, who was to give the bride in marriage.

Isabel was radiant and stately as she entered the church on the arm of Mr. Merritt. She wore a handsome dress of bluish gray trimmed in russet velvet and a matching bonnet, and carried a bouquet of white roses with streamers and bows of white ribbon. All attention centered on the bouquet, as it had been whispered that these were not the flowers Dr. Robb had sent earlier but a bouquet that had just arrived from Florence Nightingale.[3]

After the ceremony, the bride and groom departed for Oxford, where "Cliveden," the beautiful home of the William Astors, had been lent them for their honeymoon.

[2] Ethel Johns and Blanche Pfefferkorn, *The Johns Hopkins Hospital School of Nursing* (Baltimore: The Johns Hopkins Press, 1954), pp. 166–69.

[3] The ribbons and fragments of the roses are in a box in The Johns Hopkins Hospital School of Nursing Archives.

The wedding was colorfully written up in the *Hospital Nursing Supplement*, an English nursing periodical. In the journalistic jargon of the times, Isabel Hampton's marriage to Dr. Hunter Robb sounded like a fairy tale romance.[4] Accounts of the wedding were eagerly read in Baltimore. Adelaide would never begrudge a friend happiness, but this was a marriage on which she would make no predictions.

Meanwhile she had plans of her own to make. She did not want to leave Johns Hopkins. She had come to love Baltimore, its monuments and mansions, its cobblestone streets and row houses with white marble steps scrubbed by colored "waiter-men" each day, and the little bob-tailed horsecar that sometimes required two mules to get it up Hospital Hill. The city was often untidy, but the people were kind, hospitable, and content. Adelaide decided to write the trustees that she would accept the appointment on condition that she first be granted a leave of absence to visit hospitals in the United States and Great Britain.[5]

Adelaide spent her August vacation as inexpensively as possible on a short trip to Waterloo to see her father, and obtained Charlie's promise to help with money matters. In October, Isabel Hampton Robb, back from her honeymoon, stopped over in Baltimore for a week's visit. "I can never call her Mrs. Robb," Adelaide wrote her father. "Now she is back in Cleveland wrestling with the servant girl problem, and with the drawbacks of a ready furnished house as well as marketing in a strange city. Sometimes I feel sure she must wish herself back among her girls in the training school."[6]

On December 13, Adelaide received formal notice from the trustees of her appointment as superintendent of nurses and principal of the training school, effective September 1, 1895. Her salary would be $1,200 per year. In the interim she would be given a leave of absence and would be free to carry out her travel plans.[7]

Helena Barnard, a graduate of the class of 1892, was recalled from Royal Victoria Hospital, Montreal, to take over the administration of the hospital services and the training school during Miss Nutting's absence.[8] As soon as Miss Barnard was settled into the routine,

[4] Quoted in Johns and Pfefferkorn, *The Johns Hopkins Hospital School of Nursing*, pp. 94–96.

[5] Adelaide Nutting (Baltimore) to Vespasion Nutting (Waterloo, Quebec), October 30, 1894, MAN Papers.

[6] *Ibid.*

[7] "Minutes of the Board of Trustees, The Johns Hopkins Hospital, December 11, 1894." The Johns Hopkins Hospital School of Nursing Archives.

[8] Henry M. Hurd, "Sixth Report of the Superintendent, The Johns Hopkins Hospital, for the year ending January 3, 1895," *ibid.*

Adelaide began her tour of American and Canadian hospitals. On her way north she visited Mrs. Robb for several weeks in Cleveland. She found her well established in a fine home. Isabel was evidently very happy, had been welcomed by an interesting social circle, and was already taking a place in the community. She was much interested in Adelaide's plans for visiting hospitals and going to England. They fitted in very well with her own. Dr. Robb expected to attend some medical meetings on the Continent in the summer, and perhaps the three of them could get together in London. Isabel would enjoy piloting Adelaide about the hospitals in London and introducing her to British nursing friends. They talked of American nursing and the way in which a federation of alumnae associations could advance the cause of nursing and attract educated and superior women. Lavinia Dock came for a weekend and the three women held another of their informal and unofficial planning sessions.[9]

Adelaide joined Mrs. Robb at the Second Annual Meeting of the American Society of Superintendents of Training Schools for Nurses in Boston on February 3, 1895, where she met nursing leaders with whom she would work for the next thirty years. Linda Richards, who had been elected president at the meeting in New York, presided.[10] She appealed for greater uniformity in standards and training. Mrs. Robb read a paper on "The Three-Year Course in Connection with the Eight-Hour System." A third year of study, she believed, would be especially valuable to those going into nursing administration. Ever alert to the educational aspects of nurses' training and the dangers of the labor of student nurses being exploited, she insisted that under the present system a third year was necessary to protect the health of the young student nurse and to equip her properly for nursing the sick. Miss Dock and others reported on alumnae organizations, benefit funds, and central directories. Adelaide was named to a committee along with Mrs. Robb, Agnes Snively, Lavinia Dock, Louise Darche, and Edith Draper to investigate and report at the next convention on the three-year program and the eight-hour plan. Adelaide and Mrs. Robb were also placed on the Curriculum Committee.[11]

During the next few months Adelaide traveled, visited hospitals, observed, took notes, read, and planned, and managed to work in

[9] Isabel M. Stewart, "Conversations with Adelaide Nutting, Chalfonte-Haddon Hall, Atlantic City, New Jersey, April, 1940," MAN Papers.

[10] Mary M. Roberts, *American Nursing: History and Interpretation* (New York: Macmillan, 1954), p. 9.

[11] American Society of Superintendents of Training Schools for Nurses, *Second Annual Report* (Harrisburg, Pa.: Harrisburg Publishing Co., 1897).

visits with members of her family in Waterloo, Ottawa, and St. John's. By the time she returned from England, she expected to have her courses reorganized and vitalized, and her goals for The Johns Hopkins School, as well as the steps by which she hoped to attain them, outlined. Not only would she carry out the unfinished plans of Isabel Hampton, but she would advance ideas of her own.

After a brief visit with Minnie and Gilbert, young Ambrose and little Armine, Adelaide boarded the S.S. Corean bound for Glasgow. The Robbs, who were spending the earlier part of the summer in Berchtesgaden, Germany, expected to arrive in London on July 10. While Dr. Robb was hobnobbing with medical men, Isabel and Adelaide would visit hospitals and shops. Adelaide had also promised her brother-in-law, Gilbert Gosling, to look up his brother, Ambrose Gosling, and his wife in London. The latter part of July, Adelaide's brother Jim, active in the governor general's Foot Guards, would come from Ottawa with the Bisley Rifle Team, and, after the matches on the Aldershot range, she planned to do some sightseeing with him.[12]

The voyage to Glasgow was uneventful, and Adelaide enjoyed sitting on the deck in her chair, reading, and sleeping. On the ship, one of Gilbert's friends, Sir Herbert Murray, who had banking interests in Newfoundland, and four young men from St. John's insisted on seeing that she was entertained. At first she was annoyed, then amused, and finally decided that Sir Herbert was "really an old dear," although she doubted if his daughters would call on her in London as he said he would ask them to do.

The second Friday night at sea, lights were sighted off the north of Ireland. Since they would land too late on Saturday for her to get a train to London from Glasgow, Adelaide decided to go up to Edinburgh for Sunday. Sir Herbert told her about an inexpensive hotel, and, to her surprise, one of the St. John's boys decided to go along, look after her luggage, and sightsee with her. They visited the Castle, Holyrood, Arthur's Seat, and walked along High Street.

Adelaide thought how Min would love prowling along High Street from Castle Hill to Canongate, "every inch teeming with historical interest." With all the enthusiasm of a first-time tourist, Adelaide tried to imagine Boswell walking arm-in-arm with Johnson up the narrow street with its seven- and eight-story buildings, its armorial

[12] Isabel M. Stewart, "Conversations with Adelaide Nutting, Chalfonte-Haddon Hall, Atlantic City, New Jersey, April, 1940"; Adelaide Nutting [London] to Armine N. Gosling (St. John's, Newfoundland), July 5, 12, 28, and 31, 1895; and obituary, "James P. Nutting," Saturday Globe (Utica, N.Y.), May 17, 1902; MAN Papers.

bearings over the doorways dating from the sixteenth century, and its pious inscriptions exhorting all who lived within or passed by to a virtuous life. "Surely never was so quaint, so beautiful, and so interesting a city as Edinboro which one just has to love, Old Town and New Town stretching side by side." As for the hotel Sir Herbert had recommended, she awakened the next morning with several suspicious spots on her arms. However, the unpleasantness of a cheap hotel, bed bugs, and third-class rail accommodations did not lessen her enthusiasm for travel.[13]

Almost immediately after she arrived in London and went to the home for nurses which Mrs. Robb had recommended, the Ambrose Goslings called and took her to dinner, then to the Alhambra, where they were "enchanted by the flying ballet and edified by some very excellent wrestling in the Greek and Roman style." The day after she arrived, Sir Herbert Murray called to see her and took her to Lord's Crickett Ground, a century-old playing field, to see the English national game of cricket. In Hyde Park they "saw the great show of thousands of equipages, prancing horses, and elegantly dressed women" driving up and down as if on parade. Later in the evening she joined Sir Herbert and his daughters, Isabel and Mina, for dinner at their home in nearby Warwick Square. She visited the Tower of London with the Robbs, had tea with them, and shopped with Isabel. Walpoles was having a sale on linen. Isabel bought some lovely things, and Adelaide longed to get some for Min, but feared as it was that she would not have enough money to get home.

Adelaide resolved not to burden Min with accounts of the hospitals she visited and so confined her letters to the sights and events her sister would have enjoyed. In London, she had the not uncommon experience of tourists, that of discovering an old, half-forgotten friend among the throng. Across the room at Holborn's Restaurant she saw Donald McMaster. Her first impulse was to go over and speak to him. The brief glimpse brought forth a flood of memories—her mother, the flat on O'Connor Street, Sunday evening tea, debates in the House of Commons, toboggan parties, receptions, and balls at Rideau Hall. Mother Nutting would have welcomed Donald McMaster as a son-in-law. Looking back to those Ottawa days, Adelaide saw much that was shallow and unreal. Only her mother emerged—constant and loving. Adelaide had not seen Donald McMaster since his marriage five years

[13] Adelaide Nutting (Edinburgh) to Armine N. Gosling (St. John's), July 7, 1895; and Adelaide Nutting (London) to Armine N. Gosling (St. John's), July 11 and 12, 1895; MAN Papers.

before to Virginia deFord of Baltimore. He would not expect to see her, and she decided not to speak to him.[14]

On Sunday, July 28, Adelaide went with Ambrose Gosling to a small chapel attached to the Foundling Hospital, where they heard some beautiful music. With Jim and three members of his team she explored London—Westminster Abbey, the Lyceum, the National Gallery, the General Post Office, and the Cheshire Cheese. At Liberty's she helped one of the men select a piece of silk for his wife.[15] One afternoon they went up the river to Kew Gardens and had dinner at Earl's Court.

Early in August, Adelaide and Jim set off on a walking tour to Oxford, thence to Warwick, to North Wales, and finally to Chester. "I find I am able to do several miles daily over London pavements," she wrote Min, "so do not anticipate any difficulty on the Queens highway."[16]

On the voyage home, Adelaide read over her notes, reassessed herself, and made plans for the work she was soon to begin. Her horizon had been broadened, her perception of nursing needs had become more keen, and she was eager to get started. On September 24 she resumed her work at Johns Hopkins Hospital. She found the morale and discipline of the hospital school excellent, doubtless a carry-over from Miss Hampton's passion for uniformity and Miss Barnard's determination not to vary the pattern.

Adelaide decided to submit the first phase of her master plan without delay. It embodied three departures for the school: first, the three-year course, which would divide the student nurses into three classes, junior, intermediate, and senior, with only one class being admitted each year; second, a reduction of the working day to eight hours; and third, the withdrawal of all student allowances, the money thus saved to be devoted to improving the educational facilities. She claimed no originality for the ideas. Discussions on them at two national conventions of the American Society of Superintendents of Training Schools for Nurses had been highly favorable. The third year was essential for training in administrative work. Of the 101 graduates of the Hopkins Training School from 1891 through 1895, 11 were now serving as

[14] This incident is recalled when Adelaide again unexpectedly meets Donald McMaster in Ottawa in February, 1898. Adelaide Nutting (Baltimore) to Armine N. Gosling (St. John's), [Winter, 1898], *ibid.*

[15] Capt. William P. Anderson (Ottawa) to Adelaide Nutting (Baltimore), March 11, 1896, *ibid.*

[16] Adelaide Nutting (London) to Armine N. Gosling (St. John's), August 1, 1895, *ibid.*

superintendents of hospitals. Adelaide reinforced her arguments with statistics from the surveys made by the national committees on the three-year plan and the eight-hour day. From the 111 hospitals responding out of the 154 questioned, working hours varied from 15½ in most hospitals to 17; three hospitals had reduced their hours to 10½, 29 hospitals to 9½, and two of the more progressive had set up an eight-hour duty. After presenting the statistics, she asked some penetrating questions. "What are training schools?" "Are they charitable institutions?" "Are pupil nurses to be reduced to servitude?" Her answers were simple and positive: "The hours should be limited to eight wherever possible, never more than nine, and the day organized for study, work, and class. Less work, more education is needed."[17]

Dr. Hurd was skeptical at first, but, shown the advantages to the hospital of having a longer hold on the services of the students and of giving them better preparation for nursing, he agreed to endorse the plan and to submit it to the trustees. In presenting the proposal he included Miss Nutting's arguments and statistics. A committee was to be appointed immediately to investigate and to make recommendations.[18]

The Third Annual Meeting of the American Society of Superintendents was held in Philadelphia, February 12, 13, and 14, 1896. Among the topics discussed were qualifications for membership, alumnae associations, libraries for nursing schools, nurses' registries, a national uniform, the need for an official organ of the nursing profession, and the nursing of patients in their homes by student nurses. Mrs. Robb was unable to attend the meeting, but Miss Nutting's provocative address on "Hours of Duty" compensated for her absence and marked the emergence of a new leader. Miss Nutting had carefully marshaled her facts from the larger hospitals and from many of the smaller ones from Maine to California and from Illinois to Louisiana. Clearly, forcefully, and concisely she presented the data.

Adelaide Nutting implored that training schools be considered educational institutions, not service adjuncts to hospitals. She questioned how much of the physical work performed by students was educational. As for hours she said:

[17] Of the 111 hospitals responding to the questionnaire, 97 were American, 14 were Canadian; 25 were in New York, 18 in Pennsylvania, and 13 in Massachusetts.

[18] Henry M. Hurd, "Seventh Report of the Superintendent, The Johns Hopkins Hospital, for the year ending January 31, 1896," The Johns Hopkins Hospital School of Nursing Archives.

There is no other work sufficiently like nursing to serve adequately for purposes of comparison, but . . . it may be said fifty-six to sixty hours a week are considered fair working hours for the laboring man. I believe I am right in stating that few industries require their employees to work more than ten hours daily and their Sundays are free. We can not actually compare industries with training schools, nor wage-earners with pupils receiving their training in an educational institution but we can state that a pupil in a training school may work harder to receive her training than a laboring man to support his wife and family; for here we find in one of the most difficult and responsible careers a woman can undertake, that her only method of receiving a certain kind of education is not to work sixty hours per week, but a number of hours varying from that number to 105 hours.

In those schools in which the very shortest hours are adopted, nurses are working at least nine hours a day, at work which taxes the physical strength of the strong even in no small degree; of the moderately strong, to the utmost. After nine hours of hard physical labor, the nurse comes off duty—to what?—to rest? To get out of her uniform and away from the trying atmosphere of the sick-room, and into the fresh air? Not at all, but to go to her room which may be shared with a stranger, and try to bring the energies of a tired mind resident in a tired body to bear upon whatever problems her theoretical work may present. Having thus taken up her hour or hours supposed to be for rest and recreation, are her evenings free? We find they are not. For here a class or a lecture, or possibly two of each, or perhaps relief work in a ward while a member of another class is at a lecture, occupies her, and thus two or three, or it may be four, evenings in a week are taken up. If this be the picture of a day in a school in which the work is thought to be easy, what must be that in those schools where the working day is not nine, but eleven, twelve or thirteen hours long, and where study and attendance at lectures is still compulsory.[19]

Adelaide told her audience it was time people realized that training schools were educational institutions. She pointed out the dangers of reducing students to servitude. Fearlessly she asserted that in many instances it was not for the purpose of giving more and better training that they were kept on duty so long, but rather that the amount of service to the hospital might be increased and the working force of the institution be kept at a minimum. As a rule the number of student nurses was less than proportionate to the number of patients. Such attempts at economy were detrimental to student nurses and patients alike.

Adelaide challenged her fellow superintendents to look into the matter and to decide how much physical labor was required for train-

---

[19] American Society of Superintendents of Training Schools for Nurses, *Third Annual Report* (Harrisburg, Pa.: Harrisburg Publishing Co., 1897).

ing without overfatigue and without infringing on other duties. She did not leave her audience to grope for a formula; she left them a brief, concise recommendation.

> *First,* working hours in the wards should never exceed nine hours, and preferably eight; *second,* hours set aside for rest and recreation should not be infringed upon; and *third,* when an increase in theoretical instruction became necessary or advisable, either there should be a corresponding decrease in the practical work, or the length of the training period should be extended.[20]

In this, her first speech before the national body, Adelaide Nutting established herself as a potential leader within the nursing profession. She was thorough and pointed in her research, her reasoning was sound, and she provided supporting evidence for every generalization. In the discussion relative to the training period, she again committed herself unequivocally to the three-year plan under the existing hospital school system and severely condemned the all-too-common practice of sending student nurses from the hospitals into homes to care for private patients. The alternative of sending a graduate nurse accompanied by a student nurse into the homes of several patients each day was far better educationally and was a safeguard to the health of the student.

In its business meeting the Society of Superintendents cast a unanimous vote against sending student nurses on private duty outside the hospital. Miss Nutting was again appointed to the Committee on Hours, and in the election of officers for the coming year she was chosen president. The next meeting would be held in Baltimore.[21]

In March, 1896, Adelaide wrote her father: "The changes in my work which I expected to have carried out at least partially by this time are still in prospect, but they are not mere visions and I am confident are only delayed—the lengthened course of three years, the shorter hours on duty, non-payment of pupils." The private wards were filled to overflowing. She had not had time to finish a book she had started reading on the trip home from England in September. As for work and self-denial, "It is the only way to success—to put my nose to the grindstone September first and not take it off for eleven months though I dearly love a good time and my own particular kind of fleshpots. . . . When people write articles calling this the model

---

[20] Johns and Pfefferkorn, *The Johns Hopkins Hospital School of Nursing,* pp. 113–15.

[21] American Society of Superintendents of Training Schools for Nurses, *Third Annual Report.*

sick-house of the world, my hair rises on end to think of all that is expected of me which I am not going to be able to accomplish." Spring was late and she could write of no "balmy breezes and blooming magnolias." Baltimore had just emerged from the worst snow storm of the season. "This is [a] curious unreliable climate and I shall like to be back in my own country which I shall accomplish just as soon as possible." She was looking forward to a visit at Easter from Mrs. Robb, who would bring the baby with her. "She knows so well how not to interfere with my work."[22]

On April 14, 1896, the Board of Trustees authorized the superintendent of the hospital and the superintendent of nurses to carry out the third-year plan. Dr. Hurd and Miss Nutting proceeded to enforce the new instructions immediately. Seven probationers protested indignantly to the trustees. Five were assured that they would be given their diplomas at the end of two years if they passed their examinations; the other two decided to complete the full three years. The new circular announcing the third year and the discontinuance of allowances also stated that the probationary period had been extended to two months and that student nurses would be required to be on duty not less than eight hours daily and to devote two additional hours to lectures, classes, or study.[23]

The new superintendent had other problems that worried her. She wanted to be a firm disciplinarian but a just one. Her monthly journal for April, 1896, records incidents which doubtless caused her sleepless nights and anxiety. On April 8 a nurse was dismissed for having generally proved unreliable. Five days later a nurse was dismissed for making a false statement about her age and previous occupation. A junior nurse was suspended from duty because of charges made by persons outside the school; she was given an opportunity to clear herself, but, failing this, was dropped from the rolls.[24]

As spring wore on, Adelaide found herself restless, sleepless, nervous, and exhausted. One afternoon, while she was talking to Dr. Osler in the corridor, a student nurse hurried by. Adelaide stopped the girl to inquire what she had learned on the ward that day. The student, startled and unable to think of anything to reply, rushed on without answering. "Sister Adelaide, Sister Adelaide," Osler com-

[22] Adelaide Nutting (Baltimore) to Vespasion Nutting (Waterloo), March 18, 1896, MAN Papers.

[23] Johns and Pfefferkorn, *The Johns Hopkins Hospital School of Nursing*, p. 109.

[24] Adelaide Nutting, "The Johns Hopkins Hospital Monthly Report (April, 1896)," The Johns Hopkins Hospital School of Nursing Archives.

mented, "over-wrought and over-taught, over-taught and over-wrought."[25]

In early May, Adelaide reached the end of her physical and spiritual reserves and in a moment of desperation sent a letter of resignation to the trustees. It was read on May 8, and the secretary was instructed to write a letter expressing deep regret at her action and appreciation for her great services to the hospital.[26]

With a break in the hot, muggy weather, Adelaide felt refreshed and began to have regrets. To her joy and peace of mind, Dr. Hurd and the trustees requested that she reconsider, promising that in September, when classes began again, she could have another assistant. Adelaide asked that her letter of resignation be withdrawn. Remembering her responsibilities for the meeting of the Society of Superintendents in Baltimore in February and all her dreams for Hopkins, she was chagrined. She would not renege.

[25] Johns and Pfefferkorn, *The Johns Hopkins Hospital School of Nursing*, p. 121.

[26] "Minutes of the Board of Trustees, The Johns Hopkins Hospital, May 8, 1896," The Johns Hopkins Hospital School of Nursing Archives.

IX

The Wider View, 1896–1898

Adelaide Nutting's resolution to stay on at Hopkins was strengthened by a visit with her sister in St. John's, Newfoundland, and by letters from Isabel Robb. During the summer, when classes were not in session, she made careful plans for the next year's work. Ada Carr, who had been assistant superintendent since 1894, took over more of the work associated with hospital services. Miss Nutting worked out the details of the new curriculum and handled most of the correspondence with prospective students. There were 1,143 requests for circulars in 1896, and 160 young women applied for admission. Of the 61 accepted as probationers, 35 entered, and three years later 27 graduated.[1]

Adelaide found herself becoming very enthusiastic about the three-year program. The Medical School also had plans for the School of Nursing. Because it needed additional clinical experience for its students, an outside obstetrical service was organized under the direction of Dr. J. Whitridge Williams, Dr. Kelly's assistant in gynecology. An intern, accompanied by a medical student and a nurse, usually a student, would attend the woman in her home and remain for eighteen hours after the delivery. Adelaide had never liked the idea of sending students out of the hospital on private duty and had sought to end the practice. She saw possibilities in the new obstetrical service; if the demand became great enough and the public became educated to the idea, a maternity ward might be set up in the hospital, and the students could gain the necessary clinical experience there.

Adelaide felt a new sense of command as she worked into the new course of study and made plans for the superintendents' meeting to be held in Baltimore. If in the past she had faced her tasks with feel-

---

[1] Henry M. Hurd, "Eighth Report of the Superintendent, The Johns Hopkins Hospital, for year ending February 1, 1897," p. 16, The Johns Hopkins Hospital School of Nursing Archives; Ethel Johns and Blanche Pfefferkorn, *The Johns Hopkins Hospital School of Nursing* (Baltimore: The Johns Hopkins Press, 1954), pp. 380, 383.

ings of temerity and inadequacy, she now faced them with confidence and humility. No longer did she feel she was only a few pages and a few paces ahead of her students. She seemed to have caught a new vision of nursing, and she longed to bring her students up to her own professional height, where they too might make realities of dreams.

The third-year plan held much for the students' growth beyond the confines of the classroom and the ward. Adelaide wanted the young women who took their training at Johns Hopkins to be interesting, refined, and cultured persons. She wanted them to do well in their classes and to be conscientious in the performance of their duties, but she wanted them also to go beyond their assignments, to read and think for themselves, and to avail themselves of the cultural opportunities Baltimore afforded, its concerts, art galleries, and theater.

The thirty-six-month course provided for six months each in surgical, gynecological, and private wards, two months each in obstetrical, pediatric, and infectious wards, one month each in the diet school and gynecological operating room, six weeks in the general operating room, and one week in the dispensary, with the rest of the time being spent in whatever direction it was most needed. Nine weeks were allowed for vacation.

During the first year, "juniors," as they were called, were given practical training in the medical, surgical, and gynecological free wards, weekly demonstrations, and class instruction. The course work consisted of elementary materia medica, anatomy, physiology and hygiene, cookery and dietetics, practice and theory. In the intermediate year, students continued their practical work in medical, surgical, and gynecological nursing in the free wards, but they also worked in the private wards, the children's ward, the infectious ward, and the dispensary. Their classes consisted of instruction in the care of medical, surgical, and gynecological patients, infectious diseases, urinalysis, and massage. In the senior year, students were given practical training in the operating room, dispensary, maternity and children's wards, and further training in areas where more nurses were needed or where a nurse's experience had been limited. Occasionally seniors were placed in positions of responsibility if their progress and ability warranted that trust. Lectures and class work followed the outline of the year's work. Miss Nutting always gave the lectures on ethics and the history of nursing. Although staff physicians continued to lecture from time to time, Miss Nutting thought it desirable to bring in outside speakers who were qualified to discuss special types of nursing, such as those from the Baltimore Instructive Visiting Nurse Service, recently organized by Evelyn Pope, and the Henry Street Visiting Nurse Service, which Lillian Wald had begun in New York.

The withdrawal of allowances to students and the placing of senior students in charge of wards was regarded as sound by Dr. Hurd and the trustees, for it cost less to provide students with textbooks and uniforms, and the salary of a head nurse could be saved when a student nurse acted in that capacity.[2] In lieu of the allowances, a sum of money would be set aside for scholarships.[3]

On a wider front, leaders of nursing sought to improve the status of nurses and the nursing profession. As Adelaide prepared to launch the three-year plan, Lavinia Dock, who had transferred from the Illinois Training School for Nurses in Chicago to the Henry Street Visiting Nurses Association in New York, was working on a plan to organize all nurses of America. Edith Draper had pointed out the need for such an organization at the Chicago meeting in 1893, and subsequently Louise Darche had spoken at length on the matter at an early meeting of the Society of Superintendents. The superintendents had deferred action, realizing that a national organization embracing the whole nursing profession would best emerge through a federation of alumnae associations. Miss Dock investigated the laws under which professional organizations could operate and reported to the Society of Superintendents meeting in 1896 that national bodies made policy and were a great moral force, but that the real work must be done locally. Medical schools, she observed, did not lead the march of progress but received their impetus from the professional organizations. As nurses, she said, "We labor under the very serious practical disadvantage of having no recognized standard of work or requirements." In the interest of standards it seemed expedient to concentrate on a different type of national organization, a federation of alumnae associations.[4] Of the 225 training schools for nurses in existence in the United States and Canada at that time, only 40 had organized alumnae societies.

After gaining the endorsement of the Society of Superintendents, Miss Dock arranged for a meeting to be held at Manhattan Beach, New York, on September 2, 3, and 4, 1896, for the purpose of organizing the graduate nurses of the United States and Canada. The various

[2] Johns and Pfefferkorn, *The Johns Hopkins Hospital School of Nursing*, pp. 108–11.

[3] *Ibid.*, pp. 111–12.

[4] American Society of Superintendents of Training Schools for Nurses, *Third Annual Report* (Harrisburg, Pa.: Harrisburg Publishing Co., 1897).

alumnae societies were each invited to send a representative and a delegate.

Ten schools, represented by nine superintendents and nine graduate delegates, were present when Miss Dock called the meeting to order. Among those present were Miss Nutting and Mrs. Robb. The eighteen women were in complete agreement over the purpose of an alumnae federation and the value of such an organization, but they found it difficult to decide on a name. Finally, by a rising vote, "The Nurses Associated Alumnae of the United States and Canada" was chosen. Committees were appointed to report the following day with prepared statements on object, eligibility, and membership. The structure was modeled after that of the American Medical Association. One superintendent insisted that a code of ethics be included in the object.

There had been discussion of a code of ethics whenever nursing leaders gathered. A few schools had phrased their own. Lystra E. Gretter had been chairman of the committee that prepared an oath called the Nightingale Pledge, first administered to the graduating class of the Farrand School of Nursing, Detroit, in 1893. It bore a striking resemblance to the Oath of Hippocrates long administered to graduating classes of medical schools:

> I solemnly pledge myself before God and in the presence of this assembly to pass my life in purity and to practice my profession faithfully. I will abstain from whatever is deleterious and mischievous and will not take or knowingly administer any harmful drug.
>
> I will do all in my power to maintain and elevate the standards of my profession and will hold in confidence all personal matters committed to my keeping, and all family affairs coming to my knowledge in the practice of my calling.
>
> With all loyalty I will endeavor to aid the physician in his work, and devote myself to the welfare of those committed to my care.[5]

At the Third Annual Meeting of The Johns Hopkins Nurses Alumnae Association Mrs. Robb suggested that a code of ethics be adopted and was immediately asked to serve as chairman of a committee to formulate such a code. At the next meeting, on June 4, 1896, the committee submitted a code based on that of the Illinois Training School, the National Code of Medical Ethics of 1847, and Dr. Austin Flint's commentaries on the National Code.[6]

As adopted, the Hopkins Nurses' Code covered not only the duty

[5] Agnes G. Deans and Anne L. Austin, *The History of Farrand Training School for Nurses* (Detroit: Alumnae Association of Farrand School for Nurses, 1936), pp. 25–27.

[6] The committee drawing up the Hopkins Alumnae Code consisted of Mrs. Robb and three members of the class of 1894, Katherine C. deLong, Alice B. P.

of the nurse toward the physician, the patient, fellow nurses, the school, and the public but the duty of the physician to the nurse and the duty of the public to the nurse. The principles enunciated in the Hopkins code were representative of those that were to shape the ethics of the nursing profession for the next half-century. The nurse's first duty was to carry out the physician's instructions, never to criticize him with patient or friend, and to accord him respect for his higher professional position. Regardless of personal pleasure, a nurse should never refuse a call to a sick person or neglect to perform her duty to the patient kindly and humanely, making allowances for the caprices of the sick, avoiding too great an intimacy with the patient, and always respecting his confidence. It was the duty of the nurse to be loyal to her school and to wear her pin and uniform whenever in service. Unless known to be unreliable, another nurse was never to be criticized before doctor or patient. A nurse was obligated to alleviate suffering in times of epidemic, even at the jeopardy of her own life, and should be willing to give of her time to nursing the poor. The physician, in turn, should accord loyalty and support to the competent, trustworthy nurse, never criticizing her in front of patient or family, and should see that she gets rest, relief from duty, and pay. The public should discriminate between the qualified trained nurse and the ignorant and untrained.[7]

Although the history-making group at Manhattan Beach was not insensitive to ethics, it concentrated on drafting a constitution and on eligibility, and bravely attacked the matter of finances. It was decided that each affiliating alumnae association would be asked to pay an annual fee for each twenty-five members or under and that each individual would be expected to pay a minimum of two dollars to her local alumnae association. There was discussion of state organizations and of the work that could be done on the local level relative to registries and hours of duty. It was decided that the delegates and representatives would reassemble when the Society of Superintendents met in Baltimore, at which time they would take action on the constitution and elect officers.[8]

Conover, and Mary W. Heriot. The Medical Code of 1847 was based on the code written by Thomas Percival, who attempted to distinguish between medical ethics and medical etiquette.

[7] The Johns Hopkins Hospital Training School for Nurses Alumnae Association Code of Ethics, adopted June 4, 1896, manuscript, The Johns Hopkins Hospital School of Nursing Archives.

[8] *Proceedings of the Convention of Training School Alumnae Delegates and Representatives from the American Society of Superintendents of Training Schools for Nurses*, Manhattan Beach, N.Y., September 2–4, 1896.

When the new students entered Hopkins in October, 1896, Adelaide Nutting found that inaugurating the third-year plan was simpler than she had anticipated. Georgina Ross, a Hopkins graduate in the class of 1894, was appointed second assistant and was given charge of the first-year students and the Nurses' Home. With classes and lectures going smoothly, Adelaide turned her attention to the meeting of the Society of Superintendents to be held in Baltimore in February, 1897. President Gilman and Dr. Hurd entered enthusiastically into the plans for the convention.

President Gilman provided for meeting rooms in Donovan Hall and for a luncheon in McCoy Hall. The trustees sponsored a reception at the Nurses' Home, to which the medical staff, their wives, and Baltimore friends of the superintendents and associated alumnae nurses were invited. The Arundel Club, of which Miss Nutting was a member, placed its facilities at the disposal of the nurses, and Dr. and Mrs. Osler had a tea in their home for visiting superintendents and nurses. Mrs. Charles Bonaparte invited the visitors to Bonaparte House to view the family treasures, and Mr. Henry Walters opened his gallery of fine paintings to them. Special rates were obtained at Baltimore's best hotels, the Rennert, the Mt. Vernon, and the Stafford, where those attending the convention paid only a dollar a day for their rooms. Because administrators and nurses normally paid their own expenses to professional meetings, this reduced cost was a significant factor in determining attendance.

February 1 dawned bright and clear. The *Baltimore Sun* gave generous coverage to the meeting and reported more than fifty in attendance. Lavinia Dock came down early from New York to greet old friends, to check arrangements, and to give Adelaide the encouragement she would miss from Isabel, for family matters in Cleveland prevented Mrs. Robb from attending the meetings.

As Adelaide looked out over the audience and recognized so many of her former students and friends, nervousness left her and she felt a strange sense of calm and exultation. After the greetings from President Gilman, Dr. Hurd, and others had been made, she proceeded to give her own address, which the *Baltimore Sun* described as sounding the "keynote of high aim and strenuous endeavor."[9]

Adelaide's remedy for keeping undesirable persons out of the nursing profession was the same as that of the medical profession—namely, lengthening the period of training and raising the standards. She advocated fewer and better training schools. She specifically en-

[9] Clipping from the *Baltimore Sun* [February 3, 1897], scrapbook, National League of Nursing Archives, New York, N.Y.

dorsed the three-year plan for training nurses as one way of avoiding possible future overcrowding in the profession.

The Society of Superintendents went on record as approving nine-hour day duty and twelve-hour night duty for graduate nurses. This was as far as the leaders felt they dared go at that time. Lavinia Dock read a letter from the Matrons' Council of Great Britain and Ireland announcing plans for an international congress of nursing to be held in London in connection with the International Congress of Women in 1898, and inviting the Society of Superintendents to cooperate by sending representatives. Miss Mary Agnes Snively was elected president for the following year, and it was announced that the next meeting would be held in Toronto. Meanwhile, at the Arundel Club, the nurses were meeting and completing the organization of the Nurses Associated Alumnae of the United States and Canada, approving a constitution, and attending to other matters left over from the Manhattan Beach conference. Isabel Hampton Robb, Bellevue, class of 1883, was elected president, and Helena Barnard, Hopkins, class of 1892, was elected secretary.[10]

When the last superintendents and nurses had departed, Adelaide sat down to review the days' events. The meetings had gone well. The tour of the hospital had been a success from the moment the guests entered the rotunda, where all had paused before Stein's splendid copy of Thorwaldsen's marble statue "Christus Consolator," the recently installed gift of trustee William Wallace Spencer.[11] The tea in the Nurses' Home had been well attended, and Mrs. Gilman, Mrs. Hurd, and the trustees' wives were gracious hostesses. Adelaide thought her student nurses had never looked nicer or better groomed in their blue uniforms and their crisp white aprons and caps. They seemed proud to be a part of nursing. There was a growing feeling of solidarity among the superintendents, an awareness of common problems, a crystallization of purpose and goals that could be attained through unity. An international organization of nurses was about to emerge.

The convention had been splendid from beginning to end. Now there were only the tag-ends, the post-convention tasks, to attend to, the personal notes to those who had made the convention so pleasant,

[10] American Society of Superintendents of Training Schools for Nurses, *Fourth Annual Report* (Harrisburg, Pa.: Harrisburg Publishing Co., 1897).

[11] At the opening of The Johns Hopkins Hospital in 1889, President Daniel Coit Gilman said he hoped that some friend would place beneath the dome a copy of Thorwaldsen's "Christus Consolator." In 1896 the copy by Stein was brought over from Copenhagen. Johns and Pfefferkorn, *The Johns Hopkins Hospital School of Nursing*, pp. 321–22.

an azalea to the Gilmans, and a special bunch of violets, Adelaide's own favorite flower, to Mrs. Gilman and Mrs. Osler.[12] Adelaide reflected that she had allowed herself to accept the vice-presidency of the Society of Superintendents for the coming year. At any rate, her responsibilities would be fewer, and, of course, she would attend the meeting in Toronto. She might even take off two or three extra days and visit Jim and Claire and the boys in Ottawa. Although the convention was a year away, she found herself dreaming of winter in Canada—the cold, invigorating air, the crunch of thick, powdery snow, sleighs and blanketed horses, and sleigh bells.

The third-year plan was a success, and the eight-hour day for student nurses, though honored perhaps more in the breach than in the observance, was nevertheless a step forward. Devoted as Adelaide Nutting was to duty and the profession, she did not regard nursing as a cult requiring human sacrifice. She believed that nurses, perhaps more than any other group of workers, needed recreation to take them away from disease both physically and mentally.

In this connection, the library was one of Adelaide's early concerns. As a student nurse she had been surprised to learn that the hospital did not subscribe to a daily paper. As Dr. Osler's head nurse, she had contrived with him to get a small bookcase for the men's ward and then had begged the doctors for books and magazines for the convalescent patients to read. At the opening of the hospital, Dr. Billings and President Gilman had referred to a library, which was to be outfitted with books and magazines, but no special quarters had been designated, and with the precarious state of the Hopkins endowment no allocation of funds had been made for the purchase of books.

Isabel Hampton had paid for books out of her own salary and she had encouraged her nurses to subscribe to magazines and share them. One of her purposes in organizing the Journal Club had been to bring in a store of contemporary nursing materials. As a student nurse, out of a slender stipend of twelve dollars a month, Adelaide had managed to buy not only textbooks but a few other books and an occasional magazine. At Miss Hampton's direction some bookshelves had been placed along the wall of the classroom on the ground floor of the Nurses' Home, and soon the room began to take on something of the appearance of a library. The doctors, the trustees, their wives, and friends of the hospital were asked to donate books they no longer wanted to the Nurses' Library. Among the first books presented was

[12] Elizabeth Gilman (Baltimore) to Adelaide Nutting (Baltimore), [February, 1897], scrapbook, National League of Nursing, New York, N.Y.

a copy of Florence Nightingale's *Notes on Hospitals*, sent to Hopkins in March, 1875, at Miss Florence S. Lees's request for the use of the trustees. Adelaide contributed her own copy of Miss Nightingale's *Notes on Nursing*. In 1892 Dr. Osler presented a copy of his *Practice of Medicine*, just off the press. The next year, when Lavinia Dock's *Materia Medica*, Isabel Hampton's *Nursing: Its Principles and Practice*, and Miss Boland's *Handbook on Invalid Cookery* were published, copies were placed in the library. Diana C. Kimber published her *Textbook on Anatomy* in 1894 and donated a copy to the Hopkins Nurses' Library. In 1895 the Oslers contributed twenty-five volumes, and other physicians were inveigled into making similar gifts. Students began to leave behind their copies of Hawthorne, Scott, Stevenson, Mathew Arnold, Wordsworth, and Lowell. Patients returning home sent books back to their favorite nurses. The library began to take on a literary as well as a professional air.

Adelaide, always interested in history, was delighted when books on Ancient Greece, Rome, the French Revolution, or the conquest of Peru were presented. Soon the library contained more than 250 volumes. Adelaide read as widely as time would permit. A light and fitful sleeper, she often read far into the night, always with a pad and pencil at her side so that she might record some fact, phrase, or aphorism that pleased her. She became an inveterate hoarder of newspaper clippings, which varied from scientific information and articles on nursing to household hints, particularly those that might be of value for institutions.

During the early years of her superintendency, the student nurses stood somewhat in awe of Adelaide Nutting. She seemed tall and aloof in her dark uniform, relieved by only the narrow white collar and cuffs. The purple paisley shawl that she wore through the corridors on wintry days only added to her stateliness and seeming aloofness. She appeared meticulous and businesslike, and the students regarded her discipline as strict and inflexible.

Discipline was a topic to which Adelaide gave much thought. Among her papers were many penciled notes on the subject:

> Discipline—the higher meaning is where interest in the achievement of an idea or work becomes so paramount that rules are routine, accepted without question. . . .
> To maintain harmony and equilibrium of individual or group life is the main object of discipline.[13]

[13] Adelaide Nutting, "Discipline," MAN Papers.

At the first meeting of a class of probationers, Adelaide frequently remarked, "This institution stands for two things: German science and West Point discipline."[14]

Clara Noyes, a first-year student, once asked whether she might go home for a weekend. "Do you feel you have been in training long enough to ask a favor of such proportions," Adelaide replied, "one that entails such far-reaching adjustment of other people's plans?" Miss Noyes had supposed it to be only a simple request. "Simple!" Adelaide had echoed. "Are you then not aware that the senior nurse would have to be on duty all Sunday morning, that you yourself on your return would have to assume charge of all the wards on Sunday afternoon? Do you think that as yet you are capable of such responsibilities?" Clara Noyes changed her mind about going home. Years later she wrote, "This experience inculcated a sense of proportion, a realization of the importance and dignity of [her] chosen profession and a respect for authority worth numberless week-end trips and unearned pleasures."[15]

In September, 1897, an incident involving discipline caused Adelaide much anxiety and raised a considerable furor in the hospital. A second-year student nurse refused to care for a patient who had been found to have leprosy. The girl was told the consequence of refusing service to this patient and was given until the first of the year to reconsider. Meanwhile, the matter was referred to the trustees. In January, when the girl again refused assignment to the isolation ward if it involved any service to this patient, she was sent home for "disobedience to orders." Adelaide's decision was upheld, and the affair, disturbing at the time, had a salutary effect upon the training school.[16]

The reputation of The Johns Hopkins Hospital and Training School continued to grow. Demands for obstetrical services in the hospital led to the establishment of a maternity ward in the fall of 1897, and, at about the same time, the former bathhouse was converted into a children's ward with fifteen cots, with a senior student in charge. Now that clinical facilities for maternity and pediatric cases were available in the hospital, student nurses no longer had to go outside the hospital. Adelaide Nutting and Isabel Hampton had scored their point.

14 Ruth Brewster Sherman, "Random Memories of Adelaide Nutting," *The Johns Hopkins Nurses Alumnae Magazine*, April, 1949, p. 57.

15 Clara D. Noyes, "M. Adelaide Nutting: Some Reminiscences," *Red Cross Courier*, April 15, 1905.

16 Johns and Pfefferkorn, *The Johns Hopkins Hospital School of Nursing*, p. 122; see also Adelaide Nutting, "Annual Report of the Superintendent, The Johns Hopkins Hospital School of Nursing, 1897–1898," The Johns Hopkins Hospital School of Nursing Archives.

With the expansion of services within the hospital, it was obvious that the nursing staff would have to be increased. Adelaide received hundreds of applications each year, but she was reluctant to increase the number of students because accommodations in the Nurses' Home were already overcrowded to the point that personal comfort, quality of work, and discipline were jeopardized. Despite the institution's financial plight, the trustees took action and had the floors over the officers' dining room and the pharmacy converted into twenty-eight small bedrooms; ten of the third-floor rooms were set aside for use by night nurses. All rooms in both the home and the annex were shared by two persons except those reserved for officers and head nurses.[17]

The calls for Hopkins graduates were further evidence of the prestige of the Hopkins Training School. There were not enough Hopkins graduates to supply the demand, however, especially that for administrative and teaching positions. This posed a challenge. Many graduate nurses at this time preferred private duty, and those who quickly accepted administrative positions were quite bewildered by the variety of services and judgments they were expected to render, from the merits of laundry and sterilizing equipment, bookkeeping, and personnel management to developing a training school. An unidentified nursing leader of the period alleged that when five doctors got together they started a hospital and that when they hired a day nurse and a night nurse they decided to hire a third nurse and make it a training school.

In desperation these young graduates turned to their former teachers for assistance on teaching and administrative procedures and institutional management. Adelaide Nutting's mail bulged with requests: "May I come and talk with you?" "I hate to impose but could you spare me a couple of hours next week-end?" "The doctor here is most unreasonable, may I come and talk the matter over with you?" She could never turn a deaf ear to them. Remembering her own feelings of inadequacy, she listened patiently, and long into the night she wrote, giving counsel, comfort, and inspiration. Eleanor Wood (Johns Hopkins, 1901), scarcely twenty-four hours on the job as superintendent at Bryn Mawr, a fifty-bed hospital, wrote Adelaide that upon arrival she had been told she was expected to start a training school.[18]

Adelaide was convinced that nurses needed broader education and less repetitive clinical practice. The preparation for nursing was as

[17] Johns and Pfefferkorn, *The Johns Hopkins Hospital School of Nursing*, pp. 117–18.

[18] Eleanor Wharton Wood (Bryn Mawr, Pa.) to Adelaide Nutting (Baltimore), October 2, [n.d.], MAN Papers.

important as education for medicine, law, or teaching. Lavinia Dock, who was visiting Hopkins, agreed and dispatched a copy of the *Proceedings of the Fourth Annual Convention of the American Society of Superintendents of Training Schools for Nurses of the United States and Canada* to the U.S. Commissioner of Education, William T. Harris, with the request that it be included in his annual report. He replied that it could not be included in his forthcoming report but that he wished to be kept informed of the society's work; he enclosed labels so that future reports might be sent postage free.[19] Lavinia smiled as she filed the labels. "He will hear from us, whether or not we hear from him." Little did she realize that a new voice had been enlisted in the cause of nursing education.

For some time, when Adelaide, Isabel, Lavinia, Anna Maxwell, and other nursing administrators chanced to meet, they discussed the needs and possibilities of postgraduate study for teachers of nursing and hospital administrators; to them this seemed just as normal as the preparation for teachers of history, home economics, and vocational subjects. The longer Isabel Robb thought about the matter, the clearer she saw a practical curriculum emerge. With no feeling of presumption, she wrote to the chairman responsible for the program of the upcoming convention of the Society of Superintendents in Toronto and asked to be permitted to read a paper.

[19] William T. Harris, Office of the U.S. Commissioner of Education (Washington, D.C.) to Lavinia Dock (New York), May 12, 1897, *ibid.*

X

Education versus the Training of Nurses, 1898–1900

February 7, 1898, found Adelaide, her friend, Georgia Nevins, and other American superintendents of training schools for nurses en route to Toronto, Canada, for the Society of Superintendents' annual convention. Despite the weather, "all thaw, rain, and sleet," there was a gay and expectant air about the travelers. By this fifth meeting the superintendents' convention was beginning to take on aspects of a reunion as well as a crusade, and members who had attended previous meetings greeted one another as friends. Inside the station they put on their "arctics," or overshoes, and outside they raised their umbrellas to protect their new winter bonnets as they hurried to take hansom cabs or horsecars to the hotels and hospitals where they were to be guests.

The meetings, scheduled for February 8, 9, 10, and 11, were held in Auditorium Hall of the Normal School, St. James Square. The Canadian superintendents wished to make their American colleagues welcome and were prepared to dispense Dominion hospitality with a lavish round of luncheons, teas, dinners, exhibits, hospital tours, and receptions. Once the official greetings were over, the convention settled down to routine business, the reading of papers, and discussions on such down-to-earth subjects as hospital laundries, ward management, diet kitchen, the perennial matter of ethics, the third-year plan, the need for a nursing journal, and nurses' registration. Adelaide Nutting took an active part in the discussions. When asked the relation of character to ethics in the training school, she replied unhesitatingly:

> We can train women as nurses but we can not change the character. We may not be able to discover the faults in character early; they may come out afterwards to our great regret and grief, and we should be very careful about signing our names to diplomas even after pupils have reached the degree required by the school and have come to the last

months of their career there. We do not stand in the position of colleges and universities. They do not vouch for character but only for a certain degree of training or schooling. We stand in a different and peculiar position. We assume a moral responsibility for the character of the nurses we send out.[1]

As vice-president, Adelaide presided over the closing session of the convention. The last paper presented was Isabel Robb's "Qualifications for Membership in the Superintendents' Society." Mrs. Robb lamented the inadequate preparation of superintendents. Today's students would be tomorrow's superintendents. Why not provide nurses with education that would qualify them for supervisory and administrative positions? The uniformity of curriculum and high standards so greatly desired by the Society of Superintendents could best be secured, she believed, through a postgraduate program which emphasized problems of administration and nursing education. It might be patterned after some of the courses of study devised for school administrators and teachers. Mrs. Robb outlined a plan for a central board of examiners from the Society of Superintendents which would study the problem of nursing education on the postgraduate level. There was no time for discussion of the paper, but Adelaide moved that a committee be appointed to consider Isabel Robb's proposal. After the motion carried, Mrs. Robb was asked to head the committee.[2]

The Committee on Education was to be one of the most significant committees in the history of nursing. Isabel Robb had clearly stated the problem and outlined a possible solution. It remained for the Society of Superintendents to implement it.

Adelaide left Toronto on Friday afternoon for a three-day visit with Claire and Jim in Ottawa. It was her first winter visit to Canada in several years, and she found the crisp cold air refreshing and the old scenes heartwarming. There had been a heavy snowfall in Ottawa. It blanketed the streets and rooftops and piled high on the branches of trees and the fence around the Parliament buildings.

It was good to see Jim and his boys again. Harold would soon be twelve, and Keith was five and a half. This time Adelaide was able to bring them presents. Claire set out her best china and freshly polished silver and seemed so preoccupied with cooking that Adelaide inquired "why there was so much a-do." Claire then explained that they were

---

[1] American Society of Superintendents of Training Schools for Nurses, *Fifth Annual Report* (Harrisburg, Pa.: Harrisburg Publishing Co., 1898), p. 49.

[2] Mary E. P. Davis, Maud Banfield, and Lucy Walker, all of Philadelphia, were named to the committee and served with Mrs. Robb, Miss Nutting, and Miss Richards. *Ibid.*

having a party for her. "I am not going to have you go back to Baltimore and have you say that you did not see any of your old friends."[3]

Undoubtedly Jim had remembered the party so many years ago when Mother Nutting had invited the Chesleys, the McLymonts, the Huntons, Jim Cunningham, Jack Christie, and the teachers from the Ladies College and had served them oyster patties, charlotte russe, and claret cup. Claire invited many of these same people. Afterward, Adelaide wondered whether she had grown away from them or they had grown away from her. The bond of friendship which once had drawn her to them belonged to the irretrievable past. Only Jim remained constant, older but unchanged.

Adelaide spent "one delightful day in Ottawa listening to the debate in the House on the Klondike Railway bill."

> I rubbed my eyes to find out if I was really myself or another when on turning to speak to Jim I beheld Donald McMaster standing just behind, a smiling astonished mortal whom I had not spoken to for many years and last saw at the Holborn Restaurant in London. . . .
> I left Ottawa in the midst of a really magnificent snow storm in which I revelled mind and body.[4]

Back in Baltimore she found

> a depressing accumulation of work of every kind awaiting. . . . It is simply appalling to have so much expected of one. . . . to run the school, doctors, friends and relations of patients and the patients themselves and try not to starve absolutely the other side, that loves books and music and nature, is an ingenious task which I fail to perform daily.

Her "other side" was immediately appealed to, however, by three afternoon lectures on Coleridge, Shelley, and Keats by William Knight of St. Andrews University, Scotland.[5]

Then, on February 15, the U.S. battleship *Maine* was sunk in the harbor at Havana, Cuba. A chauvinistic press clamored for intervention in the Cuban civil war. "Remember the *Maine*" became its battle cry. Diplomacy failed, and April 25 found the United States at war with Spain. President McKinley called for volunteers.

Facing an imminent invasion, the Medical Department of the U.S. Army began to expand its facilities and to recruit additional physicians. More to be feared than Spanish guns were typhoid, malaria, smallpox, dysentery, and yellow fever. Surgeon General George M.

---

[3] Adelaide Nutting (Baltimore) to Armine N. Gosling (St. John's, Newfoundland), [February, 1898], MAN Papers.
[4] *Ibid.*
[5] *Ibid.*

Sternberg, who had had yellow fever and had written extensively on the bacteriology of the disease, issued a call for "immunes" to accompany the troops as "contract" surgeons. Because yellow fever had run rampant in the South in 1897, immune physicians were not difficult to find.[6] There was no army or navy nurse corps. The American Red Cross, under the direction of Clara Barton, who founded it in 1881, was loosely organized and interested chiefly in disaster relief. On the state and local level, however, a few Red Cross societies, such as the New York Auxiliary No. 3, had become very much interested in nursing.[7]

Army medical officers were not friendly to women in the services, some on "general principles," and others because they did not believe the military establishment could provide proper accommodations. When tropical fevers broke out in Cuba and an epidemic of typhoid swept through the camps in the United States, the hospital corpsmen, composed of many raw recruits, were unable to handle the situation, and Clara Barton's Red Cross nurses were unable to provide the army's needs. The Medical Department then advertised for contract nurses. Many women who responded were untrained and unreliable, and few had administrative ability. Defects in nursing organization and discipline, as well as appalling death rates, brought protests from the public.[8] Isabel Robb, president of the two-year-old Associated Alumnae, sought authorization to place the services of the organization at the disposal of the army in developing a more effective system and supplying competent nurses for key positions.[9]

Other organizations, including the Daughters of the American Revolution, also volunteered to recruit nurses. When Mrs. Robb asked for an interview with the surgeon general, she was advised that on the previous day Dr. Anita Newcomb McGee, vice-president of the Daughters of the American Revolution, had been appointed to take charge of the army nursing service. Although a comparatively young organization, the Daughters of the American Revolution was patriotic,

[6] Harvey Cushing, *Sir William Osler*, 2 vols. (Oxford: Clarendon Press, 1925), 1:468.

[7] Mary M. Roberts, *American Nursing: History and Interpretation* (New York: Macmillan, 1954), pp. 28–29.

[8] Surgeon General George M. Sternberg commented seriously and somewhat sadly that female nurses were expensive luxuries. The War Department received requisitions for bureaus, rocking chairs, and other items unknown under a male regime. Unidentified clipping, The Johns Hopkins Hospital School of Nursing Archives.

[9] Isabel M. Stewart and Anne L. Austin, *A History of Nursing from Ancient to Modern Times: A World View* (New York: G. P. Putnam's Sons, 1926), pp. 203–4.

active, well financed, and had an efficient office in Washington, while the Associated Alumnae had no such resources. Dr. McGee, alert and energetic, set high standards morally and professionally. During the summer of 1898, she and her committee reviewed more than 8,000 applications from women, both nurses and non-nurses, who wished to serve their country. Dr. McGee accepted only those nurses who had been approved by the directors of the training schools from which they graduated.

Because Dr. McGee had had no previous experience in hospital organization, nursing leaders thought the appointment should have gone to a qualified nursing superintendent; they supported their case by citing what had been accomplished in the British army when Florence Nightingale and her nurses had been given charge of all of that country's military nursing services. Despite Clara Barton's opposition, prominent persons in the New York chapter of the Red Cross successfully brought pressure to bear on the administration in Washington so that Anna C. Maxwell of New York Presbyterian Hospital, Mrs. Lucy W. Quintard of St. Luke's, and several other experienced superintendents who had volunteered were allowed to take their own trained staffs into the wards of the typhoid hospitals. Their valiant demonstration evoked high praise from the medical officers and Dr. McGee, but it came too late to decrease much of the appalling mortality. The actual fighting lasted less than two months, but the struggle with typhoid and yellow fever continued long after the smoke of battle had cleared away and Dr. McGee had been appointed acting assistant surgeon general.[10]

When the war ended, Dr. McGee expressed her appreciation of the heroic nurses, of the services rendered by registrars and superintendents of hospitals, and of the religious orders—Sisters of Charity, of Mercy, and of the Holy Cross—which had permitted members to sign up as contract nurses.[11] In order that the nation never again be unprepared to nurse its armed services properly in war or in peace, Dr. McGee began working on plans for a permanent nursing corps. On December 8, 1898, she addressed a letter to Adelaide Nutting.

Dear Madam:

Will you kindly inform me the least salary which the Army could offer to nurses, the terms being enlistment for three years, after a proba-

---

[10] *Ibid.*, pp. 203–5; Roberts, *American Nursing*, pp. 29–30; Portia B. Kernodle, *The Red Cross in Action, 1882–1948* (New York: Harper & Bros., 1949), p. 19.

[11] George M. Sternberg (Washington, D.C.) to Dr. Anita Newcomb McGee (Washington, D.C.), September 9, 1898, National Archives, Washington, D.C.

tionary course and the additional compensation being food, lodging and an allowance for a prescribed uniform.

We wish to obtain a good class of nurses but do not want to make the salary any higher than is absolutely necessary to effect that purpose. The details just mentioned are not yet decided upon.

Any advice or suggestions . . . will be appreciated.

Very sincerely,

Anita Newcomb McGee
Acting Assistant Surgeon General
U.S.A.[12]

Adelaide replied that good nurses were receiving from $21 to $25 per week for private duty and that the demand was greater than the supply. Nurses in charge of hospital work of varying degrees and responsibilities were paid from $50 to $100 per month. Head nurses were paid from $30 to $40 per month and in all institutions were supplied with comfortable rooms, board, and laundry. She suggested that Dr. McGee draw her own inferences.[13]

In December, 1898, the executive committee of the Associated Alumnae and a number of influential lay women met at the New York Hospital Training School for Nurses and laid plans for submitting a bill to Congress which would provide for a permanent army nurse corps. The corps would be responsible only to the military authorities and would be free from the control of voluntary organizations such as the Red Cross and the Daughters of the American Revolution. It would be directed by a nurse, not a physician. Adelaide Nutting was appointed secretary of a subcommittee to organize committees of nurses in the various states, to keep them informed of the progress of the bill, and to urge them to press upon their representatives and senators the need for a properly organized army nurse corps.[14]

In Baltimore, Adelaide arranged for an open meeting on the bill to be held at the Arundel Club and made a special effort to see that influential people of the city, and members of the Hopkins Hospital staff and Medical School attended. She carefully outlined every step of the meeting. She asked Miss Elizabeth King, long prominent in social and philanthropic affairs, to state the purpose of the meeting, and then

[12] Anita Newcomb McGee (Washington, D.C.) to Adelaide Nutting (Baltimore), December 8, 1898, The Johns Hopkins Hospital School of Nursing Archives.

[13] Adelaide Nutting (Baltimore) to Dr. Anita Newcomb McGee (Washington, D.C.), ibid.

[14] Ethel Johns and Blanche Pfefferkorn, The Johns Hopkins Hospital School of Nursing (Baltimore: The Johns Hopkins Press, 1954), p. 19.

asked Dr. Johnson, a respected physician, to preside for the remainder of the evening and to introduce the various items she had set up for the agenda. Miss Margaret Astor, a nurse, gave an account of her observations and work in Cuba. Georgia Nevins came up from Garfield Hospital in Washington to outline the history of the bill. There were remarks by Dr. Osler, Dr. I. E. Atkinson, Dr. Welch, and Skipworth Wilmer, prominent attorney and trustee of The Johns Hopkins Hospital. After some concluding comments, Miss Nutting proposed a resolution favoring the bill. It was seconded by Dr. Osler, as prearranged. The resounding "ayes" indicated that the groundwork had been well laid.[15]

Adelaide Nutting also persuaded the trustees of The Johns Hopkins Hospital to go on record in favor of the bill. Twenty-three Johns Hopkins graduates had volunteered and been sent to various camps and hospitals. Four were in charge of hospitals.[16] Dr. Osler went to Washington and laid the case before Dr. Sternberg, the surgeon general, and influential members of the Senate.[17]

The bill finally came before Congress in 1900. Miss Nutting appeared with her committee before a hearing of the Committee on Military Affairs. Dr. Welch spoke in behalf of the nurses' proposal; there was opposition on the part of many members of the medical profession, however, and the bill failed to pass.

The Society of Superintendents and the Associated Alumnae were disappointed but not discouraged. They strengthened their lobby and worked for another bill. Meanwhile, the army itself was undergoing reorganization, and, at the request of the surgeon general, Dr. McGee wrote the section of the Army Reorganization Act of 1901 which established the "Army Nurse Corps, Female," and stipulated that the direction of the service be under a graduate nurse.[18]

With the establishment of the Army Nurse Corps, Isabel Robb turned her attention to bringing about a liaison between the Associated Alumnae and the American Red Cross. The goal was to have every graduate nurse become a member of the Red Cross and thus be ready at the call to aid suffering humanity.

[15] Adelaide Nutting, "Notes for meeting to be held at Arundel Club" and rough draft of resolution in behalf of the Arundel Club supporting the army nurse corps bill (n.d.); Adelaide Nutting (New York) to Lavinia Dock (Fayetteville, Pa.), December 31, 1920; MAN Papers. See also Johns and Pfefferkorn, *The Johns Hopkins Hospital School of Nursing*, p. 118.

[16] Johns and Pfefferkorn, *The Johns Hopkins Hospital School of Nursing*, p. 120.

[17] William Osler (Baltimore) to Adelaide Nutting (Baltimore), November 24, 1899, The Johns Hopkins Hospital School of Nursing Archives.

[18] Roberts, *American Nursing*, p. 30.

Adelaide Nutting, who had spent much time on the army bill, now began reworking the Hopkins curriculum to give the third-year students an enriched background and sounder preparation for nursing. There were many new developments in nursing for which she wanted her graduates prepared—notably, industrial, visiting, and school nursing. In 1893, Lillian Wald and Mary Brewster had started a nursing service on the lower East Side of New York that was to be the forerunner of the famous Henry Street Settlement and the New York Visiting Nurses' Association. Three years later, in January, 1896, the Instructive Visiting Nurses' Association was founded in Baltimore, with Adelaide Nutting's classmate, Evelyn Pope, its sole nurse for the first six months. In 1894, Boston became the first city in the United States to institute medical inspection in the schools. Three years later this practice was started in New York. London gained its first school nurse in 1898. Before many years passed, the school nurse would become an integral part of the American educational system.[19]

In 1899, Adelaide Nutting inaugurated a brief series of lectures on social and public questions through which she hoped to alert students to the possibilities for their intelligent and useful participation in the community. Such topics as "Organization of Charities," "Rescue of Children from an Unfavorable Environment," and "Functions of Municipality and State" were discussed. The lectures were so worthwhile that she hoped to make them a definite part of the third year of study.[20]

By this time the third-year plan was well established and student allowances had been discontinued. The eight-hour duty also had been approved, although demands within the hospital often made it difficult to enforce. Miss Nutting's next innovation would be a six-month preparatory course for students before they were allowed in the wards. Adelaide believed there was something incongruous and fearful about sending a young woman into the wards, uninformed as to sanitation, asepsis, and hospital procedures.

> In my judgment the course of instruction for the first year should be so altered as to permit of a certain preliminary training of the pupil before she enters the wards of the Hospital. This training might cover a period of six months with distinct advantage to the pupil and should embrace a practical study of household duties and administration and of cookery for invalids.

[19] *Ibid.*, p. 660.
[20] Henry M. Hurd, "Eleventh Report of the Superintendent, The Johns Hopkins Hospital, for the year ending January 31, 1900," The Johns Hopkins Hospital School of Nursing Archives.

All necessary study of anatomy and physiology and of materia medica, should form the earliest training and instruction given to a pupil. Such a change would better further development of the educational ideals in the training of nurses which this School has at all times advanced. It would in some measure correspond to the general accepted methods of teaching in other professions, notably that of medicine where it is considered neither wise nor safe for student or patient that theory and practice should begin together.[21]

It had not been difficult to convince the trustees of the desirability of the three-year plan, for it had increased the number of student nurses available for nursing services. The preparatory course would do the opposite. Because the financial condition at Hopkins continued to be precarious, Miss Nutting decided to wait for a more propitious moment to make this request for change.

Adelaide made a point of keeping track of the nursing graduates, of their progress, successes, and failures. She reported to the trustees the success and reputation the graduates enjoyed. Twenty-four Hopkins women were in charge of hospitals in 1900. Among the larger of these were a 400-bed hospital in Naples, Italy; Garfield Hospital, Washington, D.C., 150 beds; Winnipeg General Hospital, 250 beds; New England General Hospital, Roxbury, Massachusetts, 165 beds; and St. John's Hospital, St. John's, Newfoundland, 120 beds.

Through her work with the Society of Superintendents and the Associated Alumnae, Adelaide Nutting was becoming a well-known figure in American nursing. Her work on committees was outstanding. She could be depended upon to make careful studies, summarize data, and present facts and recommendations concisely, forcefully, and unemotionally. Between the annual meetings she did her homework conscientiously, and, when she spoke, nurses and superintendents listened.

After the Toronto meeting in 1898, Isabel Robb began to draft a practical solution to the problem of graduate training for administrative positions in hospitals and training schools. Although much of the committee work had to be done by correspondence, Isabel and Adelaide managed to get together and work out a curriculum which they thought, with the exception of certain professional courses, could be taught by the faculties and with the facilities of schools already in existence. They then submitted it to the other members of the committee.

Adelaide Nutting and Isabel Robb had read much in the papers

[21] *Ibid.*

about Teachers College when it affiliated with Columbia University in
1898. Beginning as an experiment in preparing teachers for the practical arts, it had become a university school for the scientific study of
education and the training of leaders in fields not covered by existing
teacher-training institutions.[22] Teachers College had four goals: general culture, special scholarship, professional knowledge, and technical skill. Dean James Earl Russell envisaged not only a college education but a "training which would enable the student to see the
relationships existing everywhere in the various fields of knowledge,
even the unity of all knowledge, . . . liberal enough to inspire respect
for knowledge, broad enough to justify independent knowledge, ac-
curate enough to beget a love of truth."[23]

Working from a catalog, Isabel and Adelaide outlined "A Possible
Course at Teachers College for a Training Class for Administrative
Positions in Nursing," which would embrace courses already scheduled in psychology, biology, domestic science, physical science, and
special lectures on subjects pertinent to nursing education. Next they
had an interview with Dean Russell. They told him there was no reason why the principles that applied to teachers of teachers in the
fields of practical arts, domestic science, manual training, woodwork,
shop work, and school administration should not apply also to
teachers in nursing education. With the staff it had brought together,
they believed Teachers College had some obligation to the nursing
profession. To Dean Russell's question, "Is there a nursing profession?" they replied that there was a vocation of nursing and that they
hoped to make of it a profession.

At first Dean Russell could see no connection between nursing and
teaching. Isabel and Adelaide took him to St. Luke's Hospital at 8 P.M.
They met a class of twenty or thirty girls who had had twelve hours
of duty on the floor. They were reciting aloud verbatim from Gray's
Anatomy, the page listing the bones of the human body. Dean Russell
was convinced. Here was a teacher, in woeful need of knowledge of
how to teach, drilling overworked students who were the victims of
ignorance and exploitation.[24]

[22] Isabel M. Stewart, "Three Decades of Nursing Education, Teachers College,
Columbia University," in Methods and Problems of Medical Education, 21st ser.
(New York: Rockefeller Foundation, 1932), p. 1.
[23] Lawrence A. Cremin et al., A History of Teachers College, Columbia University (New York: Columbia University Press, 1954), p. 36; see also James E.
Russell, "The Function of the University in Training Teachers," Columbia University Quarterly 1 (1898–99): 323–42.
[24] "Thirtieth Anniversary Celebration of the Nursing Education Department,
Teachers College, Columbia University," Nursing Education Bulletin 2 (1929): 12.

The course outlined by Isabel and Adelaide was acceptable to Dean Russell. With the title "Hospital Economics," it would come under the administration of Miss Helen Kinne, director of the training for teachers of home economics. If twelve students could be secured for the course, the dean estimated that the cost of the specialized instruction could be absorbed by allocating to the program $75 from the $400 paid by each student for board, room, and tuition. He was willing to undertake the course for as few as six students, but the deficit would have to be made up by the Society of Superintendents. He asked about the possibility of the society's endowing a chair for $50,000, should the arrangement become permanent.

When the Sixth Annual Convention of the Society of Superintendents assembled at the Academy of Medicine in New York on May 5, Isabel Robb proposed that a board of examiners be appointed by the society to receive the names of candidates for the course and to endorse them after carefully examining their certificates and the recommendations of the principals of the schools from which they graduated as to their general fitness to become superintendents. The candidates would study for eight months at Teachers College and then spend from three to five months on private duty. After this year of preparation, having passed the required examination, each candidate would receive a certificate as evidence of being qualified for the position of superintendent of a hospital or training school. The certificate would be signed by the dean of Teachers College and by members of the society's Board of Examiners. The cost to the student would be about $400, for tuition, board, lodgings, and laundry.

Animated discussion followed the reading of the proposed course of study. Miss A. A. Hintze of the Women's Medical Hospital, Philadelphia, rose to speak. "If we can carry out this further educational training, we shall reach a unique place. I move this association sanction this plan and that the Chair be authorized to appoint a committee with power to act."[25] Several voices quickly seconded her motion. Isabel Robb explained that the curriculum was not final and that the plan would be purely experimental for one year. At first Dean Russell had been unwilling to try the course for less than two years. Mrs. Robb suggested that Social Reform Movements might be a required course instead of an elective, while Adelaide Nutting insisted on a course in sociology. A member of the District Nursing Board in Baltimore had once complained to Adelaide: "What a pity that your nurses

[25] American Society of Superintendents of Training Schools for Nurses, *Sixth Annual Report* (Harrisburg, Pa.: Harrisburg Publishing Co., 1900), pp. 58–59.

know so little beside nursing. They should study municipal and civil affairs before they can be valuable to the community in other ways." As a result, Adelaide had brought lecturers on social problems to Johns Hopkins, among them Jane Addams from Hull House in Chicago.

Isabel Robb proposed two ways of financing the course: twelve scholars at $400 each, or an endowment of $50,000. An endowment would be an appropriate commemoration of twenty-five years of nurses training in America. For the first year of the course, the society pledged $1,000, although its annual income was less than half that amount.[26]

When the convention ended, Isabel Robb and Adelaide Nutting turned to finding nurses who had the money and inclination to take the course. Copy for the announcement to come from Teachers College was sent at once to Dean Russell. The committee prepared mailing lists, but the circulars failed to arrive. In mid-July, in desperation, Mrs. Robb asked what had happened to the announcements. The dean replied that he was sorry the circulars were late, but that they would go on with the course "if only one student shows up to take it."[27]

On June 22, Anna L. Alline, of the Brooklyn Homeopathic Hospital and Training School for Nurses, sent an inquiry to Mrs. Robb. She had attended Iowa State Normal for two years and had taught for six years in Plymouth County, Iowa. She held a life certificate in teaching. Linda Richards, America's first trained nurse, had signed Miss Alline's nursing school diploma and now approved her for the course.

The circulars finally got into the mail, but there were few responses. Isabel Robb was disposed to attribute the lack of inquiries to the delay in having the circulars printed. Later she was thankful the delay had forced Dean Russell's commitment that the course would go on if only one candidate appeared.

The September 9, 1899, issue of *Nursing Record and Hospital World* carried a detailed announcement of the course in Hospital Economics to be given at Teachers College. It cited the purpose of the course, listed the personnel of the Department of Home Economics and the Board of Examiners, and described the requirements for admission, the eight months of study, the period of private duty, and the certificate to be awarded to those graduating. In lieu of a diploma from an approved high school, a qualifying examination might be

[26] *Ibid.*

[27] James Earl Russell (Kidderson-on-Lake Cayuga, N.Y.) to Mrs. Hunter Robb (Cleveland, Ohio), July 17, 1899, Department of Nursing Education Archives, Teachers College.

taken. In the English examination, special attention would be given to spelling, grammar, punctuation, and paragraph structure. Candidates for the examination in 1899 were expected to have read Dryden's *Palamon and Arcite*; Pope's *Iliad*, Books I, VII, XII, and XXIV; *Sir Roger de Coverley Papers*; *The Spectator*; Goldsmith, *Vicar of Wakefield*; Coleridge, *Rime of the Ancient Mariner*; Cooper, *Last of the Mohicans*; Lowell, *Vision of Sir Launfal*; Hawthorne, *The House of the Seven Gables*; Shakespeare, *Macbeth*; Milton, *Paradise Lost*, Books I and II; Burke, *Speech on Conciliation*; Carlyle, *Essay on Burns*; and Meyers, *Ancient, Medieval, and Modern World*. In the mathematics examination, candidates would be tested especially in fractions, percentages, and the metric system.[28]

It is not known whether any nurses were frightened away from the qualifying examination by the formidable list of classics, but, when Teachers College opened in the fall, only two students, Anna Alline and Aurelia Gorman, were registered for the course in hospital economics.[29] Both held satisfactory high school diplomas and fitted into classes with prospective teachers of the household arts, manual training, and general education. They would learn principles and make their own application to nursing. To fulfill the requirement of practice teaching, Miss Alline and Miss Gorman gave six lectures on home nursing to the seniors in the Department of Domestic Science, with Miss Kinne serving as critic.[30]

Lectures on nursing subjects were provided by the Society of Superintendents' Committee on Education. Early in the year Dr. John S. Billings gave two two-hour lectures on "Hospital Construction: Ventilation and Sanitation"; then Miss Maud Banfield, superintendent of Polyclinic Hospital, Philadelphia, and Miss Lucy Walker, superintendent of Pennsylvania Hospital, Philadelphia, each gave one lecture on "Hospital Administration"; in April, Adelaide Nutting gave two lectures on the "History of Nursing." Isabel Robb concluded the series in May with two lectures on "Training School Organization." Only Dr. Billings was paid for his services.

The Committee on Education, greatly worried about the financing of the course, literally went out begging for funds. Dean Russell turned back $75 from the fees paid by the two students, Mrs. White-

---

[28] "Teachers College, Columbia University: Course in Hospital Economics," *Nursing Record and Nursing World*, September 9, 1899; see *ibid.*

[29] James Earl Russell, "Account of the Beginnings of the Nursing Education Department" (Speech given on October 30, 1924, at the Thirtieth Anniversary Celebration of the Nursing Education Department, Teachers College), *Nursing Education Bulletin* 2 (1929): 1.

[30] Adelaide Nutting, memorandum (n.d.), MAN Papers.

law Reid gave $200, a trained nurse sent $100, the alumnae associations of Hopkins and Bellevue made gifts, and the individual superintendents, although earning only between $1,200 and $1,500 a year, contributed generously.[31]

Miss Alline and Miss Gorman seemed happy in their studies, although at times it was difficult for them to translate the psychology course into a sickroom situation. The superintendents' Committee on Education was loath to abandon the project, believing that another year would bring an increased interest on the part of nurses who wanted to advance in the profession and also a greater willingness to contribute on the part of loyal superintendents who desired to see their successors better trained. Dean Russell was becoming more and more impressed with nurses' training as a field of education. In February, 1900, he wrote to Isabel Robb, inquiring whether the Society of Superintendents could raise $1,000 to underwrite the hospital economics course for the coming year. "Personally," he wrote, "I am disposed to have great faith in the undertaking. . . . With a pledge of $1,000 a year for the support of such a department, I believe our Trustees would have no hesitation in inaugurating the work in a thorough and systematic manner." He then offered to speak at the next nurses' convention.[32] Before that meeting in April, he wrote to Adelaide Nutting about the possibility of her coming to New York to direct the course. When she declined, he asked the opinion of the committee about inviting Miss Alline to stay on as manager of the course, giving nursing lectures, conducting field trips to hospitals and nursing centers, and assisting Miss Kinne.

No papers were read at the Seventh Annual Convention of the Society of Superintendents in New York on April 30, May 1, and May 2, 1900, but the society's reports and business were of far-reaching significance. Then, speaking on "The Function and Purposes of Teachers College," Dean Russell stressed the way in which it could be of service to nursing education.[33]

Anna Alline and Aurelia Gorman, who had accompanied Dean Russell to the convention, reported on their experiences. Miss Alline felt better prepared for either hospital or training school administration. She believed that many superintendents and doctors were poor

[31] American Society of Superintendents of Training Schools for Nurses, *Seventh Annual Report* (Harrisburg, Pa.: Harrisburg Publishing Co., 1900), pp. 37–38.

[32] James Earl Russell (New York) to Mrs. Hunter Robb (Cleveland, Ohio), February 10, 1900, Department of Nursing Education Archives, Teachers College.

[33] James E. Russell, in American Society of Superintendents of Training Schools for Nurses, *Seventh Annual Report*, pp. 10–17.

teachers because they did not know how to teach. She had found the study of diet especially helpful, but she discounted the course in psychology. Miss Gorman agreed and said that she, too, had learned many new methods.

From the reception given the remarks of Dean Russell and the students, it was evident that the Society of Superintendents did not want to abandon the course in hospital economics. The society's membership now numbered 126 superintendents. Someone suggested that if each superintendent pledged to give or to secure a donation of ten dollars the finance problem would be solved.

As yet, not a single application had been received for the coming year, but Isabel Robb insisted that things were looking up for nursing. Fifty-five schools had now lengthened their course to three years. It was thought that the long list of readings may have discouraged applicants, so the preliminary qualifying examination for admission to the hospital economics course was waived.

Lavinia Dock proposed that the Society of Superintendents and the Associated Alumnae form a federation of nurses and affiliate with the National Council of Women in order to become eligible for representation at the meeting of the International Council of Women in London in July and participate in the organization of an International Council of Nurses. The superintendents approved the idea and referred it to the Associated Alumnae. Lavinia Dock's willingness to serve as a representative at her own expense was applauded.

Adelaide Nutting, Isabel Robb, and Lavinia Dock remained in New York for the annual meeting of the Associated Alumnae. The proposal for a federation of nurses was quickly endorsed and Miss Dock became American nursing's representative at the meetings in London. Miss Nutting reported the status of the bill for an army nurse corps, and Mrs. Robb pleaded the cause of the Teachers College course in hospital economics, the need for state organizations of nurses, and registration.

Sophia Palmer and Mary E. P. Davis presented plans for a nursing journal, a goal of nursing since the congress at the Chicago World's Fair in 1893. The Committee on Ways and Means of Producing a Magazine was reorganized, and Miss Davis, who had just resigned as superintendent of the University of Pennsylvania Hospital, was made chairman. Sophia Palmer, superintendent of the Rochester City Hospital, Rochester, New York, had been interested in the project from the beginning, and she, Adelaide Nutting, and Isabel Robb also were appointed members of the committee.

Miss Palmer and Miss Davis were good businesswomen and

wanted to start the magazine as soon as possible. Of the four methods of producing a magazine which the committee had explored, a stock company was considered preferable. The committee had even proceeded to solicit subscriptions to the magazine and sales of stock to nurses and alumnae associations. It was determined to keep control of the magazine within the profession. Five hundred fifty subscriptions to the periodical had been secured and more had been promised. The committee admitted it had exceeded its authority, but capital was needed, and there seemed to be no other way of starting the magazine. Subscribers to the magazine and purchasers of stock had been discreetly advised that, if the magazine did not materialize, no one should expect a return.

The need for a journal was urgent. The development and promotion of standards for the rapidly increasing number of nursing schools and the need for legal controls over the practice of nursing demanded an organ through which nurses and superintendents could communicate with one another and build a true profession. Again, the nurses gave their unqualified approval.[34]

Years later, reading an account of the course, Adelaide penciled in the margin, "No money, nothing but ideas, convictions and faith."[35]

[34] Roberts, *American Nursing*, pp. 41–47.
[35] M. A. Nutting, "Brief Account of the Course in Hospital Economics," *Teachers College Record*, May, 1910, pp. 1–6 (also in MAN Papers).

XI

Unfinished Business, 1900–1902

As Adelaide turned to the correspondence,[1] hospital reports, and sundry items that had accumulated in her absence, she pondered her reply to Dean Russell's offer. Although she enjoyed teaching and believed there would be fewer stresses and strains at Teachers College than at Hopkins, she did not know whether she was ready to leave Baltimore. If the changes she dreamed of for Hopkins were not put into effect, such an opportunity might not come again. She recognized the possibilities of the hospital economics course at Teachers College, but felt that her way was not clear to leave Johns Hopkins. Her answer to Dean Russell on May 10 stated that things were looking up at Hopkins and that she would therefore decline his offer.[2] Helen Kinne, director of the Home Economics Department, Teachers College, wrote that she was disappointed that Miss Nutting had decided not to come to Teachers College. She feared that the hospital economics course might be jeopardized by her decision. "Is your decision for all time, or may we some day ask you again?"[3]

Miss Kinne's letter did not require an immediate reply, and Adelaide laid it aside. She was happier in Baltimore than in any other place she had ever lived. She had a comfortable apartment in the Nurses' Home, a dependable staff, and many friends—the Oslers, the Hurds, the Gilmans, Elizabeth King, and the stimulating women at the Arundel Club. Many of her students lived nearby. Hopkins had given her much; she owed it to the hospital to stay on. The preparatory course would have to be properly launched, and she wanted to help Dr. Osler in his crusade against tuberculosis, of which there was much in Baltimore. Someone had to carry forward the organization of

[1] William T. Dixon (Baltimore) to M. A. Nutting (Baltimore), May 9, 1900, MAN Papers.

[2] Adelaide Nutting (Baltimore) to James E. Russell (New York), May 10, 1900, *ibid.*

[3] Helen Kinne (New York) to M. A. Nutting (Baltimore), May 26, 1900, *ibid.*

nurses in Maryland so that later the goals of national registration and professionalization might be achieved. She would still go to New York to give lectures in the hospital economics course, but she was not ready to take over the management of it.

Eleven graduate nurses applied and were accepted for the hospital economics course at Teachers College in 1900, but three withdrew before classes began, one became ill, and only six remained to complete their work. Anna Alline, who had taken the course the year before, agreed to manage the program, to offer an elective in home nursing to seniors in the Home Economics Department, and to conduct field trips for $400, a sum which the Society of Superintendents would have to raise. Miss Alline wrote longhand monthly reports which were relayed as "round robins" to members of the Committee on Education. Adelaide gave her lectures on December 5, and Miss Alline wrote Miss Maud Banfield, chairman of the Committee on Education, that the students had enjoyed the lectures very much and were greatly pleased with her.[4]

In October, 1900, the first issue of the *American Journal of Nursing* appeared. It was a sixty-four page magazine whose feature articles dealt with private nursing, hospital and training school items, the care of children, foreign correspondence, official reports of nursing organizations, food and dietetics, sanitation and hospital construction, education, subjects of current interest, progressive movements, and prophylactics. Advertising would be limited to sixteen pages and to the front and back covers.

As a superintendent, a stockholder in the enterprise, and a nurse, Adelaide Nutting looked over the new journal critically. It represented a milestone in the history of American nursing. On the whole, J. B. Lippincott Company had done a creditable piece of publishing, and Sophia Palmer, as editor, deserved a letter of congratulation by return mail. As Adelaide had expected, Lavinia Dock's article, "What We May Expect from the Law," was provocative. Who else could have been entrusted with firing the opening gun for state organization and registration? One by one Lavinia had listed the obstacles in the way of achieving a real nursing profession: the exploitation of student nurses, long hours, the lack of uniformity in standards of training, the six-week and correspondence schools of nursing. The article concluded with some constructive recommendations: state organizations, salaried graduate nurses in private hospitals, postgraduate work in specialty

---

[4] Anna L. Alline (New York) to Maud Banfield (Philadelphia), December 12, 1901, Department of Nursing Education Archives, Teachers College.

hospitals, and the rotation of students from a large central school to various hospitals for specialized training.[5] Isabel Robb devoted most of the education section to the hospital economics course at Teachers College.[6]

Judging by its first issue, the *American Journal of Nursing* promised much. Adelaide regretted that the pressure of work at the hospital and her precarious health had forced her to decline a position in the Department of Prophylactics. She had no real misgivings, however; she had paid $100 for a share in the company, had been one of the five persons who had pledged $100 more to get the presses rolling, and had written countless letters to prospective subscribers and advertisers. Only two older and larger hospitals outranked Hopkins in the number of alumnae subscribers to the magazine. Later she hoped to write an article and to solicit more subscriptions.

The preparatory course at Hopkins was now Adelaide's prime objective. Years later Mary Bartlett Dixon recalled a conversation with her before entering the training school:

> I may accept you for one reason. I can not develop our school unless I have the understanding and active support of the Board of Trustees. Your father is President of the Board and through you, as a student of this school, I believe I can demonstrate the reasonableness of one of my most important plans. I am speaking of the basic training of students over some months before they are called upon to assume ward duties and responsibilities. If you are accepted as a probationer, the morning after you arrive you will have to go into a ward completely unprepared for the work that will confront you. I am sure you will encounter great difficulties and I am equally sure your head nurse will encounter through you even greater difficulties for she is a very busy person and has not the time to teach you.

When Adelaide finally accepted Mary Dixon, she admonished her:

> You are about to enter the School of Nursing of a very great hospital. We are all of us here working together day and night, year after year, to give our patients the best possible care and service. You will be a small cog in a very great wheel but always remember a cog, however small is of vital importance.[7]

[5] Lavinia Dock, "What We May Expect from the Law," *American Journal of Nursing*, October, 1900, p. 11.
[6] Significantly, vol. 1, no. 1, of *Teachers College Record* made no reference to the hospital economics course. Perhaps the administration regarded the future of the course too uncertain to warrant publicity.
[7] Mary Bartlett Dixon Cullen, "Remembrances of Mary Adelaide Nutting," *The Johns Hopkins Nurses Alumnae Magazine*, April, 1949, p. 50.

A crisis in the domestic management of the hospital provided Adelaide with an opportunity to advance her proposal. She talked at length with Dr. Hurd, the hospital superintendent, after which he indicated her suggestion might be a solution to two problems, domestic work in the hospital and more effective preparation of student nurses. On October 19, 1900, Dr. Hurd proposed to the trustees of the hospital that there should be a "reorganization of the domestic work in the Nurses' Home whereby all branches of it should be placed under the direction of the Superintendent of Nurses," and in November he was authorized to make such changes as would "facilitate the preliminary training of nurses in housekeeping."[8] On February 1, 1901, the Nurses' Home was removed from the charge of the matron of the hospital and placed under the control of the superintendent of nurses. Adelaide had hoped to begin the preparatory course immediately, but, because of the time involved in reorganizing the entire household, training the new maids, and getting everything in good running order, she decided to wait until the second division of the class entered in October.

Sixteen students were admitted to the first preparatory course, and by December the program was off to a good start. The idea was not really new, having been in use in British schools for several years and to a certain degree in the Waltham Hospital in Massachusetts. In all the professions except nursing, instruction preceded practice. It seemed strange that anything as vitally important as nursing should be the exception.

Probationers would now enter twice yearly in groups of from sixteen to eighteen. They were assigned to various departments of the training school household, where they were taught by practical experience the best methods of housekeeping and of selecting, preparing, and serving foods. They were trained also in the surgical supply rooms and in the preparation of all types of dressings. Their afternoons were given over to study and classes. The complete course in anatomy, requiring about nine hours a week, was to be completed during the first six months. Other subjects studied during this period were hygiene, materia medica, and elements of practical nursing. All food served to the students and graduate nurses was prepared in the new model kitchen in the Nurses' Home, largely by the probationers under the direction and supervision of special teachers, Emma Shedley and Mary Peacock, both graduates of Drexel Institute. Miss Ross was in charge of the home.[9] For the sake of identification, and to protect

[8] Ethel Johns and Blanche Pfefferkorn, *The Johns Hopkins Hospital School of Nursing* (Baltimore: The Johns Hopkins Press, 1954), p. 124.
[9] *Ibid.*, pp. 124–27.

them from being asked to do things they were not prepared to do, the probationers wore pink uniforms with white cuffs and white aprons. The upper classes referred to them as the "pinkies."[10]

Adelaide continued to teach classes in ethics and the history of nursing, but her direct contact with the student nurses was largely limited to her morning and afternoon rounds of the wards. Many legends grew up about her. To some of the student nurses, she seemed aloof, stern, severe, yet none questioned her sense of justice. After most were out of school and saw her in perspective, affection replaced awe. They sought her advice.[11]

Although Adelaide insisted on high standards at Hopkins, her demands for quality did not blind her human understanding. A young student nurse on early night duty once administered the wrong dose of medicine. The girl felt sure that this blunder would jeopardize her future, that no one would trust her again, and that she would never regain confidence in herself. At the close of the year, she was given a scholarship for general proficiency. When she expressed amazement at being thought worthy of the honor after having made such a mistake, Adelaide reassured her that it would not be just to allow one error to mar any capable student's career.[12] Recalling the incident years later, Effie Taylor said, "Next to my mother, I loved her."

The second year of the hospital economics course at Teachers College in New York was not so tranquil as the first. The new students may not have been so well prepared as Anna Alline and Aurelia Gorman, but they were far more vocal and extremely critical. On October 22, 1900, Mary V. Sullivan wrote to Miss Nutting: "The whole class is dissatisfied. The course is too new. It needs years to perfect and complete it. The class is small and [has] to take lessons with other students. The class had a meeting and protested they wanted psychology cut out." A month later Mary Sullivan wrote again, saying that all six students were dissatisfied.[13] On December 26, 1900, Ida Palmer, sister of Sophia Palmer, editor of the *American Journal of Nursing*, voiced her complaints in a letter to Miss Banfield: "That the course is necessary and that the nursing profession will be greatly benefitted by it, I am confident but as it is at

---

[10] Jessie Black McVicar, "Preliminary Course for Nurses, The Johns Hopkins Hospital School of Nursing," *The Johns Hopkins Nurses Alumnae Magazine*, April, 1958, p. 25.

[11] Isabel M. Stewart, *Oral History*, 2 vols. (New York: Columbia University, Butler Library, 1958), 2: 209–93.

[12] Effie J. Taylor, "Miss Nutting's Contribution to Nursing Education," *The Johns Hopkins Nurses Alumnae Magazine*, April, 1949, p. 47.

[13] Mary V. Sullivan (New York) to Adelaide Nutting (Baltimore), October 22 and November 24 and 25, 1900, MAN Papers.

present there is a great deal which could be eliminated and the work condensed giving time for other subjects of equal importance." Miss Palmer thought the course in health and sanitation should be changed and shortened, that a short course in bacteriology and a few lectures on the best method of teaching materia medica would be helpful, and that nurses should be taught psychology in a class by themselves. The course on food and dietetics seemed divided and sub-divided to a minute degree. Ida Palmer did not think sociology was important and regretted that the class had decided not to send a formal statement of opinion to the Society of Superintendents' Committee on Education.[14]

Dean Russell and the Committee on Education were unmoved by the suggestion that psychology be eliminated, but the teacher in charge was advised to take into account the interests of the nursing students and their obvious limitations. Adelaide was adamant about the systematic study of society, its structure, and its organized patterns of collective human behavior, which she considered essential to the nurse as well as to the superintendent. She had little patience with people who were not willing "to stretch their intellects." All her life she had been reaching for things beyond her first comprehension. She had studied and struggled with meaning, and she knew the thrill of grasping an idea.

The criticisms of the Teachers College course were well aired at the superintendents' convention in Buffalo, New York, September 16 and 17, 1901, and a special board was named to investigate the charges. The board's decision was presented at the next meeting:

> Students must be made to clearly understand that the course is in no sense intended as a post-graduate course in practical nursing and that it does not supply anything in the practical branches but that it is an advanced course for such trained nurses as are already expert in all branches of practical nursing and who can give proof of this adequate training, of maturity of mind, of capacity for advanced work, and of earnestness of purpose.[15]

Miss Alline, Dean Russell, and the staff were fully supported.

Back in New York, Grace Dodge, philanthropist and benefactor of Teachers College, was quietly observing this new departure in nursing education. She had originally advised Dean Russell to give the hospital economics course a trial. Now she insisted that it be continued

---

[14] Ida R. Palmer (New York) to Maud Banfield, (Philadelphia), December 26, 1900, *ibid.*

[15] American Society of Superintendents of Training Schools for Nurses, *Eighth Annual Report* (Harrisburg, Pa.: Harrisburg Publishing Co., 1901).

and, if possible, that Miss Nutting be brought to New York to direct it. When Adelaide had decided against coming to Teachers College in 1901, Miss Dodge had said, "We will ask her again." Dean Russell knew that when Miss Dodge wanted something very much she would either provide the money herself or induce someone else to give it.[16]

The summer of 1901 was crammed with activity. In addition to screening and notifying applicants of their admission, and writing literally hundreds of letters in behalf of the *American Journal of Nursing* and the hospital economics course at Teachers College, Adelaide prepared two papers: "Household Economics in the Training School for Nurses," which she presented at the Third Annual Conference of Home Economics Teachers at Lake Placid, New York; and "The Hospital and the Community," which she sent to be read at the Society of Superintendents' meeting in Buffalo.

Through the Home Economics Department of Teachers College, Adelaide had been invited to the Lake Placid conference sponsored by Mr. and Mrs. Melvil Dewey. In her paper she pointed out the importance of diet and the proper preparation of food for the sick, especially vital now that visiting nurse services were growing. She recommended that, within the hospital, non-resident workers be employed for definite hours at specified rates of payment. The meeting's discussions were stimulating and forward-looking, and Adelaide became a good friend of the Deweys and of Ellen H. Richards of the Massachusetts Institute of Technology. She would return to other conferences at Lake Placid. A few years later, when Mrs. Richards organized the nation's first Home Economics Association, Adelaide played a significant part in the planning.[17]

During the summer of 1901, Adelaide entertained many distinguished doctors and their wives, as well as nurses who wished to visit the famous hospital on their way to or from the World's Fair and the International Congress of Nurses in Buffalo. She did not attend any of the professional meetings, but remained available to meet foreign visitors and conduct them on a tour of the hospital and training school.[18]

[16] James B. Russell (New York) to Mrs. Hunter Robb (Cleveland, Ohio), March 30, 1900; Grace H. Dodge (New York) to Maud Banfield (Philadelphia), n.d.; and Isabel M. Stewart, "Notes," [1916]; MAN Papers.

[17] Katharine Fisher, "Adelaide Nutting and Home Economics," 1958, *ibid.*

[18] Visiting delegates and nurses attending the International Congress of Nurses and the superintendents' convention wore scarlet bows with the name of their country stitched in white on one end. Special arrangements were made for entertaining foreign visitors at hospitals in Boston, New York, Philadelphia, Buffalo, Chicago, Washington, D.C., San Francisco, and Montreal. *American Journal of Nursing*, June, 1901, p. 677.

Conventions were expensive, and, after spending $100 for *Journal* stock, contributing $100 to the first issue, and making a substantial contribution to the hospital economics course at Teachers College, Adelaide did not feel financially able to attend. From time to time she sent money to her father and to Jim for help with his growing boys. She was also saving toward a trip to Europe. She was intrigued by old and rare books and occasionally made a purchase which was the envy of Dr. Welch and Dr. Osler. She was especially interested in books by and about Florence Nightingale, and within twenty-five years her collection of Nightingaliana would be the finest in America.

As Adelaide read and reworked her lectures, she became increasingly aware of the need for a textbook on the history of nursing. She read all that she could find on the subject in the Baltimore libraries and often visited the Library of Congress and the Surgeon General's Library in Washington. When she was in England in 1895, she had looked up the history of St. Bartholomew's Hospital, St. Thomas' Hospital, and the Edinburgh Infirmary. She had started out only to prepare a few lectures and had not thought seriously about writing a book until about 1902. The numerous sources of her outlines and lectures were so scattered as not to be available to the rank and file of nurses, if indeed they had time, energy, or inclination to pursue the subject. Thus she decided to outline various chapters for a book. Parts of a number of chapters were already written. The scope of the book increased as she thought about it, however, and she wondered whether she would ever get it written. About this time Lavinia Dock, traveling in Europe, wrote an interesting account of a visit to Pastor Theodor Fliedner's Deaconess Home at Kaiserwerth on the Rhine. Adelaide replied, "We must have a history of nursing. Will you help me write it?"[19] Lavinia had vision and wrote with zest and sparkle. She agreed to do research while abroad.

Before definite plans were drawn up, Adelaide had another of her perennial bouts with cold, physical exhaustion, and near pneumonia. Once more Dr. Osler advised that a trip to Europe—a sea voyage and complete rest from the worries and responsibility of the hospital, the *Journal*, and the Teachers College course—was what she needed. For the time being, she must lay aside her plans for organizing the Maryland nurses, her work with the Baltimore Visiting Nurses and the anti-tuberculosis campaign.

The first week in April, 1902, Adelaide boarded the German S.S. *Lahu* bound for the Mediterranean. She hoped to spend the spring

[19] Adelaide Nutting, "Notes for Story of Life," MAN Papers; Lavinia Dock, "Writing the History of Nursing," *The Johns Hopkins Nurses Alumnae Magazine*, April, 1950, p. 59.

months leisurely in Italy, then go north into Switzerland and France, and across the channel to England, booking passage to Halifax in mid-July. After a long visit at her sister's home in St. John's, Newfoundland, she would return by way of Montreal and Waterloo for a brief visit with her father, Charlie, and Lizzie. In Italy she planned to see Grace Baxter, a Hopkins graduate of 1895, and Eleanor Wharton Wood, class of 1901, and in France would visit another graduate, Mary Cloud Bean, who was staying with Mrs. Samuel McClure, a cousin of Dr. Hurd, wife of the editor of *McClure's Magazine*, and a former Hopkins patient. She looked forward to sightseeing in London with her fourteen-year-old nephew, Ambrose Gosling, now a student at Forrest School, near Epping Forest.[20]

Adelaide was so exhausted by the time she reached the dock in New York that she wished for nothing but quiet and solitude aboard ship. The *Lahu* was not a steady craft, however, and Adelaide's cabin was directly over the propeller, which did not contribute to a relaxing journey. The ship started to roll as it left the harbor and kept rolling so continuously that it was ten days before Adelaide could summon courage and strength even to write a letter.

Of the 160 passengers, she found some quite interesting: a young sculptor, a pupil of St. Gaudens, now on his way to Paris for further study; a New York coffee merchant who boasted 500 percent profits; an old German shopkeeper and his wife on a visit to the fatherland; a young professor from the University of Michigan on a five-month holiday; and two charming Philadelphia women who knew some of Adelaide's Baltimore friends.[21]

Adelaide delighted in travel, visiting places she had read about, and reliving the great moments of history. She longed to share her experiences with those she loved, and wrote long letters describing the country, the people, art, architecture, and unusual facets of the various cultures. Meticulously she related the details of the journey from Gibraltar to Rome, to Switzerland, to France, and on to England.

Grace Baxter, a former student, met her at the dock in Naples, guided her through customs, and took her to a hotel overlooking the Bay of Sorrento. The view from her window included Capri and Mt. Vesuvius. She thrilled to the blue sky, the bluer waters of the Mediterranean, and the soft salmon pink of the houses, which seemed to stack one atop another on the steep hillside.

[20] Adelaide Nutting (Rome) to Armine N. Gosling (St. John's, Newfoundland), May 6, 1902; Adelaide Nutting (Luzern, Switzerland) to Armine N. Gosling (St. John's), May 25, 1902; and Adelaide Nutting (Divonne, France) to Armine N. Gosling (St. John's), June 7, 1902; MAN Papers.

[21] Adelaide Nutting (aboard the S.S. *Lahu*, en route to Sicily) to Armine N. Gosling (St. John's), April 13, 1902, *ibid.*

With the young coffee salesman who had been at her table on board ship, Adelaide visited Pompeii, Vesuvius, Sorrento, and Capri.[22] Grace Baxter took her on a number of drives. The twenty-mile drive over the hills from Sorrento to the Gulf and on to Amalfi was the one she enjoyed most. Adelaide also visited Miss Baxter's hospital, where the young nurses presented her with a large bouquet of roses.

Adelaide visited art galleries, museums, and historical sites. She was delighted to find some sculpture by Michelangelo in Naples.[23] From Rome she wrote her sister that his great spirit still seemed to be brooding there. She started out after breakfast each day, visiting church after church, St. Peter's, the Vatican, and gallery after gallery, walking until footsore and weary, and even then she felt she had only begun to see Rome. She spent two mornings in the Forum and regretted that she could not spend weeks studying the recent excavations. She found much that was exciting, the Alban Hills, Hadrian's Villa, the Coliseum, the Arch of Constantine, "still splendid though built in the year 312," the Catacombs, the ground over which St. Paul must have traveled often, the Appian Way, and the remains of the old aqueduct beyond.

In Florence she stayed with Grace Baxter's mother, a writer and authority on Italian architecture. Here she was joined by Eleanor Wood, who traveled with her to Venice and Milan. Adelaide was "conscious of Byron almost every minute in Venice" and regretted that she did not have a copy of his *Letters* with her; she would have liked to verify many things—the Palasso Mocenigo, where he lived for so long, the home of Desdemona, the Lido, where he galloped his horse up and down the sands, and the Armenian Monastery, with his inkstand and quills and his signature on the register.[24] She had to tear herself away from Venice and could spend only a day in Milan, where she visited the great cathedral. Then, with Miss Wood, she hastened to the Alps by the St. Gotthard Railway and on into Switzerland.[25]

After some "splendid days in the high Alps about the Matterhorn and a drive over the mountains and through the Valley of Chamonix and around Mont Blanc," they arrived in Geneva, where they relived the Protestant Reformation. Afterward they took a steamer up the

[22] Adelaide Nutting (Rome) to Armine N. Gosling (St. John's), May 1, 1902, *ibid.*

[23] Adelaide Nutting (Rome) to Armine N. Gosling (St. John's), May 6, 1902, *ibid.*

[24] *Ibid.*

[25] Adelaide Nutting (Luzern, Switzerland) to Armine N. Gosling (St. John's), May 25, 1902, *ibid.*

river to Divonne, where they were to be the guests of Mrs. McClure and her nurse and companion, Mary Cloud Bean.

Adelaide had hardly a chance to grasp the beauty of Divonne when Mrs. McClure handed her a letter from her brother Charlie. She quickly opened it and started to read. Suddenly it seemed as if her heart had stopped beating and her whole body was numb with shock. Jim, her younger brother, had died of pneumonia on May 8.[26] Mrs. McClure's physician promptly put Adelaide to bed, took her pulse, and noted her pale nails and wan face. She was prostrated not by grief alone; her body had been starved to nourish her brain. He prescribed two months in Divonne, with complete rest and nourishing food.

To get home to Claire and the three little boys as quickly as possible was Adelaide's first desire. The baby was only four and a half months old. Charlie's letter had been so pitiful; he had loved Jim more than anyone on earth.[27] When it was not possible to get an earlier passage home than she had originally planned, Adelaide resolutely decided to go on to Paris with Miss Wood and then to give young Ambrose a holiday in London, though she feared she would have little heart for amusements.[28]

In Paris, while Eleanor Wood attended to some business, Adelaide stayed near the Latin Quarter in a queer old hotel built for George IV when he came to Paris; its chief merit now was its comparative inexpensiveness. She visited the Louvre, where she saw "a few hundred more statues and miles of paintings," the Place de Concorde, the Arc de Triomphe, the Champs-Elysées, the Bois de Boulogne, Luxemburg Gardens, and Notre Dame, but she admired far more St. Étienne de Mont and found it hard to pass by the bookstalls on the left bank of the Sienne.[29]

[26] James Peasley Nutting (born August 1, 1856; died May 8, 1902) was educated at Waterloo Academy. In 1877 he became a Post Office employee in Ottawa, then transferred to the Department of Trade and Finance, where he advanced to chief clerk. Jim was identified with athletics, as a member of the Ottawa football team and as a runner; he belonged to the governor general's Foot Guards, and in 1895 represented the corps on the Bisley Team. He was a member of Christ Church Cathedral. Jim married Claire Lizzie Sinclair on September 16, 1885; they had four sons: Harold Headley Sinclair, Keith, Kenneth Hunt (died in infancy), and Bruce. Jim Nutting was buried in Beechwood, Ottawa. *Saturday Globe* (Utica, N.Y.), May 17, 1902; *Waterloo Advertiser*; *Journal of the Seventh Session of the Diocese of Ottawa* (Ottawa: Paynter & Abbott, 1902), p. 92.

[27] Adelaide Nutting (Divonne, France) to Armine N. Gosling (St. John's), June 7, 1902, MAN Papers.

[28] Adelaide Nutting (Divonne, France) to Armine N. Gosling (St. John's), June 11, 1902, *ibid.*

[29] Adelaide Nutting (London) to Lizzie H. Nutting (Waterloo, Quebec), June 25, 1902, *ibid.*

Adelaide had two weeks in London before the S.S. *Siberian* sailed on July 5. She and Miss Wood had reserved rooms at St. Andrew's House, a small but comfortable clubhouse for nurses. London was crowded with visitors pouring into the city for the coronation scheduled for June 26. Sir Herbert Murray came shortly after her arrival, invited her to stay at his home, and offered to get tickets for the coronation. Knowing that he had many relatives and friends who would expect the privilege of his hospitality during coronation week, she said she would come for a few days afterward. The King, however, had an emergency appendectomy, and the coronation did not take place until August 9, long after Adelaide had gone on to St. John's.

Young Ambrose managed to come into London for a few days of sightseeing, and one of the things that stood out in his memory forty years later was a trip in a hansom cab with his aunt to 10 South Street, Park Lane, where he sat and talked to the cabbie while Adelaide went to pay her respects at the door of Florence Nightingale's home, even though she would probably not be able to see her.

With Diana Kimber, Adelaide visited hospitals and other nursing leaders. She inquired about the progress British nurses were making relative to registration and hours. Browsing in old bookshops and museums, she carefully avoided the places she had gone to with Jim.[30]

In St. John's, Adelaide thrilled to see Minnie and Gilbert and the children. Minnie looked tired, but the children were healthy and happy. Armine was eleven, and Adelaide's namesake, Frances Adelaide, was six; Arthur Charles, the surviving twin born the previous August, was strong and alert and smiled for everyone. Somehow he would always be his aunt's favorite. The family was delighted with the gifts Adelaide brought and paid rapt attention as she told of her travels and her visit with Ambrose in London.

Adelaide and Minnie had long talks alone about their family, their mother, their brother Arthur, who had died the year before in western Canada, and Jim. They longed to comfort Claire and her boys, Charlie, and their father, now eighty-six. Loss and grief, years and distance, seemed to draw the two women closer and to strengthen their love for each other.

After a few days in Ottawa with Claire and the boys, Adelaide went to Waterloo. Soon it was September and time to return to Hopkins.

[30] *Ibid.*

XII

A Busy Interlude, 1902–1904

Back at her desk, in black uniform and white cap, Adelaide greeted her staff. It was good to be home again. She thanked those who had written letters of condolence and sympathy and then turned to the correspondence that had accumulated. Dr. Hurd dropped in and reported that all had gone well in her absence. He added, however, that he wished to talk to her about the preparatory course, which was not paying its way and was a drain on the hospital budget.

While away, Adelaide had tried to put everything relating to the hospital out of her mind. Although she had made notes about the hospitals she saw and old books pertaining to the history of nursing, she had spent most of her waking hours absorbing the beauties of nature and communing with the poets and the greats of art, literature, and history. Before she left Baltimore, she had written a paper on "The Education of Nurses: The Preparatory Course," which was to be read at the superintendents' convention in Detroit, and then had promptly dismissed the matter.[1] She had asked to be relieved of all responsibilities concerning the Education Committee when she went abroad, but supposed she would be asked to serve again because of her deep interest in the hospital economics course.

The mail undoubtedly included a letter from Sophia Palmer and Mary E. P. Davis about the *Journal*, and one from Mrs. Robb about the Teachers College course. Although Isabel had resigned as chairman of the Education Committee when her baby was born, she agreed to give lectures to the hospital economics students, despite the difficulty of traveling from Ohio to New York.[2] Adelaide wondered

[1] American Society of Superintendents of Training Schools for Nurses, *Ninth Annual Report* (Harrisburg, Pa.: Harrisburg Publishing Co., 1902).
[2] American Society of Superintendents of Training Schools for Nurses, *Eighth Annual Report* (Harrisburg, Pa.: Harrisburg Publishing Co., 1901), p. 18; see also Isabel H. Robb (Cleveland, Ohio) to Maud Banfield (Philadelphia), MAN Papers.

whether being a wife and mother was as gratifying to Isabel as she had anticipated. Isabel had never liked sewing and by her own confession detested cooking. Yet she was a charming hostess, and Dr. Robb, who could well afford a cook and servants, encouraged his wife in her work in behalf of nursing. Adelaide thought how much she owed Isabel for her inspiration, her confidence, and her dreams.

There would be a letter from Lavinia Dock, perhaps two. She would probably read Adelaide's paper at the Society of Superintendents' meeting in Detroit. Certainly she could interpret the Hopkins program if any questions were asked. Before going abroad again Lavinia would want to know more of the details of the history of nursing they planned to write.

As soon as the new class was launched in the preparatory course and the classes for the upper students were well under way, Adelaide turned to the plans for organizing Maryland nurses and to the passage of laws regulating license and practice. Registration of nurses had been a primary objective of American nursing organizations since the plan was advanced at the International Council of Nurses in London in 1899.[3]

In 1900 there were 432 training schools for nurses in the United States, and from them 3,456 nurses were graduated.[4] These schools were rapidly organizing their alumnae and affiliating with the Associated Alumnae. When the Associated Alumnae applied for incorporation under the laws of the state of New York, it was advised that Canadian membership was not permissible and that the Canadian nurses should form their own association. The name of the original organization was then changed to the "Nurses Associated Alumnae of the United States." Incorporation would be essential if the organization were to publish a journal or own property in New York, and in 1901 this was effected. The national organization urged alumnae of the various states to form state associations. At the third annual convention of the Associated Alumnae in 1900, Isabel Robb appealed for state registration.[5]

Within two years the graduate nurses of four states were organized and working for state registration; in 1903, acts governing the practice of nursing were passed first in North Carolina, then in New

[3] Isabel M. Stewart and Anne L. Austin, *A History of Nursing from Ancient to Modern Times: A World View* (New York: G. P. Putnam's Sons, 1926), p. 201.

[4] Mary M. Roberts, *American Nursing: History and Interpretation* (New York: Macmillan, 1954), p. 110.

[5] Blanche Pfefferkorn, "Nursing Organizations in the United States: Their Origin, Purpose, and Some of Their Results," *The Modern Hospital* 8 (1917): 1–2.

Jersey, New York, and Virginia. Adelaide hoped to organize Maryland nurses. By 1903 fourteen hospitals in the state had training schools for nurses; eleven of these were in Baltimore.[6] Adelaide invited seventeen nurses from the various Maryland hospitals and training schools to an informal meeting to discuss the formation of a state organization of nurses. Fourteen nurses came.[7] After discussing the merits and procedures of organization, the group called a meeting for December 14, 1903, and all graduate nurses of the state were invited to participate in the organization of the Maryland State Association of Graduate Nurses.

About four hundred nurses attended the December meeting in the Arundel Club auditorium. After a word of greeting and stating the purpose of the meeting, Adelaide introduced the president of the Arundel Club, Mrs. William Ellicott (the former Elizabeth King), Judge Henry Harlan, president of the hospital board, and Dr. William H. Welch. A committee had previously drafted a constitution for consideration as soon as organization was effected. Sound legal advice had been secured in drawing up the document, and there was very little about it that required extensive amendment. When the constitution was accepted, the body proceeded to elect officers. Adelaide was elected president.

The same committee that had drawn up the constitution had also been working on a bill providing for registration of nurses to be presented to the Maryland legislature. This bill would authorize the Maryland State Association of Graduate Nurses to nominate twelve members, five of whom the governor would choose to constitute a board of examiners. Of the first appointees, one would serve for one year, two for two years, and two for three years; thereafter each member would hold office for three years. The Board of Examiners was to choose a president and a secretary-treasurer. The secretary would receive $100 plus travel expenses, while other members would

[6] The following Maryland hospitals had training schools in 1902: Johns Hopkins Hospital; Union Protestant Infirmary (became Union Memorial in 1920); Maryland Homeopathic Hospital (closed in 1914, later reopened); Maryland General Hospital (directed first by Sisters of Charity, later by the Methodists); Church Home and Infirmary (Episcopal); St. Agnes Hospital (started by Sisters of Charity); Franklin Square Hospital and Training School (originally National Temperance Hospital); Western Maryland School of Nursing; United Charities Hospital, Cambridge; Baltimore City Hospital; Barnard Sanitarium (became Biedler-Silliman Sanitarium in 1907); St. Joseph's Hospital (Sisters of the Third Order of St. Francis); Frederick City Hospital. *Twenty-fifth Anniversary of the Maryland State Nurses Association: A Historical Sketch, 1903–1928*, (Baltimore: J. H. Furst Co., 1928).

[7] *Proceedings of the Maryland State Association of Graduate Nurses* (Baltimore: J. H. Furst Co., 1905).

receive $5 per meeting and travel expenses. Salaries and travel costs were to be paid from the fees received, and nothing was to be paid out of the state's treasury.[8] If the bill passed, three years after its passage all nurses desiring to practice in the state of Maryland would have to pass qualifying examinations set up by the Board of Examiners and to pay a registration fee of $5.

The newly organized state association of graduate nurses quickly endorsed the proposed legislation, and Adelaide Nutting as president was authorized to see that nurses and members of the legislature were circularized as to the merits of the bill. The committee had done its work well, and no changes were made in the original draft. It passed in both houses and was signed by Governor Edwin Warfield on March 25, 1904.[9] Adelaide insisted that credit for securing the legislation belonged to Judge Harlan and the Maryland nurses.[10]

Shortly thereafter a board of examiners was named, and Georgina Ross was appointed state inspector of training schools for the state of Maryland. Adelaide wrote Miss Palmer of the *Journal* that because there were so few schools in the state it would not be necessary for Miss Ross to devote a great deal of time to the work: "A few days here and there for the next two or three months will cover the ground but it is a first rate step, and I am pleased enough that we have accomplished it."[11] Six hundred sixty-eight nurses were registered under the waiver and, when the first state examination was given in 1907, thirty-four nurses took it. In 1906 a bill permitting hospitals to send students and other nurses out on private duty failed because the Legislative Committee of the Maryland State Association of Graduate Nurses went into action to defeat it.

Meanwhile, Adelaide concerned herself with the preparatory course and the Baltimore Anti-Tuberculosis Campaign. After talking over the matter with Dr. Hurd, she recommended to the trustees that $50 be paid by each student for the preparatory instruction, a fee which would be returned to students not accepted for further training. The recommendation was promptly approved by the trustees, and students entering in 1904 paid tuition.[12]

Adelaide continued her battle for higher educational qualifications,

[8] Maryland, state bill no. 172 (1904).

[9] *Twenty-fifth Anniversary of the Maryland State Nurses Association.*

[10] M. A. Nutting (Baltimore) to Sarah F. Martin (Baltimore), March 28, 1904, MAN Papers.

[11] Adelaide Nutting (Baltimore) to Sophia Palmer (Rochester, N.Y.), December 2, 1904, *ibid.*

[12] Adelaide Nutting, "Some Results of Preparatory Instruction," *American Journal of Nursing*, June, 1905, p. 585.

asserting in an article published in the October, 1904, issue of *American Journal of Nursing* that "nursing is one of the few branches of education where more emphasis is placed on age, height, weight, and freedom from family ties and less exacting about educational qualifications."[13]

Since returning from Europe in 1902, Adelaide had scarcely had a day to call her own. When vacation time came in August, 1903, she spent a week of it on business in New York, New Bedford, and Boston, and then hurried on to visit a friend who lived at Islesboro on a large island off the coast of Maine. She was delighted with the view of the Maine mountains across the bay, and looked forward to a quiet rest. The day after her arrival, however, her hostess was taken ill with a severe fever. When two trained nurses came from Boston, Adelaide decided to finish her vacation in Waterloo.

> I had intended to come here for a week later feeling I must try to have a look at Father but a fortnight here is more than enough. Charlie and Lizzie are as kind as possible and I can get out to drive every day, but an unfathomable, irresistible gloom always settles on me the moment I come to the place where we spent so many horrible years, where Mother worked and suffered, where we lived out our sordid and miserable days of childhood and youth. It is all alike hideous, yet I find myself being pulled back here year after year, family affection becoming too strong a tie to resist.[14]

The new class had barely entered Hopkins when the time came to go to Pittsburgh for the superintendents' annual convention. This was the first time in three years that Adelaide had been able to attend, although she had sent a paper to be read at Detroit and a formal report to the Buffalo meeting. This time it was her pleasure to read to the assembled superintendents a letter from the students taking the hospital economics course, in which they expressed appreciation for the privilege that was theirs in taking a course so valuable and helpful.[15]

In a discussion of current events as a subject for the training course, Adelaide strongly defended its inclusion, saying that nurses needed to be informed of what was going on in the world, especially in such matters as the war against tuberculosis, laws for the protec-

[13] M. A. Nutting, "Suggestions for Educational Standards for State Registration," *ibid.*, October, 1904, pp. 13–25.

[14] Adelaide Nutting (Waterloo, Quebec) to Armine N. Gosling (St. John's, Newfoundland), September 14, [1903], MAN Papers.

[15] American Society of Superintendents of Training Schools for Nurses, *Tenth Annual Report* (Harrisburg, Pa.: Harrisburg Publishing Co., 1903), p. 15.

tion of women and children, tenement houses and sweatshops and their relation to health, and the trouble in the Far East. Pointing up the meaning of the struggle between capital and labor, she said, "Nurses must be good citizens."[16]

When the question of continuing the hospital economics course and the increasing need for funds came up, Adelaide suggested: "the way out of that difficulty will come when we have a college of our own in which all branches of nursing, preparatory as well as graduate shall be taught, with such a college and good hospital facilities we could teach hospital administration as it is not now dreamed of. . . . We should all look forward to this." Meanwhile, there was the Teachers College course. The Society of Superintendents' treasury could not be tapped forever; an endowment was imperative. It was suggested that an appeal be made to the Carnegie Foundation to finance the Teachers College graduate nursing program.[17]

The convention's general discussions indicated a tendency toward raising the educational requirements and lowering the age limits for admission to nursing schools. At Hopkins the circular for 1903–4 stated that "applicants must not be under twenty-one years of age."[18] Newly enacted laws in New York, Virginia, North Carolina, and New Jersey were alike in specifying an age requirement of twenty-one years and a diploma from a recognized school of nursing as prerequisites for a license to practice. The superintendents were unanimous in opposing correspondence schools of nursing. The Executive Council also refused to take as a member of the society any superintendent who sent student nurses out to nurse in private homes. The Society of Superintendents was beginning to be a power in advancing the profession; its leaders were mapping the objectives that would engage the combined forces of superintendents and nurses. Among these objectives were city directories for nurses, nursing school inspection, public health legislation, and insistence upon training in a general hospital, rather than in a specialized hospital, as a prerequisite for registration.

Adelaide was especially interested in the work of visiting nurses among the poor and needy. Baltimore had had a visiting nurse service since 1896, and the reports these nurses made were a sad commentary on the city's general health and sanitary conditions. Dr. Osler and Dr. Welch had long advocated radical reforms. The water supply

---

[16] *Ibid.*, p. 24.

[17] *Ibid.*, p. 43.

[18] In 1922 the statement was changed to read "applicants must not be under twenty years of age." Ethel Johns and Blanche Pfefferkorn, *The Johns Hopkins Hospital School of Nursing* (Baltimore: The Johns Hopkins Press, 1954), p. 218.

stood in constant danger of contamination, sewage disposal was inadequate, filth lay in the streets, stench arose in certain localities, and rats roamed the alleys. Typhoid, tuberculosis, pneumonia, and infectious diseases took a heavy toll among the sick poor of Baltimore.[19]

Typhoid was on the decline, however, and now Osler was crusading against tuberculosis. As early as 1899 he estimated that there were from eight to ten thousand cases in Baltimore alone, of whom only a possible 5 percent could receive treatment in sanitariums. He believed an active campaign to enlighten the public was the only way to conquer the disease. Assisted by a gift from two Baltimore women, he had Blanche Epler and Adelaide Dutcher, medical students, follow to their homes all consumptive patients who came to the Hopkins dispensary. Their report led him in 1900 to organize the Laennec Society, a group of medical professors and practitioners who met monthly to advance their study of tuberculosis. Dr. Welch, president of the Baltimore Board of Health, aided and abetted Dr. Osler when he challenged the mayor of Baltimore and the city government to take action to improve health conditions; it was 1903, however, before a visiting nurse was employed to give attention exclusively to the tubercular poor.[20]

Inspired by the International Tuberculosis Congress in Berlin in 1901, Osler, Welch, and friends hoped to dramatize the subject by holding a tuberculosis exposition in Baltimore in January, 1904. Almost from the beginning, Adelaide took part in the planning. She would present a study of nurses engaged in a house-to-house visitation of tubercular patients. She believed this was the best method of caring for tubercular patients and that it was of inestimable value to the patients' families and friends.[21]

After the Pittsburgh convention in October, Adelaide began to investigate the work being done by visiting nurses. Because no general source was available, she was forced to write hundreds of letters to nursing directories, alumnae associations, boards of health, and individuals. After reading copies of the New York Tuberculosis Committee, she wrote Lillian Wald of the Henry Street Visiting Nurse Service, asking for copies of other reports. "It seems to me typical of woman's work that such masses of it should be of the kind which is unrecorded by anybody except, I hope, by the recording angel." Ex-

[19] Harvey Cushing, *Sir William Osler*, 2 vols. (Oxford: Clarendon Press, 1925), 1: 380–81.
[20] *Ibid.*, pp. 535, 570.
[21] M. Adelaide Nutting (Baltimore) to Sophia Palmer (Rochester, N.Y.), January 3, 1904, MAN Papers.

pecting to be in New York the next week, she concluded, "I do hope I shall have a chance to shake hands with you."[22]

The Tuberculosis Exposition was held the last week in January, 1904. There were public lectures by noted medical leaders in the fight against tuberculosis, and exhibits lined the long corridors and entrances of the university's McCoy Hall and the walls of the assembly room. Statistical charts showed the prevalence and distribution of tuberculosis in the United States, particularly in Maryland, by age, sex, occupation, race, and heredity. One section, devoted to tenement houses, sweatshops, and factories, indicated the improvement that had been made through recent revisions of laws and other reforms. There were plans and elevations of every variety of hospital, tent, sanitarium, and sleeping shack. A house and home hygiene exhibit featured verandas, wheeling and reclining couches, and a model sickroom marked by simplicity, cleanliness, homelikeness, and stressing the protection of others.

In her address Adelaide pointed out that "tuberculosis visiting" was the outgrowth of an impulse set in motion by the medical profession. Chicago had sixteen nurses regularly visiting 408 families; in Philadelphia fourteen nurses visited 65 families; in Baltimore five nurses visited 110 families; and in Washington, D.C., seven nurses visited 144 families. During a period of nine months, one nurse from the Grace Forman Vanderbilt Clinic met 339 families; in four months the Boston Visiting Nurse Society visited 245 patients in their homes.

To care for a tubercular patient in a hospital in 1904, it cost not less than $1.00 a day, although most hospitals charged from $2.00 to $2.50 a day. In a year a visiting nurse could reach 500 patients. "Hospitals," Adelaide said, "reach the consumptive few, the visiting nurse, the consumptive many." Dr. Osler estimated that 98 percent could be cared for in their homes.

The nurse, Adelaide went on to say, must instruct families in such matters as fresh air, nourishing food, rest, care of sputum, and the use of paper cups and sanitary tissue. She advocated the use of wheeling chairs, open trolley car rides, and single beds, and described how roofs and fire escapes might be used to give the tubercular patient fresh air. She stressed good food and advised nurses to study diet in the homes they visited, cautioning obstetrical nurses to be alert to signs of tuberculosis in mothers. Poor food—poor in quality, quantity, and mode of preparation—she warned, contributes to the disease.[23]

[22] M. Adelaide Nutting (Baltimore) to Lillian Wald (New York), January 8, 1904, *ibid.*

[23] M. Adelaide Nutting, "Visiting Nurses in the Homes of Tubercular Patients, Baltimore," *American Journal of Nursing*, February, 1904.

The exposition was a success in every way,[24] but, before the hospital staff had a chance to settle back into the usual routine, Baltimore was struck a hard and sudden blow that was seriously to affect the future of the hospital. On Sunday, February 7, 1904, at about 11:00 A.M., a fire broke out in downtown Baltimore and swept through the city, raging until Monday evening. No damage was done to the hospital, but great clouds of smoke and showers of sparks blew over the buildings from the flaming city below.[25] The fire proved most disastrous to the real and lease-hold property belonging to the hospital. Sixty-four stores, warehouses, and office buildings, widely separated, and having an assessed value of more than $1,250,000, were destroyed. The loss, only partially covered by insurance, came at a time when the hospital's financial situation was far from stable.

It was a solemn group of nurses and students that met for prayers that cold, wintry Monday morning. Adelaide was deeply moved by the spirit of loyalty and devotion that pervaded the group. Every student nurse was eager to help, and the graduate nurses offered to stay at their posts without charge as long as they were needed. Several of the physicians of the hospital volunteered to surrender their salaries for a time or to assume the expense of laboratories to maintain unimpaired the usefulness of the hospital.[26] Letters poured in to Adelaide from the alumnae, offering sympathy, cheer, and help.

Still immersed in the gloom brought by the fire, on February 17 Adelaide received word that her father, Vespasion Nutting, had died in Waterloo in his eighty-eighth year. Armine was too far away, and Adelaide dared not make the trip, so Charlie laid him beside their mother, who had passed away twenty years before. One by one the ties of home and family were being broken.

The depression which threatened Hopkins was relieved by the gift of half a million dollars from John D. Rockefeller. When the announcement was accompanied by the statement that this very liberal donation had been made because of Mr. Rockefeller's opinion of the high character of the work the hospital and the medical school were doing in medical instruction and research, including the training of nurses, hope rose in the training school.

The third week of March, Adelaide lectured in Philadelphia. She scarcely had a minute to work on the history that she and Lavinia Dock had started. She promised a paper on "Educational Standards

[24] The National Organization for the Study and Prevention of Tuberculosis, founded in 1904, is now the National Tuberculosis Association.

[25] Cushing, *Sir William Osler*, 1: 630.

[26] Johns and Pfefferkorn, *The Johns Hopkins Hospital School of Nursing*, p. 133.

for State Registration" for the Associated Alumnae convention in June, although it would have to be read by someone else. Because of a growing weariness, she asked to have the summer off. Since Miss Dock had resigned the past year, Adelaide had been serving as secretary of the Society of Superintendents, and, with her work for the Education Committee and the lectures at Teachers College, she began to wonder whether another breakdown might be in the offing.[27] She hoped she could maintain the deception of health and energy and not completely collapse before June 29, when she planned to sail for Newfoundland and a summer's visit with Minnie, Gilbert, and the children.

With commencement over, Adelaide was on her way. It was good to be at sea again. She breathed deeply of the cool salt breeze. How relaxing it was to be free of air that was always faintly tinged with the odor of chlorine, bichloride of mercury, or carbolic acid. Something about the roll of the ship made her want to do nothing, not even read or think. As the ship neared Halifax, however, she began to think more and more about her sister's family. Ambrose was still at school in England. Armine was now thirteen, Frances Adelaide was eight, and Charles Arthur was three. Elizabeth Gilbert, born the previous September, had lived only a few months. Adelaide loved them all, but her heart went out to Arthur; something unexplainable made her lavish affection upon him as if to compensate for the loss of his twin.

Life was unusually quiet that summer in St. John's. Minnie and Gilbert were active in church and community affairs, but when Adelaide came they saw to it that she was free to do only the things she chose to do. She read books aloud with Minnie, and, an expert with a needle, helped Minnie with her sewing and with bits of fine embroidery and stitchery for the cathedral bazaar in September. As they sewed, they recalled the beautiful garments their mother had made.

Gilbert joined them in the evenings, and after the children had gone to bed they read aloud and talked of books and travel. Gilbert had worked hard and prospered. He now had the means to indulge his love of books and history and had begun a valuable collection of first editions. He was interested in writing a biography of Sir Humphrey Gilbert. Adelaide encouraged him and so did his friend Dr. Wilfred Grenfell. Grenfell had been a guest in Minnie and Gilbert's home a number of times when Adelaide had been there. To raise funds for his numerous philanthropic projects, he had been lecturing in the

[27] Ada Carr (Newport, R.I.) to M. A. Nutting (Baltimore), April 9, 1904, MAN Papers.

United States and Canada, and was especially desirous of lecturing in Baltimore so that he might look into the hospitals and methods used there. Adelaide often sent Minnie books and magazines that she thought appropriate for the hospitals and libraries he was establishing in those isolated villages.[28] It was good to meet people who had dreams and the strength and courage to fulfill them.

The Goslings enjoyed picnics quite as much as Adelaide did, and after church on Sunday they packed a picnic basket, put it in the carriage, and drove up into the hills, where they spread their meal under the pine trees. The crunch of the needles under their feet and the warm fragrance of pine brought back memories of the Shefford hills.

In a moment of confidence, Adelaide told her sister that her health might not long permit her to continue the work she was doing. "Gilbert and I always have a home for you," Minnie answered.

[28] Armine Nutting Gosling, William Gilbert Gosling: A Tribute (New York: Guild Press, 1935), pp. 35–37; Adelaide Nutting (Baltimore) to Dr. Wilfred Grenfell, January 8, 1903, MAN Papers.

XIII

Time of Decision, 1905–1906

Although Adelaide had been away from the hospital all summer, she did not expect it to be difficult to slip back into the routine. She was grateful for a dependable staff, many of whom were graduates of the school and had been promoted from one position to another. Aside from correspondence, there would be little to do before settling down to a winter of teaching, supervising, and writing.

On her desk lay a letter from Dr. Osler, who with his family had been spending the summer in England. Before Adelaide reached the end of the second sentence, tears came to her eyes.

Dear Miss Nutting,

   I hate to think that the break in our school circle should have been at this weak link but it seems to have been ordained. I could not resist the temptation for an easier life and the academic surroundings of Oxford. I dare say I shall often look back with regret to the Johns Hopkins Hospital and my active life but I have much to do if my health remains and there are arrears of work to be made up, which I could never have accomplished in Baltimore. I hope my successor will appreciate as much as I do what the Training School has done for the Hospital. I do not leave until June so we have another session's work together.

Sincerely yours,

William Osler[1]

What would Johns Hopkins be like without Dr. Osler? Dr. Hurd and members of the staff dropped in to ask if Adelaide had heard the news. "Hopkins without Dr. Osler?" they echoed. "Incredible."

On October 5 the new surgical building, with its clinical amphi-

---

[1] William Osler (Pointe à Pic, Quebec) to Adelaide Nutting (Baltimore), August 19, [1904], MAN Papers.

theater, was formally opened. To Adelaide the highlight of the day came when Dr. Osler presided at the dedication of a tablet to the memory of Jesse W. Lazear of Baltimore, a graduate of the Academic Department of The Johns Hopkins University and of the Medical School of Columbia University, and a former resident physician of the hospital. As a member of the Yellow Fever Commission in Cuba, he had let a stray mosquito from a yellow fever ward sting him on the hand. Twelve days later he was dead.[2]

Large as it seemed, John D. Rockefeller's gift following the Baltimore fire did little more than relieve the financial strain on the hospital and restore it to its former position. Any hope that Adelaide might have entertained for expansion and improvement of educational facilities was doomed. The funds allocated for graduate nurses were so reduced that upper-class student nurses had to be placed in charge of wards before they were prepared to assume such a responsibility. Adelaide was determined that the supervisory and teaching staff not be cut back at the very time when it should have been expanded. The ever-growing reputation of the medical staff brought more and more private patients who demanded special nurses. Adelaide told the trustees that the hospital no longer had enough of its own graduates for special duty, and that she would be obliged to call in nurses from other schools, where the training might not be the same; this, she said, would reflect on the hospital and the school. There were many young women applying for entrance to the Hopkins Training School, but the Nurses' Home and the temporary annex could not accommodate any more students.

In desperation she worked out a plan by which third-year students might do special nursing in private wards, with the revenue derived to be set aside for building purposes. She estimated that the services of ten student nurses at $21 a week would bring in $10,000 a year, and that, deducting $300 for each girl's maintenance, the net return would be $7,000.

This self-liquidating plan was never put into effect. In December, 1905, Helen Skipworth Wilmer, a recent graduate of the training school, contributed $30,000 for the construction of an addition to the Nurses' Home as a memorial to her father, Skipworth Wilmer. Her generosity and Adelaide's pleas moved the trustees to provide an additional wing similar to the Wilmer memorial. When completed, each nurse would have a single room with a commodious closet, and

[2] "Opening of Surgical Building and New Clinical Amphitheatre of Johns Hopkins Hospital, October 5, 1904," *The Johns Hopkins Hospital Bulletin*, December, 1904.

there would be adequate dining rooms, sitting rooms, and kitchens.[3] Construction did not begin at once on either structure, but the gift and the appropriation caused Adelaide to rejoice and embark on new plans for the educational program and more effective nursing.

Adelaide's interest in the *Journal* continued, and from time to time she contributed articles, news items, and suggestions on policy. She was indignant when Dr. Alfred Worcester, a Waltham, Massachusetts, physician, took what she considered an undue interest in nursing affairs. On October 14, 1904, she wrote Miss Palmer that she once thought this doctor "a good and kind man somewhat inclined to meddle in woman's affairs and so far as nursing affairs mounted on a hobby and riding it hard." "What would the medical men think," she asked, "if we stepped out of our ranks to try to manage their affairs, and why should we be forever loyal to them as a body when so many medical people observe no loyalty to us but on the contrary hamper and hinder our best work and development in every available way?"[4]

Later Adelaide wrote Miss Palmer that while in New York she had managed to see a nurse who was influential with McClure's publishing house and would get them to drop all advertisements for correspondence schools of nursing after the current contracts expired. She also asked that the next issue of the *Journal* carry an announcement of the *History of Nursing*, which she and Lavinia Dock were writing, lest a certain Waltham physician think she had gotten that idea from him too.[5]

At the annual meeting of the Maryland State Association of Graduate Nurses at the Arundel Club on December 30, Adelaide, in her address as president, pointed to the organization's accomplishments in its first year: the nurse registration law and the appointment of an inspector and a board of examiners. The two goals to which the nurses should now direct their attention, she believed, were a central directory and nurses in the public schools. Because more graduate nurses were engaged in private duty in homes than in hospital wards, it was important that persons desiring nursing services should know where to look for them. In addition, by means of a directory, unemployed nurses could make their availability known. School nurses could detect chronic conditions of eyesight and hearing,

[3] Adelaide Nutting (Baltimore) to Armine Gosling (St. John's, Newfoundland), December, 1905, MAN Papers.
[4] M. A. Nutting (Baltimore) to Sophia Palmer (Rochester, N.Y.), October 14, 1904, *ibid.*
[5] M. A. Nutting (Baltimore) to Sophia Palmer (Rochester), November 4, 1904, *ibid.*

nose and throat, as well as symptoms of contagious diseases, thereby reducing the danger of epidemics.

Ill with a relapse of pleurisy two weeks later, Adelaide wrote her sister an account of the meeting.

> Stenographer every morning, nice women reporters often, and interviews of all sorts and conditions, people to get my program in proper shape. I got the President of the New York Board of Health down, and other dignitaries up, and brought forward the question of nursing in the public schools in a splendid meeting. The reward of our efforts is that in this morning's paper, it is announced that a medical inspector and a trained nurse will begin work experimentally in some of the public schools at once. You see it is worthwhile to work like a galley slave.[6]

Adelaide was delighted to learn that Minnie and Gilbert were vacationing in England. As she wrote to her sister she relived her own visits there.

> It is a comfort to know you have crossed the wide ocean and are enjoying the fulfillment of our childish dreams. I can picture you and Gilbert going about from gallery to gallery and enjoying the things one starves for here—and in spirit every day I make some sort of journey with you. . . . Jim and I spent three or four entire days in Westminster Abbey. . . . I prowled about into the cloisters there, and into all sorts of queer old corners, and I love to remember my searchings and surprises. . . .
>
> St. Margaret's just next is where Isabel Hampton made the mistake of her life and married Dr. Hunter Robb. Florence Nightingale sent her a bunch of roses on that regrettable occasion.[7]

There was a frequent exchange of letters between Adelaide and Lavinia Dock after they decided on the joint authorship of a history of nursing. From Europe Lavinia kept Adelaide informed of the progress she was making on the research and, knowing of Adelaide's frail health and her tendency to overwork, she felt now and then duty-bound to send sisterly advice.

> For the sake of self-preservation give up the state work and if you must the *Journal* directorship . . . and did you tell Miss Palmer the book would be ready in a year? I had at least a three year period in my mind. Never in the world could we finish in a year if we both worked very hard. Don't for heaven's sake, strain your nerves for such tensity of action. . . . And can't you give up the secretary work of the Superintendents' Society? There is so much writing.
>
> There are a number of old warhorses out of a job just now, are there not? Can not some one of them take it up to employ their leisure hours?

[6] Adelaide Nutting (Baltimore) to Armine Gosling (London), January 12, 1905, *ibid.*

[7] Adelaide Nutting (Baltimore) to Armine N. Gosling (London), January 13, 1905, *ibid.*

You must cut down your nerve-racking expenditures or you will go bankrupt.

Yes, I will help to write or collaborate or whatever you like. I will, for instance, write up lots of the modern stuff. But finally you must put the finish touch on all because your literary style is really distinguished, admirable. What I had thought was, a good deal might be done next winter. I will not undertake regular work at the Settlement. Truth to tell, I feel a little too old to carry the bag.

Lavinia promised to read the French and Spanish sources but felt frustrated that she did not know more languages.[8]

By mid-January the old symptoms of exhaustion appeared again, and Adelaide, facing the dire possibilities, began to withdraw from some of her many activities. She began with the Board of Directors of the *Journal*. Writing Isabel McIsaac, she explained: "It seems selfish of me to desert the ship at this time and . . . nothing less than a fear of another breakdown would keep me from continuing the work I have begun. . . . I think if I can take matters a little more quietly for another year, I can get back where I was on returning from Europe two years ago." She listed the help she had given during the past year: conducting *The Johns Hopkins Nurses Alumnae Magazine* and assisting with the *Journal of Nursing*; incessant work with the Society of Superintendents, which she must carry on until May; because of Lavinia Dock's absence, the correspondence of the American Federation of Nurses with the National Council of Women; collecting for and forwarding the work done at Teachers College; organizing the Maryland State Association of Graduate Nurses and getting the bill for registration through the legislature. "I have been riding for a fall which I grieve to say I have had and can not recover from."[9]

After several weeks rest in Summerville, South Carolina, Adelaide returned to Baltimore. By April she was serving on a committee soliciting for a gift for Dr. Osler and helping to plan a farewell party for the Oslers to be held at the Nurses' Home. She made a hurried trip to Washington to attend a meeting of the Society of Superintendents Council, and on May 25 gave her annual address at the nurses' commencement. The class of thirty-eight nurses was the largest ever to graduate from The Johns Hopkins Training School.

Classes were not in session during the summer, and Adelaide spent as much free time as she had apart from the nursing services on the *History of Nursing* manuscript. After two years in Europe, Lavinia

[8] Lavinia L. Dock [Austria] to Adelaide Nutting (Baltimore), January 13, [1906], *ibid.*

[9] M. A. Nutting (Baltimore) to Isabel McIsaac (Benton Harbor, Mich.), January 11, 1905, *ibid.*

Dock would soon return from London, and Adelaide did not want her to think she had fallen down on her share of work on the history.

Over the years Adelaide had seen to it that the library of the training school acquired a substantial collection of books dealing with nursing history. In December, 1905, she organized a history of nursing club, hoping that the head nurses and senior students would not only enjoy the study and gain a better background for their profession but that they might even wish to add to the collection.

At the new club's organization meeting, Adelaide referred to the unique collection of rare books on nursing being brought together in the training school library, a collection which should ultimately be of interest to others. Dr. Florence Rena Sabin of The Johns Hopkins Medical School also spoke. Dr. Sabin was greatly admired by everyone connected with the hospital. One of the first women to graduate from the Hopkins Medical School, she was the first woman on its faculty. She commended the formation of a club which would give attention and labor to such a purely thoughtful side of nursing work. "The story of the lives and work of these women, and sometimes men," she said, "could hardly fail to be of much help and inspiration. The kind of inspiration that in a commercial day like the present, is sorely needed."[10]

When the matter of a name for the club came up, Adelaide asked the privilege of suggesting one. After reading excerpts from Dr. Osler's address on "Science and Immortality," she concluded that "we ourselves perhaps have a good claim to be permitted to style ourselves Teresians." Osler had once referred to Baltimore's little band of district nurses as disciples of St. Theresa. After the election of officers, a program arranged by Miss Nutting was presented. Ada Carr, head nurse, read a short paper on "St. Theresa," and Elsie Lawler read three short sketches, "Fabiola, Paula and Olympia."[11] Once each month for the next twenty years Hopkins nurses would assemble for an evening's excursion into the history and romance of nursing.

In December Adelaide realized her health was breaking. She had been president of the Maryland State Association of Graduate Nurses in 1904 and 1905, and, when she resigned, she had been elected president for life.[12] She saw no escape from extra professional obligations except to leave the hospital and nursing and resolved to resign when

[10] "Book of the Society of the Teresians," The Johns Hopkins Hospital School of Nursing Archives.

[11] Ibid.

[12] Twenty-fifth Anniversary of the Maryland State Nurses Association: A Historical Sketch, 1903–1928 (Baltimore: J. H. Furst Co., 1928), p. 30.

the current year was over. If she secretly hoped Dean Russell would again invite her to Teachers College, she did not confide it even to her sister. "I am anxious to put in a splendid year of work—the home stretch, you know—and after that you must be prepared to have me on your hands. I'll do the family mending, and earn my salt and that's all I shall need really. But I must make my exit with the lights up and the band playing."[13]

Adelaide's letter to Armine had scarcely reached Newfoundland before a long letter arrived from Annie W. Goodrich, superintendent of the New York Hospital Training School for Nurses. Miss Goodrich had just talked at length with Dean Russell about the hospital economics course. "Is there any possibility of you ever being willing to consider taking over that position?" she wrote Adelaide. "For sake of the profession?" Dean Russell believed that he would have no difficulty in obtaining a salary that she would consider. Moreover, the work would be very light the first year, so she could take up other things. Miss Goodrich implored that Adelaide not say no positively until she had had a chance to talk with her on the subject.[14]

Adelaide thought the matter over. Perhaps this was the answer to her dilemma. The one-year curriculum in hospital economics had been extended to two years in 1903. Miss Alline was leaving to become state inspector of New York nursing schools, and it was vital to the future of the course that someone take charge who was fully equipped. In fairness to The Johns Hopkins Hospital and Training School, Adelaide went immediately to Dr. Hurd to tell him what she was considering.

Shortly after this she became ill with diphtheria. Georgina Ross cared for her in her apartment until she was able to travel to Atlantic City to recuperate. Dean Russell came there and pressed her for an answer.[15] On April 19 she had a long talk with the dean, and the following day she sent her resignation to Dr. Hurd to be presented to the Board of Trustees.[16]

Dr. Hurd replied at once. Although he regretted to see her leave, he had feared for the past two years she had been taxing her strength "beyond the limits wisdom would set as the bounds of the possibili-

---

[13] Adelaide Nutting (Baltimore) to Armine N. Gosling (St. John's), [December, 1905], MAN Papers.

[14] Annie W. Goodrich (New York) to Adelaide Nutting (Baltimore), January 9, 1906, ibid.

[15] Ethel Johns, "Interview with Miss Josephine Waldhouser, 'Teenie,' October 25, 1948," The Johns Hopkins Hospital School of Nursing Archives.

[16] Adelaide Nutting (Atlantic City) to Henry Hurd (Baltimore), April 20, 1906, MAN Papers.

ties of any person." In her new work he believed that she would be happier, healthier, and equally useful in the end.[17]

At the annual meeting of the Society of Superintendents, Dean Russell and Miss Goodrich announced that Miss Nutting would take over the chair of Hospital Administration at Teachers College. Soon letters began to pour in. Helen Kinne, director of Domestic Science, was elated. "I am glad that you realize the great opportunity that we have here. It is my opinion that something can be done here that has not been accomplished anywhere."[18] David Coit Gilman, former president of Johns Hopkins, wrote, "You will be missed more than tongue can tell by Baltimore but the opening to which you are called is important, unique and one for which you are most qualified and I congratulate you on this well earned distinction."[19] Lavinia Dock posted a note from Washington, D.C., where she was working on the History of Nursing: "Dear Adelaide, So you've decided. Well, I am terribly sorry to see you leave JHH. I always wanted you to be there continuously to shine and enjoy the fruits of your labors. Yet this thing is so special I could not advise you not to take it."[20] In early June a letter came from Dr. Osler in England, "The news of your defection came as a great shock but I am sure that you have taken the right course."[21] He expressed pleasure that she was to have her portrait painted and the wish that Hopkins could have one of Isabel Hampton as she looked in the old days. A week later Mrs. Osler sent her congratulations and invited Adelaide to visit them on her forthcoming trip abroad.[22]

In May the Baltimore Sun carried a feature article reviewing Adelaide's accomplishments at Hopkins during the eleven years she had been in charge of the hospital services and the training school. Significant improvements listed were (1) the change from a two-year to a three-year course, (2) the eight-hour day, (3) non-payment of student nurses and the substitution of scholarships for worthy and needy pupils, (4) the preparatory course, and (5) lowering the age of admission to twenty-one years. The Sun also took note that the alumnae of the school were employing Cecilia Beaux, of Philadelphia,

[17] Henry M. Hurd (Baltimore) to Adelaide Nutting (Baltimore), April 1, 1906, ibid.

[18] Helen Kinne (New York) to M. A. Nutting (Baltimore), April 26, 1906, ibid.

[19] Daniel Coit Gilman (Baltimore) to Adelaide Nutting (Baltimore), [Spring, 1906], ibid.

[20] Lavinia L. Dock (Washington, D.C.) to Adelaide Nutting, (Baltimore), [1906], ibid.

[21] William Osler (Oxford) to Adelaide Nutting (Baltimore), June 1, 1906, ibid.

[22] Grace R. Osler (Oxford) to Adelaide Nutting (Baltimore), July 15, 1906, ibid.

to paint Miss Nutting's portrait. The article concluded, "Miss Nutting, very modest, gives all the credit for Hopkins' notable school to Mrs. Robb."[23]

The reporter might have added that lecturers received a fee, that postgraduate courses were in the process of development, that students from other schools were granted certain affiliating privileges, and that public health services had been initiated. Upon reading the article, Adelaide questioned the eight-hour day as a *fait accompli*, saying it had "proceeded much more circumspectly."[24]

Commencement Day, May 24, 1906, was a poignant occasion for Adelaide. Since she would not be presenting another class for its diplomas, her commencement address would in a sense be her own valedictory. Fifteen years before, she had taken her place on the wide stairway beneath the great rotunda and had listened as Dr. Osler commended Hopkins' first graduating class to useful and happy lives, "having been initiated in the Great Secret—that happiness lies in the absorption in some vocation that satisfies the soul; that we are here to add what we can to, not to get what we can from life."[25]

Standing in the presence of the 1906 graduating class of thirty-two earnest young women, their parents, and friends, Adelaide traced the progress of nursing during that interval.

> Fifteen years ago the thirty-five training schools in this country furnished little in the way of opportunity for institutional work and district nursing was in its infancy, it had indeed begun to work in but two of our cities. The latest records show about 1500 hospitals and the thirty-five training schools we had in the year 1890 are now numbered at 867. The two or three District Nursing Associations have grown to 220, occupying between five and six hundred nurses.[26]

She spoke of the new demands on nursing as advances were made in medicine, surgery, neurology, and psychiatry, and of the growing awareness of the public in matters of social welfare and health, especially tuberculosis. She estimated that there were perhaps three

[23] Clipping from the *Baltimore Sun*, [May, 1906], Adelaide Nutting's Scrapbook, *ibid.*

[24] Ethel Johns and Blanche Pfefferkorn, *The Johns Hopkins Hospital School of Nursing* (Baltimore: The Johns Hopkins Press, 1954), p. 152.

[25] William Osler, "Doctor and Nurse," *"Aequanimitas," with Other Addresses to Medical Students and Nurses* (Philadelphia: Blacton Sons Co., 1905), quoted in Harvey Cushing, *Sir William Osler*, 2 vols. (Oxford: Clarendon Press, 1925), 1: 352.

[26] Adelaide Nutting, "Address to Graduation Class, Johns Hopkins School of Nurses, May 24, 1906," quoted in Johns and Pfefferkorn, *The Johns Hopkins Hospital School of Nursing*, p. 154.

hundred schools where the true significance of nursing was understood and where the moral obligation of the training school was really
to educate, not merely to train, the nurse. She wished that all of the
22,000 young women currently enrolled in nursing schools might be
given training and direction by the ablest, most skillful, and highly
trained nurse-instructors, and that they might come under the influence of women of high intellect, education, culture, and the noblest
character.

The matter, as one considers it in all its phases seems to point to the
necessity of placing the training school on the basis of other educational
institutions. In the effort to give our pupils first the preparatory teaching which has become an absolute necessity and later the complete and
rounded course of training and experience which is due them, and which
the community needs of them, it has become quite clear that the work
of training schools in the education of nurses calls for a new system
and a new method of government.
Controlled by the needs of the hospital, training schools must stop
at a certain point far short of their highest efficiency. Hospitals are
founded primarily for the care of the sick. Invaluable centers for educational purposes they have become, but to carry out in its entirety an
educational system is beyond the possibility and province of the hospital.
It has gone as far as it well can go in this direction, and the training
school for nurses must turn back to the community, and ask if it has
no duty toward it. The public profits richly by the hospital training
school, and as had been shown, the need for the services of the nurse
as an important factor in the whole life of the community, seems to be
asserting herself as we have pressed her into one new avenue of work
after another often for which there has been no conscious attempt at
preparation on her part.
To make the best and the most of our training schools, the community must be as willing to give for them as for a medical school and
not leave the hospital to do it all. The small hospitals struggling pitifully,
ineffectually, with a problem of education quite beyond their grasp, are
in urgent need of nursing schools founded on a separate and independent basis in which the course of study and training will be complete,
each hospital contributing what it fairly can as a field for teaching and
receiving of the student, what she must necessarily give in obtaining her
practical training and experience. The formation of such a school is the
next step forward.[27]

To the unimaginative, Adelaide Nutting's address might have been
only an interesting essay on the history of nursing. To those who
looked deeper, it was a credo, a manifesto. A collegiate school of
nursing might not be realized at Hopkins or at Columbia, but it would
come within her time.

[27] *Ibid.*, pp. 155–56.

XIV

A Portrait and a Pilgrimage, 1906–1907

The nursing profession hailed the announcement that Adelaide Nutting was taking over the hospital economics course at Teachers College, Columbia University, as a great step forward, but to the Hopkins Nurses Alumnae the news came as a profound shock. Some of them had known no other teacher. Adelaide Nutting was the living symbol of their alma mater. Immediately the alumnae and students began thinking of how they could express their loyalty and devotion to her and to the school. When Dr. Osler had gone to Oxford as regius professor and the famous Big Four was broken up, Mary Garrett had commissioned John Singer Sargent to paint a group portrait of Welch, Kelly, Osler, and Halsted, to be hung in the Medical School.[1] The Nurses Alumnae felt no less honor was due Miss Nutting, and Cecelia Beaux, a distinguished Philadelphia artist, was engaged to paint Adelaide's portrait. It would be presented to the trustees in order that she too "might be kept in remembrance as she had lived and worked among them."

In mid-May, Adelaide received a letter from her former classmate, Susan Read, now the wife of Dr. William S. Thayer.

My dear Miss Nutting,
    I was requested this afternoon by a committee of nurses from the various classes to inform you of our wish to have a portrait of you painted for the Training School.
    This wish is an expression of our high regard for you personally, of our sincere appreciation of your years of unselfish devotion to the Training School and the Nurses, and of all you have accomplished not only in their behalf but for all the profession of nursing in which you have been a far reaching influence for all that was most progressive and best.
    Miss Cecelia Beaux to whom I wrote on the subject some months ago has just returned from abroad and will be able to give you sittings at her studio at Gloucester, Massachusetts, during the early summer.

[1] Harvey Cushing, *Sir William Osler*, 2 vols. (Oxford: Clarendon Press, 1925), 1: 673 and 2: 5, 48, 50, 78, 151.

139

The nurses seem anxious that you should wear your black uniform with the white collar and cuffs and cap for they all admire it and like to see you in it.

As we hear that you are going off for your vacation about the beginning of July we hope that you may be able to see Miss Beaux in June.

The nurses are very much interested in the portrait and I am sure that you would have been gratified by their enthusiasm.

As soon as I hear from you I will write to Miss Beaux.

Ever yours,

Susan R. Thayer[2]

On Tuesday, June 19, Adelaide arrived in Gloucester and took lodgings in a small, old-fashioned, and inexpensive hotel that Miss Beaux recommended, a quiet little house on a hill overlooking the moor. Before coming to Gloucester, Adelaide had learned that Rudyard Kipling had lived there while writing *Captains Courageous*. To her delight she now learned that she was occupying the room in which he had lived and written. This fact brought Kipling more sharply into her life, and she resolved to read his novel again.

As soon as Adelaide settled herself, she called Miss Beaux and made an appointment to see her. About eleven the next morning she walked around "the lovely little curve of shore to a point where in among a tangle of trees and shrubs" she found Miss Beaux's studio.

Miss Beaux was a woman in her early fifties, of slightly over medium height, "with blue gray eyes not widely opened, a rather large mouth, and a face longer than ordinary, a good heavy chin and jaw, . . . a pleasant friendly smile," and beautiful teeth. She smiled, greeted Adelaide, and looked at her as though she were "doing a lot of things, rejecting, accepting, and debating all in a moment." Adelaide felt sure Miss Beaux was disappointed here and there in her subject. Then she realized that Miss Beaux had expected her to come dressed for a sitting rather than in the shirtwaist, skirt, and hat she had worn. As a result Miss Beaux would do nothing and they would spend the morning getting acquainted.

Adelaide was intrigued with the house from the moment she stepped into the small entry, on into the living room with its French windows, and then a few steps down into a small cloister, paved with flagstones and partitioned off so that one could always be sheltered from the wind, yet roofless so that sunshine could be found if it were desired. The place was surrounded by shrubbery, with one or two

    [2] Susan R. Thayer (Baltimore) to M. A. Nutting (Baltimore), May 14, 1906, MAN Papers.

trees at the end and a pretty path losing itself shortly in the tangle. "What a delightful place," Adelaide wrote, "just right for a quiet breakfast and early tea, green about, water beyond, and heaven above." Miss Beaux had wanted the house to look like that of a working woman, but to Adelaide it looked more like a place in which to relax.

As they walked to the studio, Miss Beaux talked of some of her "sitters." Recently she had painted Bishop Grier, a man of great conviction and fiery zeal. Miss Beaux had hoped to paint him as such, but, after he had been standing for a time, his expression had become like that of a petulant old woman or an old pussycat. Adelaide's hostess asked her about the uniform she had promised the students she would wear. After describing the soft black silk with the narrow white high collar and cuffs, black girdle, and white skull cap, Adelaide wondered whether it might not be a little severe. On the contrary, Miss Beaux said she had always wanted to paint someone in that kind of cap and garb and thought it would do very well.

Miss Beaux related how in her childhood her grandmother and aunts had trained her in habits of frugality and simplicity, saying she believed this careful home training had had much to do with her later success. She also mentioned her quiet, retired, and companionless life in West Philadelphia, which she had always hated and meant to get out of as soon as possible. Adelaide recalled her own childhood in Waterloo but said nothing. Unknowingly, Miss Beaux had struck a responsive chord, and the two women were fast on the way to becoming friends.

The next morning Adelaide wore her uniform to the studio and carried her cap. Miss Beaux spent an hour on the pose, light, and background, trying Adelaide in a variety of positions and studying her through a small piece of paper, about two by three inches, which she had torn to resemble a frame. Then she had Adelaide stand for a while, first on one side of the room and then on the other, against a golden background, then against the gray linen background formed by the curtains at the large French windows. The last seemed to satisfy Miss Beaux. She then asked Adelaide what she usually carried in her hands. Adelaide replied that ordinarily she carried a small, red leather notebook, which was as familiar as the uniform. Miss Beaux nodded approvingly. Just the right touch of color. She would paint Adelaide's hands holding the book. Finally she posed Adelaide before the gray curtains, turning as though to walk away, then looking back. "Yes, that's pretty nice," she said half to herself.

The next two mornings, while Miss Beaux sketched her subject, she talked almost continuously, inquiring about Adelaide and her work, commenting upon anything that attracted her attention, or talking about herself and the cottage.

Each day for nearly two weeks Adelaide sat from ten o'clock until half-past twelve while Miss Beaux painted and talked. Miss Beaux told Adelaide much about her family, and how she was not allowed to go to Paris until she was much older than most students who went there to study. She said that, as a young girl, she had showed no special talent and had done nothing remarkable, simply progressing in the usual way, always doing her best to do good honest work.

Grounded on a common love of beauty, truth, and honesty, the two women in a fortnight developed a close friendship. Adelaide, who had dreaded the long hours of sitting, found such stimulating companionship in Cecelia Beaux that she left Gloucester reluctantly. She had come to look upon the portrait as something objective, not herself perhaps as she looked in the mirror, but herself as seen by another. She regretted that she had not kept a diary of each day's proceedings and conversation—the evolution of a portrait and a friendship.[3]

Adelaide spent the summer with Minnie, Gilbert, and the children before returning to Baltimore for her last months at Hopkins. She took along enough work to keep her busy for twice the length of her holiday, yet she managed to find time for picnics with the children, to read books with Armine, and to attend a few public gatherings. Armine was very active in promoting educational improvements and woman suffrage. Gilbert had been church secretary and a member of the finance committee for the cathedral that had recently been built, and was freer now to pursue another of his numerous hobbies, the study and writing of the *History of Labrador*. He had always felt great compassion for the poor fisher folk and had tried to secure better housing and working conditions for those living in St. John's. In this connection he had come out openly against federation with Canada, lest union imperil the free trade upon which their prosperity depended. Adelaide had always found her brother-in-law to be an interesting and admirable person, but now his growing political convictions, social consciousness, and intellectual curiosity made him an even more stimulating companion.

Among the items on Adelaide's summer agenda was the completion of her special report to the U.S. Commissioner of Education on the

[3] Adelaide Nutting (Gloucester, Mass.) to Armine N. Gosling (St. John's, Newfoundland), June, 1906, *ibid.*

"Education and Professional Position of Nurses," which would be included in his annual report for 1906.[4] It was a revision and an updating of the monograph she had prepared in 1904, giving the history of nursing education, nursing organizations in the United States, and state legislation affecting nursing. By 1906, Indiana, California, Colorado, Connecticut, the District of Columbia, Iowa, New Hampshire, West Virginia, and Illinois had joined the ranks of New York, North Carolina, Virginia, New Jersey, and Maryland in passing registration laws. The standards of training schools were steadily being raised. Much remained to be done, but the future of nursing education and the profession looked bright.[5]

Adelaide had also brought along several chapters of the *History of Nursing* manuscript which she wanted to put in final shape. She and Lavinia had set 1907 as the completion date, and certainly the manuscript should be ready for press before they left for Europe and the meeting of the International Council of Nurses in Paris. When they set out to write the history, Adelaide already had completed a detailed skeleton of countries, time periods, leading events, subevents, personalities, and activities to the end of the 1890s. Lavinia suggested the introductory material on "Mutual Aid." From these data they planned their chapters. Adelaide had less time than Lavinia for the actual writing, but she insisted on preparing the chapters on the French hospitals in Canada, the Spanish hospitals in Mexico, and the military orders. They wrote with self-assurance and asked no one's advice or counsel.

Adelaide read all of Lavinia's pages, suggested, criticized, added supplementary material, and gave final approval. As the chapters were finished, she had them typed and passed them on to be read by Dr. Frank Smith, Johns Hopkins' authority on grammar and rhetoric. When the first two volumes of the history were ready for the press, Adelaide and Lavinia looked about for a publisher. They knew nothing about the business of publishing, and when G. P. Putnam's agreed to take the manuscript and to give them royalties of 25 percent, on the condition that the authors pay the publication costs, they decided to look no further and began figuring how they could meet this expense.[6] To publish the history and attend the International

[4] M. Adelaide Nutting, "Educational and Professional Position of Nurses," in *Report of the U.S. Commissioner of Education for 1906* (Washington, D.C.: Government Printing Office, 1907).

[5] *Ibid.*

[6] Lavinia Dock (New York) to Adelaide Nutting (St. John's), n.d., MAN Papers; Lavinia Dock, "Writing the History of Nursing," *The Johns Hopkins Nurses Alumnae Magazine*, April, 1950, p. 59.

Council of Nurses, where she was scheduled to present a paper, Adelaide would have to borrow some money from Charlie. She had no doubts as to the success of the volumes and went confidently ahead with her plans.

When Adelaide returned to Baltimore she withdrew from social engagements and the clubs she enjoyed so much and devoted all time beyond that required by her position to the history and nursing organization demands. She missed her friends at the Arundel Club, afternoon tea with Elizabeth Ellicott, and occasional Sunday dinners with Mr. and Mrs. Charles Grasty of the *Baltimore Sun*. Adelaide had always been pleased to discuss with the editor of this distinguished newspaper matters relating to civic affairs, especially education, public health, and the prevention of disease, and he listened to her opinions with respect.[7]

Time was passing very fast. On January 30 and 31, 1907, Adelaide attended the fourth annual meeting of the Maryland State Association of Graduate Nurses, where she told of her future work at Teachers College. She appealed to her fellow nurses to join the Red Cross Volunteer Nurses and to be prepared to serve in times of emergency or disaster. For her services to the state of Maryland and Maryland nurses, she was voted honorary president for life.[8] Adelaide was as moved as she had been three years before, when these loyal nurses had insisted that her license be the first issued under the Maryland Registration Act.

On February 11, Adelaide brought as her guest to the tenth annual meeting of the Instructive Visiting Nurses Association of Baltimore Dr. Wilfred Grenfell, for whom she had arranged a speaking engagement in Baltimore. Miss LaMotte, the special tuberculosis nurse whose salary was paid by Mrs. Osler, reported on the tuberculosis work in the city, and Adelaide spoke on the great economic value the public derived from the services of the district nurse. Dr. Grenfell described the work of the Labrador missions, and, before he left the city, Adelaide helped him recruit two Hopkins graduates, Amy E. MacMahon and V. M. Macdonald, both of the class of 1903, for work in his missions.[9]

The portrait painted by Miss Beaux the previous summer was formally presented on March 30. It had previously been exhibited at the Corcoran Gallery in Washington and the Walter Rowland Galleries in Boston. At the Corcoran Gallery it had been part of an

[7] Frances K. M. Butler, "Memories of Adelaide Nutting," *The Johns Hopkins Nurses Alumnae Magazine*, April, 1958, p. 38.

[8] *Ibid.*, March, 1907, p. 22.

[9] *Ibid.*, p. 23; *ibid.*, June, 1907, p. 62.

exhibit featuring American artists. Outstanding there were the five portraits by John Singer Sargent, one being the large canvas of Doctors Welch, Osler, Halsted, and Kelly. The *Boston Transcript* commented:

> No one stands up beside Sargent in the display for he is in a class by himself. But Miss Beaux crowds him a little all the same, for in her "Miss Nutting," the portrait of a nurse for the Johns Hopkins School of Nurses, she shows quite the best performance we have on record for her. Its simplicity, directness and feminine charm are not to be mistaken, while technically it leaves nothing to be desired.

Later, when the portrait was exhibited at the Rowland Galleries, the *Transcript* described it as one of "the most remarkable characterizations of a type that has come from the brush of this exceptionally talented painter. . . . A useful and estimable personage, strong of will and very capable. The head is painted with an extraordinary certitude, candor, and comprehension."[10]

The portrait presentation was Adelaide's real farewell to Hopkins. Many friends, alumnae, and trustees attended the simple ceremony. Miss Beaux was unable to come. Adelaide's friend and classmate Georgia Nevins read Susan Read Thayer's speech presenting the portrait to the trustees. Accepting the gift for the trustees, Judge Harlan paid high tribute to Adelaide. Tracing her association with the Hopkins Hospital, and noting that she had known every nurse who graduated from the training school, he concluded by saying that no one had done more to bring dignity and importance to the profession of trained nurses.[11]

Dr. William Welch then spoke on behalf of the physicians.

> The vocation of the nurse is one of the most useful of all callings for women and it has long had an immense influence in the improvement of medical practice. If one looks back over the progress in medicine, the last one hundred years, there is no one factor bearing on the treatment of disease which has had a greater essential influence than the system of trained nursing. . . . A successful school for nurses is one of the important possessions of a well-organized hospital. . . . I know from conversations with her that she has had the most intelligent thought about the education of nurses. She has informed herself upon the history of the subject, about the methods of teaching other subjects, teaching medicine, and has by her own thought and by the application of her method contributed very importantly to the training of nurses. . . .
>
> The Medical Staff of the Hospital owes a great debt of gratitude to

[10] *Ibid.*, March, 1907, p. 26; clippings (n.d.), Scrapbook, MAN Papers.
[11] *The Johns Hopkins Nurses Alumnae Magazine*, March, 1907, p. 49.

Miss Nutting and to the nurses who trained under her. The position which the Hospital has obtained is due in no small measure to her work here.[12]

Elizabeth King Ellicott spoke briefly, stressing Adelaide's gift for friendship. Then there was tea in the Nurses' Home, followed by fond goodbyes.[13]

When the last guest had departed, Adelaide went back to look at the portrait again. Teenie, the head waitress, was standing before it, tears in her eyes. She had taken Miss Nutting her meals when she had been ill with diphtheria, and in appreciation Adelaide had given her a silk petticoat that rustled when she walked. She had never owned anything so beautiful. "Don't cry," Adelaide said, putting her arms around her. "Remember Adelaide Nutting is always your friend." She put her head on Teenie's shoulder and they both cried. Recalling the incident forty years later, Teenie treasured the memory of her having said "Adelaide Nutting," not "Miss Nutting."[14]

A few days later Dean Russell sent Benjamin Andrews, secretary of the Department of Domestic Economy, and Miss Helen Kinne, director of Domestic Science, to Baltimore to discuss the curriculum for the Department of Domestic Administration, which Miss Nutting would direct, and the plans for the building soon to be erected. Andrews was at once impressed by the wide range of interests Adelaide's apartment revealed: music, literature, rare books, and art. Adelaide talked enthusiastically of the rising profession of nursing. Sometimes she spoke almost protectively. She related that Edward Bok had come to see her, and, perching himself on a corner of her table, had proposed that she write a series of nursing lessons for home study to be published in the *Ladies Home Journal.* She considered such a step unprofessional, and her eyes flashed with indignation as she recalled the incident.

Inasmuch as she would be director of the Department of Domestic Economy, Adelaide suggested that her visitors take a look at one or two of her housekeeping inventions. In the basement they saw the sterilizing lines she had designed and a controlled live-steam outlet for cleaning garbage cans. Later they walked about the hospital and stopped to see the portrait by Miss Beaux. On the way they saw a great mass of yellow daffodils and, to Andrews' delight and amazement, Adelaide quoted Shakespeare:

[12] *Ibid.,* pp. 50, 51.
[13] *Ibid.,* p. 51.
[14] Ethel Johns, "Interview with Josephine Waldhauser, 'Teenie,' October 25, 1948," The Johns Hopkins Hospital School of Nursing Archives.

Daffodils that come before the swallow
Dare and take the winds of March with beauty.

This woman, the first nurse to become a college professor, was no ordinary nurse. Under her direction Andrews would develop such courses in applied economics as economics of the household, home finance, standards of living, educational economics, and research methods.[15]

Adelaide sailed for England on May 1, 1907. She was to present a paper at the International Council of Nurses in Paris, but she had been too busy to do any work on it before she left Baltimore, and on shipboard she was too weary to do any concentrated thinking or writing. In London she began making arrangements to visit hospitals and to interview nursing leaders and educators. She had two appointments with a member of the Board of Education, and, in talking with him, learned that he was one of a group trying to introduce into London University a three-year course to prepare women for the head of households and institutions, very much like what she was planning to do at Teachers College. "Isn't it amazing," she wrote her sister, "that the very same idea should have broken out, as it were, in two remote places at the very same time?"[16]

The weather in London was cold and gray and "ugly beyond belief." The old strep throat condition to which she was subject flared up again, and she was forced to stay in bed for a week. There were so many places and people she wanted to see—Diana Kimber; the Oslers in their new home at Oxford; and Dr. Grenfell, completing his degree at Cambridge, who had invited her to visit in his mother's home. There were days when she wondered whether she would be able to go on to Paris.

She was glad that she had seen the Ambrose Goslings and her niece Armine, who was attending school in England, shortly after her arrival. Later, half-sick, weary, and lonely, she was reluctant to go sightseeing by herself. She kept putting off work on the paper, thinking that another day she would feel more like writing.[17]

On June 15, Adelaide went to Paris, where she expected to stay at a hotel. Her friend Edith Thuresson Kelly met her, however, and invited her, along with Lavinia Dock, to stay at the Kellys' town house. Edmund Kelly was an American lawyer especially skillful in international law. He had lived in Paris for many years and had

[15] Benjamin R. Andrews, "Memo on Adelaide Nutting," to Isabel M. Stewart (n.d.), MAN Papers.
[16] Adelaide Nutting (Aisne, France) to Armine N. Gosling (St. John's) June 23, 1907, *ibid.*
[17] *Ibid.*

become quite wealthy. After the death of his wife, he had married Edith Thuresson, who had been doing private duty nursing. They had homes in Paris and in the country near Aisne.

Adelaide, still far from well, was glad to be away from the hustle and bustle of the council headquarters. The sun shone brightly in Paris, and she enjoyed the drives to and from the Kellys' home. Although she managed to attend the important meetings of the council and to preside at one of the sessions, her lingering throat condition compelled her to forego the banquets and many of the social functions. She was unable to complete her paper, but Lavinia Dock spoke on the organization of the Society of Superintendents and the Associated Alumnae of graduate nurses in America, and told how the Society of Superintendents had persuaded Teachers College, Columbia University, to establish a course in teaching and administration for hospital-trained nurses. At first it had not been thought possible for the students to do practical work in a hospital, but recently five of the largest hospitals in New York had affiliated, and now students from the hospital economics course would gain practical experience in administration, the purchase of equipment, and teaching. Lavinia went on to explain that an endowment for the chair was highly desirable but said that for the time being it seemed wise for the Society of Superintendents to hold the purse strings and control the appointment of a director.[18]

After the Paris meeting, Adelaide and Lavinia accompanied Mrs. Kelly to the Kellys' country home, Coucy le Chateau, once a famous castle, near Aisne. Living in a castle was a new experience for Adelaide, one which challenged her imagination.

> I write at this moment from the loveliest spot on earth from the tower of one of the oldest ruins and certainly the most famous, not only in France but in Europe. Just two and one half hours from Paris. . . .
>
> The place is made up of one of the towers, a good deal of ground about it, and a cluster of small cottages about which have been transformed into the most comfortable of dwellings. The great charm of the place lies in the view and the gardens. Coucy-le-chateau (as opposed to Coucy-le-Ville) consists of the ruins of this wonderfully big and beautiful castle—a tiny French village huddled within the old walls, and at the top of one of the old towers and about it Mrs. Kelly has made gardens which are a dream of beauty, especially the roses which rival anything I have ever seen even in Italy. . . .
>
> As to our conference of nurses . . . it was really stunning. Three hundred nurses from all over the country from Sweden, Holland, Belgium, and even from Finland . . . the representative of the old aristoc-

[18] Margaret Breay and Ethel Gordon Fenwick, *History of the International Council of Nurses* (Geneva: International Council of Nurses, 1931), p. 35.

racy, a Baroness von Mannerheim of Helsingfors. She is superintendent of one of the hospitals there. Ireland was represented by Lady
Hermione Blackwood who is a district nurse on the West Coast. I think
these two were the only titled ladies we own, but the general character
of the assemblage was remarkable. Mrs. Robb was there looking her
best, and a good many came from as far as California. . . .

We were splendidly received in Paris by the city officials who opened
our meeting with long speeches, and later with great formality and
splendor at the Hotel de Ville. On every public occasion, tongues were
loosened and the ceremonies set afloat, as it were, with champagne.
I never saw so much in my life.

As nursing affairs are in a rather critical stage just now in France, I
think our convention was most timely and feel sure it will prove a helpful support to the men and women who are trying to introduce into
French hospitals the nursing system that has so reformed the hospitals
of England and America. The whole religious question obtrudes here,
and the sentiment of centuries is with the religious orders and with
nursing carried on from a purely religious motive. Some of the officials,
the heads of the Assistance Publique, for instance, are entirely in favor
of our method; and everywhere we have been received with the utmost
courtesy.[19]

From Coucy le Chateau, Adelaide and Lavinia traveled to Berlin,
to which they had been invited by Sister Agnes Karll, editor of the
Untern Lazarus Kreutz, the militant organ of the German Nurses
Association, which Sister Agnes had helped to found in 1903. Sister
Agnes was an ardent feminist as well as a champion of reform in
nursing practice and training. The three women discussed the status
of all facets of German nursing—Catholic sisterhoods, deaconesses,
Red Cross mother-houses, as well as the "wild," or independent,
nurses who had either broken ties with their mother-house or taken
a short course in nursing and been licensed by a physician. In 1905,
the Federal Council of Germany had accepted the draft of an act
which would regulate the practice of nursing throughout the empire,
but the act had not yet been put into effect. Even in Prussia, where
the act was to have been carried out first, almost anyone with the
requisite hospital experience who passed the state examinations could
be registered whether or not she had graduated from a course of
training.[20] Learning firsthand from Sister Agnes of the trials and
vicissitudes of raising nursing standards in Germany, Adelaide and
Lavinia tried to lend encouragement and inspiration.

From Berlin, Lavinia Dock went to southern France to visit Dr.
Anna Hamilton at Bordeaux and to secure additional materials for the

[19] Adelaide Nutting (Aisne, France) to Armine N. Gosling (St. John's) June
23, 1907, MAN Papers.
[20] Sister Agnes Karll (Berlin) to Adelaide Nutting, [Liverpool], September 3,
1907, *ibid.*

third volume of the *History of Nursing*. A few days later, Adelaide returned to England. Meanwhile, Volume 1 of the Nutting and Dock *History of Nursing* had gone to press.

The highlight of Adelaide's trip to Europe came in London, where she spent a quiet half-hour with Florence Nightingale. She approached 10 High Street, Park Lane, with all the reverence of a pilgrim to Mecca. Miss Nightingale, sitting in her wheelchair, a light shawl about her shoulders and another over her knees, asked Adelaide to come closer so that she might not miss a word. She inquired of The Johns Hopkins Hospital and of Mrs. Robb and listened intently as Adelaide told her about nursing in America. Notwithstanding her eighty-seven years, Miss Nightingale seemed "wonderfully sympathetic as if an unquenchable spirit still shone in her eyes and filled her voice." When Adelaide rose to go, Miss Nightingale said, "No, tell me more." Later Adelaide said she had never been more profoundly affected than when Miss Nightingale pressed her hand at parting and asked her to come again. She would treasure those moments forever.[21]

On September 6, Adelaide sailed from Liverpool. In less than three weeks she would be embarking on a new career. Somewhat wistfully she thought of the old life at Hopkins. She would lay away the black uniform with the white collar, cuffs, and cap, and the red leather notebook the Teresians had given her at Christmas two years before.

Her luggage unpacked and the bags stowed away, Adelaide returned to the deck and read again the bon voyage letter Sister Agnes Karll had written.

> I'm dreadfully in the blues and there is nobody to encourage me at all. From all sides spring worries and nasty things but I am rather placid, only tired of it all.
> I will think of your new work and be so glad for every bit I can help you, dear. You only need to tell me what I can do.
> Now goodnight for today. I [felt] so dreadfully lonely when your train passed away that the tears came. You don't know what the days with you meant to me. Why don't we have more women [like] you and Miss Dock. I will always be longing for you both.
> Goodnight, a happy journey. . . . All the best and kindest wishes for your work.
>
> Yours truly,
>
> Sister Agnes[22]

---

[21] *American Journal of Nursing*, November, 1907, p. 103.
[22] Sister Agnes Karll (Berlin) to Adelaide Nutting, [Liverpool], September 3, 1907, MAN Papers.

XV

Professor, 1907–1910

On September 25, Adelaide Nutting began her work at Teachers College. Ever since her appointment as Isabel Hampton's assistant she had been alert to teaching techniques and methods that were compatible with the laws of learning. She had read all that she could find on ways of teaching and learning, while at the same time keeping up with advances in her own field and in medical science generally. Although she had not done formal academic work beyond high school and The Johns Hopkins Hospital Training School, she tried to compensate by means of a rigorous, self-disciplined program of reading, study, and public lectures. She had always enjoyed literature and history, and was fascinated by new developments in psychology and the social sciences. She eagerly awaited *The Atlantic, Harper's*, the *North American Review, The New Republic*, and *The Manchester Guardian*.

Dean James E. Russell had marked Adelaide as an asset for his emerging Teachers College when he first met her in 1899. In turn, she became equally well impressed with Dean Russell and Teachers College, a venturesome institution which, in addition to general culture, scholarship, professional knowledge, and technical skills, offered training that would enable the student to perceive the relationships existing everywhere in the various fields of knowledge.[1]

In 1907 Teachers College was a complex of five brown sandstone and red brick buildings east of Broadway, between 120th and 121st streets. Main was constructed in 1894 and subsequently Macy, Thompson, and Milbank were constructed. Horace Mann, the most recently built, housed the elementary and high schools. Adelaide was

[1] James E. Russell, "Report to the Trustees of Teachers College, Columbia University," [1900], pp. 13–14, on file at the Department of Nursing Education Archives, Teachers College; *idem*, "The Function of the University in Training Teachers," *Columbia University Quarterly* 1 (1898–99): 323–42.

assigned an office on the top floor of Thompson, in which the physical education and health work was centered.

Adelaide attended the first faculty meeting preceding registration, and was introduced with other new staff members. She was delighted with Dean Russell's interpretation of Teachers College, of its unique role in education. She met a number of the faculty whom she came to regard as the stalwart great, the rugged pioneers of Teachers College, Paul Monroe, Edward L. Thorndike, Frank McMurry, Henry Suzzalo, David Snedden, Julius Sachs, Henry Johnson, Thomas Wood, Maurice Bigelow, and Patty Hill.

At registration only two new students enrolled in the hospital economics course, but two former students were returning for the second year of work (a program Miss Alline had inaugurated in 1905) at the request of the Society of Superintendents. Students completing only the first year of work were given certificates, while those completing two full years of work received diplomas.[2]

Dean Russell had seen to it that Adelaide's schedule would be light the first year so that she might have time to become thoroughly acquainted with New York City's hospital facilities and personnel. He intimated that as enrollments and funds permitted, her work would be solely in the field of nursing education. Meanwhile, as President Nicholas Murray Butler had stated in his letter of April 21, 1906, her work would include "investigation and instruction in the management and administration of households, hospitals, asylums, dormitories, and other domestic institutions."[3]

Adelaide was grateful for every association that she had had with institutional housekeeping at Johns Hopkins, every minute spent with Rachel Bonner in the kitchen, the linen rooms, and the laundry, the long hours with Dr. Hurd going over the hospital accounts, and perhaps most of all for her mother's abiding lessons in thrift and economy. She subscribed to a clipping bureau for articles on domestic economy, laundry, cleaning, and the management of servants. She herself was an inveterate clipper of household hints and shortcuts adaptable for hospital use. Soon she was drafting courses in management which would appeal to home economics majors as well as to those in hospital administration. In addition, she arranged a series of lectures to which the public might be admitted for a small fee.

[2] *American Journal of Nursing*, July, 1907, p. 776.
[3] Miss Nutting was approved by the Trustees of Teachers College for a three-year appointment as full professor dating from July 1, 1906, at a salary of $2,500 for nine months and a leave of absence without pay during the academic year 1906. Nicholas Murray Butler (New York) to Margaret [sic] Adelaide Nutting (Atlantic City), April 21, 1906, MAN Papers.

The 1907–8 schedule included lectures on "Laundries," by Clara Noyes of St. Luke's Hospital, New Bedford, Massachusetts; "History and Social Aspects of Nursing," by Lillian Wald; "History of Nursing and Hospitals," by Lavinia Dock; "Hospital Planning," by the architect Charles Butler; "Working Essentials and Hospital Construction," by Annie W. Goodrich of Bellevue and Allied Training Schools; and "Training School Administration," by Mrs. Robb of Cleveland and Mary Riddle of Newton Hospital, Lower Newton Falls, Massachusetts.[4] Whenever possible, Adelaide called on her friends, qualified Hopkins graduates, and the resources of the Society of Superintendents for lectures. Those who had contributed so generously to the hospital economics course in the past were now determined to see the endowment go forward; they wanted to ensure that the position of chairman would always be held by a nurse.

From the number of letters written by nurses and superintendents congratulating her on the appointment and wishing her well, Adelaide was well aware that the profession stood back of her. By the same token, she must not disappoint them. As she was settling into the new work, she received a reassuring note from Lavinia Dock, written from Carcassone, France, where she was gathering material for the third volume of their History of Nursing.

My dear Adelaide—

You will be arriving in New York about noon and I am sure you will be homesick, lonely, and scared enough at first. You must go down to the Settlement early, and get a little friendly cheer, and comfort in you. Oh dear, I am agog to know how you like it, and what you will think of it all at first.

I fear there will be times when you will want to kill us, Miss Ross, and every one who ever advised you to take it—but dear girl, it is without a doubt destiny, for we shall get this chair endowed and you must hang on to it at least as long as that, even if you do not like it and that will be an objective for you to go by, in case brother Russell and the others turn out less well than you had hoped. . . .

You would be quite touched if you realized the admiration and almost reverence with which many women over here look up to you as a superintendent who has done so much for education. I encounter this quite frequently, especially among the Hollanders.

How delightful that you saw Miss Nightingale. I am dying to know what you said to her. Wonderful old lady. Do be sure to have Putnams send her the very first copy that is finished.[5]

[4] Isabel M. Stewart, Twenty-five Years of Nursing Education in Teachers College, 1899–1925 (Teachers College Bulletin, 17th ser., no. 3, February, 1926), p. 8; American Journal of Nursing, November, 1907, p. 125.

[5] Lavinia Dock (Carcassone, France) to Adelaide Nutting (New York), October 6, [1907], MAN Papers.

If Adelaide had regrets, she confided them to no one. Teachers College offered her a challenge. She was reminded of Dr. Halsted's oft-repeated remark at Hopkins, "Here, we try things." She was too busy to be lonely. At the first opportunity she went down to Henry Street Settlement to talk with Lillian Wald and arrange for her to lecture at Teachers College and for nurses from the college to visit the settlement. Adelaide, long interested in the visiting nurse, believed that the profession had a great obligation to meet in providing her with adequate preparation. She had done what she could in Baltimore to show her students how poverty, ignorance of the laws of health and sanitation, and poor living conditions among the less fortunate contributed to disease and its spread. Other nursing leaders were also aware of this, and the early issues of the *American Journal of Nursing* contained numerous articles on the subject.[6]

Lillian Wald, who had begun the first visiting nurse service in 1893 on the Lower East Side of New York, and who now directed a nursing service over a large area of the city's slums, was enthusiastic about Adelaide's proposals. She would be happy to work with Adelaide in securing better-trained personnel. She hoped for more women with the human understanding, sensitivity, fearlessness, and technical skill of Lavinia Dock. She told Adelaide that, when confronted with needy immigrants unable to speak English, Lavinia would undertake to learn enough of the family's native language to make herself understood. Adelaide smiled, for this must have been the source of Lavinia's uncanny gift for languages, which had been so helpful in the preparation of the *History of Nursing*. Miss Wald suggested that when Lavinia returned in November they must get together often.

In the late fall of 1907 the first two volumes of the *History of Nursing* were off the press and ready for distribution. Adelaide and Lavinia had made out lists of persons to whom they wished complimentary copies be sent at once. First on Adelaide's list was Florence Nightingale, then Dr. and Mrs. Osler, Dr. and Mrs. H. A. Kelly, and Isabel Robb.[7]

When the first copies arrived from Putnam's, the authors eagerly inspected the modest dark blue volumes with their thin gold lettering. They thought the frontispiece, "Hygeia, Goddess of Health," had turned out very well, that the title page was quite imposing, and that the dedication, "To all Members of the Nursing Profession," stood out neat and plain. Even the Preface read better in print.

---

[6] Adelaide Nutting, "Memorandum on the Helen Hartley Jenkins Endowment," for Isabel Stewart (n.d.), *ibid.*

[7] Adelaide Nutting, memorandum [1907], *ibid.*

As the result of this paucity of literature upon the subject, the modern nurse, keenly interested in the present and future of her profession, knows little of its past. She loses both the inspiration which arises from cherished tradition, and the perspective which shows the relation of one progressive movement to others. Only in the light of history can she see how closely her own calling is linked with the general conditions of education and of liberty that obtain—as they rise, she rises, and as they sink, she falls.[8]

Lavinia and Adelaide were proud of the rare old pictures and drawings they had been able to secure. There were fifty-eight of these in the first volume. Both were curious and impatient for the reviews and comments of critics as well as of their friends. Lavinia was especially anxious to hear what Miss Nightingale's opinion would be. As comments on the *History* arrived at Teachers College and at Henry Street Settlement, notes were exchanged. Lavinia dispatched one written by a doctor in Brooklyn and endorsed it, "Sent along by Putnams to cheer us."

It is a work well conceived and methodically arranged and gotten up in excellent taste. The authors have not confined themselves to a bare narration of facts but have illuminated the text with their own thought and personality. This quality saves the work from the dry, prosy, matter-of-fact style of the average historical writer. Moreover while recognizing the fine sentiment of humanity that has actuated the Saints and Sisterhoods in caring for the sick, the authors have risen above the platitudes of piety, the conceits of superstition, into the realm of a national and humane sentiment.[9]

Ernestine Evans wrote Putnam's that the *History* was not merely a textbook but one of the liveliest and finest histories of the woman's movement yet published, and that its interest was broad enough, its literary style so distinguished, and its account of little-known historical periods so animated that women's clubs and women students everywhere might profit by it.[10]

Genevieve Cooke, of the Fabiola Hospital, Oakland, California, and editor of *The Nurses Journal of the Pacific Coast*, wrote to Lavinia Dock:

I just wish to thank you in behalf of the profession for the labor of love, as I know it was, put into the production of the *History of Nurs-*

[8] M. Adelaide Nutting and Lavinia L. Dock, Preface to *A History of Nursing*, 4 vols. (New York: G. P. Putnam's Sons, 1907–12) 1: v.

[9] Lavinia Dock (New York) to Adelaide Nutting (New York), [1907], MAN Papers.

[10] Ernestine Evans, "Adelaide Nutting," *The Woman Citizen*, June 27, 1925, pp. 9–11.

sing. I am fascinated with it and I snatch it up each spare moment for I have been looking forward to it for a whole year. The publishers sent it last week for review and I have this day ordered three sets, one to present to a pupil nurse, one for Miss K. Fitch, and one for myself.[11]

Dr. Frank Smith, whose opinion on literary style was so highly valued at Hopkins, wrote:

> I sat down to glance it over and never let go of it for four hours. . . . I'd like to express my appreciation of the book in calm, temperate and dispassionate language. . . . I have not read one half dozen books in as many years that could be grouped with it in respect to literary quality in the exploration of a technical subject. . . . The balance and structural grace of its sentences, its propriety, its economy of expression and the richness are a continuous delight.[12]

In early February Adelaide received the eagerly awaited letter from Dr. Osler: "The history is splendid. Such a credit to you both and to the Johns Hopkins and to the profession, and to the States and to Canada!"[13]

In thanking Miss Nutting for her copy of the *History*, Sister Agnes Karll wrote from Berlin:

> That dear long letter. It is so good to know that friendship is like the light of the sun, does not depend on letters and talking to each other, but is always, sometimes behind clouds of work but it is there. I think there is a good deal of telegraphy without a wire between mankind. One does feel the kind thoughts of those one loves and they are support in black hours.[14]

Soon Sister Agnes would be translating the *History* into German. If the translation brought any profits, they were to go to Sister Agnes and her work in behalf of nursing reform, as the authors' contribution to the cause of improved nursing in Germany.[15]

Gratifying as were the reviews and the letters of friends, Adelaide

[11] Genevieve Cooke (Oakland, Calif.) to Lavinia Dock (New York), February 24, 1908, MAN Papers.

[12] Lavinia L. Dock, "Excerpts from Letters about the *History of Nursing*," *ibid.*

[13] William Osler (Oxford) to Adelaide Nutting (New York), January 28, [1908], *ibid.*

[14] Sister Agnes Karll (Berlin) to Adelaide Nutting (New York), May 13, 1908, *ibid.*

[15] Sister Agnes Karll, a former German Red Cross nurse, founded the German Nurses Association in 1903 and three years later became the editor of its militant organ, *Unterm Lazarus Kreutz.* In 1909 she was elected president of the International Council of Nurses, and presided over the congress held in Berlin in 1912. Isabel M. Stewart and Anne L. Austin, *A History of Nursing from Ancient to Modern Times: A World View* (New York: G. P. Putnam's Sons, 1926), pp. 305–8.

had no desire to sit back and complacently enjoy the fruits of past labors. She kept seeing greater possibilities in Teachers College. She studied the catalog, with its ever-increasing variety of courses, and analyzed the competency of the staff in terms of what they might bring to the Department of Household Administration and to nursing. Under her direction in the next few years, Benjamin Andrews, economist and secretary of the department, would develop such courses in applied economics as economics of the household, standards of living, consumer education, educational economics, home finance, and research methods."[16]

Through her association with the Lake Placid group, visiting nurses, and tenement inspectors, Adelaide came to believe that qualified visiting housekeepers could bring invaluable aid to homes where mothers were facing the handicaps of illness or lacked the ability to deal with household problems. Some progress had already been made along these lines. As a visiting dietitian for the Association for Improving the Condition of the Poor, Winifred Gibbs was demonstrating its value in New York City. Mabel Kittredge was establishing housekeeping centers closely related to New York's public schools, and similar housekeeping services were available in about twenty other cities and towns.[17] Adelaide gave much thought to domestic workers in homes and institutions. She was familiar with the research of Professor Lucy Salmon, *Domestic Science* (1896), and, when she discovered an economist in Washington who had made a study of the hours and wages of domestic servants, she asked him to lecture at Teachers College. Deeply impressed by what he had to say, Adelaide urged her friend S. S. McClure to have Dr. J. W. Rubinow write an article for *McClure's Magazine* on the wages and hours of domestic workers as a nationwide problem which demanded remedial action. As a result of her concern, domestic services became a subject of investigation by Benjamin Andrews. He collected all the research that had been done on the subject, organized a teaching unit on it, and subsequently wrote a chapter on it for his text.[18]

Adelaide looked upon domestic service as a labor problem with significant social implications. At Hopkins, when more graduate

[16] Benjamin R. Andrews, "Memorandum on Adelaide Nutting," to Isabel Stewart, (n.d.); and Benjamin R. Andrews (South Burlington, Vt.) to Stella Goostray (Boston), January 30, 1958; MAN Papers.

[17] Katharine Fisher, "Adelaide Nutting and Home Economics," an unpublished manuscript written at the request of Isabel Stewart and found on Miss Fisher's desk after her death. *Ibid.*

[18] Benjamin R. Andrews (South Burlington) to Stella Goostray (Boston), January 30, 1958, *ibid.*

nurses went into private duty than remained in hospital work, and when student nurses were recruited largely from servantless homes, she was careful to instruct the nurses—who might be called to nurse in homes where there were servants—on their relationships with other members of the household staff as well as with the patient and family. She told them what they could rightfully expect and what they should give in return. Consideration, kindness, cheerfulness, and respect were qualities which every nurse should constantly express.

Adelaide believed the word "servant" retained too much of its feudal character, and she tried to find a term that would convey an idea of the value and dignity of work well done. Certainly the conditions of work, the hours, and the wages for so-called domestics, when compared with those of workers in other fields, called for great improvement. The domestic worker had little association with others who were performing the same kind of service; she was usually isolated, her hours were uncertain, and free time did not afford her a normal social life. Worst of all, she was usually untrained in an occupation which required skill in a diversity of tasks—from cooking, marketing, and cleaning to caring for children and elderly persons. Adelaide endorsed the idea that more adequate training should be provided for these people, and that they should be non-resident employees paid for a definite number of hours at specified rates.

Whether one were to manage a home or take charge of the housekeeping and dietary departments of an institution, Adelaide stressed to her students the importance of organizing details and a careful work schedule, and of controlling the conditions necessary to give these details the attention they required. This called for sound business procedures, a properly working system for making transactions and controlling finances, a careful analysis of monthly and yearly expenses, budgeting, and an adequate system of accounting.

Adelaide was also alert to the impact of economic and social change on the home and community. As home crafts were replaced by industry, problems in consumption took on new significance. In the passing of home crafts and personal pride in work well done, she sensed the loss of the domestic worker's respect for the jobs he did. Somehow this must be regained.

The increase in apartment dwellers, public dining rooms, large-group households, and the changing pattern of family life brought a challenge to management. Adelaide believed that a serious obstacle in the way of effective management was that those in charge had never made a searching inquiry into better methods of work, or into the time assigned to performing various tasks, and consequently could not set up suitable standards for determining daily performance. Her attention was attracted to Frederick Taylor's time and motion studies, which were transforming industry by setting up standards for measuring a good day's work. Working with him were Frank Gilbreth and his wife, Lillian. Adelaide approached Mrs. Gilbreth about the possibility of making a similar study of household tasks, with a view toward greater efficiency and more free time for the household worker, be she an employee or a housewife and mother.[19]

Adelaide seriously considered the possibility of establishing fellowships for carrying on such research, but an event in 1909 was to redefine her position at Teachers College and to direct her energies specifically into the field of health and nursing education.

Adelaide spent Christmas, 1907, in Baltimore as the guest of her friend and successor at Hopkins, Georgina Ross. She was very happy to be back in Baltimore, and there was a gay round of teas, dinners, and receptions which she enjoyed very much. Her friends Elizabeth King Ellicott, Susan Thayer, Dr. Welch, and the Hurds were delighted to see her. Dr. Welch, now president of the American Academy for the Advancement of Science, told her that a committee of one hundred had been organized to work for a national department of health comparable to the Departments of the Interior and Commerce and Labor.

Adelaide stayed over to speak to the Teresians on January 3 about foreign hospitals and her visit with Florence Nightingale. The Teresians proudly showed her the bookcase recently given them by Teresian alumnae. The 600 volumes the society had collected were to be known as the "Nutting Collection." Among these were the autographed copies of the History of Nursing which Adelaide and Lavinia had sent.[20]

One of the important events during Adelaide's summer in St. John's in 1908 was the anti-tuberculosis convention held there. For some time, physicians throughout the towns and villages of the island and the coast of Labrador had noted an increasing number of cases of tuberculosis. Most cases were beyond arrest when they reached the physician's attention, and it was imperative that the matter be attacked from the angle of prevention. Adelaide, who had often discussed the problem with Dr. Grenfell and the Goslings, was invited to make one of the principal addresses. She chose as her subject "The Opportunity of the Teacher in the Prevention of Tuberculosis" be-

[19] Katharine Fisher, "Adelaide Nutting and Home Economics."
[20] "Book of the Teresians," MAN Papers; The Johns Hopkins Nurses Alumnae Magazine, March, 1908, pp. 11, 32, 43, 45.

cause of the unique position of leadership the teacher had in the class-room and in her contacts with the home.

> Prevention involves education at these various levels, enlightenment that gives people power to safe-guard themselves and their homes. The carefully educated nurse in her hospital has learned much that would be helpful to these people (1) the importance of personal and domestic cleanliness, fresh air and sunlight (2) composition of foods, what is suit-able and nourishing for infants and adults, which are not or are unsafe, (3) knows of dangers of certain occupations, habits, ways of living. This knowledge gives her power in the prevention of diseases. . . . She can show people the simple laws of healthful living, and how they may be applied.[21]

Adelaide asked for medical inspection in the schools, not only so that diseases might be discovered in their early stages and the contagion removed, but also so that certain physical defects, such as poor eye-sight, might be remedied. The visiting nurse, she said, follows the children to their homes to teach the mothers. In a factory the nurse checking the health of employees is a distinct economic asset. Ade-laide stressed the importance of milk depots supplying pure, fresh milk. She also noted that the visiting nurse shows the young mother how to feed a baby, wash it, dress it, and keep it clean. In June, 1908, when 125 babies died in Montreal, the newspapers called not only for a better, purer milk supply but also for nurses who would teach. The tuberculosis nurse was an agent of prevention.

The school nurse, Adelaide went on to explain, teaches in schools and through schools. Courses in physiology and hygiene find a proper place in the curriculum, and every step in the study can be given a practical application. "Skin and function" lead to the need for bathing and personal cleanliness; "lungs" to the composition of air and the need for ventilation; and "food, etc.," to a good diet and a body less susceptible to tuberculosis. Adelaide appealed for home economics in the schools in order that girls might learn the importance of the choice of food and how to prepare it. She spoke of the care of the teeth and told of free dental care for the poor in Germany, pointed out the dangers of flies and mosquitoes, and asked for clean school-rooms, exercise in the open air, clean clothes, clean bodies, clean toilets, and the proper temperature and fresh air in classrooms.

It was a simple, forceful, down-to-earth talk. Anyone who listened,

[21] M. Adelaide Nutting, "The Opportunity of the Teacher in the Prevention of Tuberculosis" (Address before the Anti-Tuberculosis Convention, St. John's, Newfoundland, July, 1908), MAN Papers.

literate or illiterate, could understand and grasp the implications of ignoring these health factors.

There were other speakers—physicians, ministers, and civic leaders —as well as well-chosen and impressive exhibits. It would not be long before St. John's had its visiting nurse.

In the fall of 1908 twenty-one nurses, three times the number of the previous year, enrolled in the Teachers College hospital economics course, but five later withdrew for financial reasons.[22]

At registration Adelaide noticed an attractive, alert, poised, refined, and mature young woman standing near the door. "Well," she said to herself, "I hope she is one of mine." The student came to her desk, and the minute she gave her name, Isabel Maitland Stewart, Adelaide recalled the correspondence. Here was another fellow-Canadian, a former school teacher who had studied at Winnipeg Collegiate Institute. After teaching in rural and small-town schools, she had enrolled in the Winnipeg General Hospital Training School for Nurses. On completion of the course, she had done private duty, become a supervisor, and then had spent a brief period in district nursing.[23]

Isabel Stewart was impressed by Adelaide Nutting's memory. Had Miss Stewart not written articles for the *Canadian Nurse*, and had she and Ethel Johns not started the *Winnipeg Alumnae Journal*? Isabel smiled. It was through reading articles by Miss Nutting in the *American Journal of Nursing* that she had decided to study at Teachers College. She had spent the past summer in England and Scotland with a sick aunt. She told Miss Nutting she had not seen Florence Nightingale, who now saw members of her own family only by appointment, and who, because of her age and difficulty in hearing, was almost never seen by strangers, even for a few minutes. Isabel had, however, gone to see Mrs. Fenwick, founder of the *British Journal of Nursing*, in her office in London.[24]

If Adelaide was delighted with her new student, Isabel Stewart was equally pleased with her teacher. Miss Nutting seemed to inspire frankness and honesty, and Isabel was led almost at once to confess to her, "I do not want to be an administrator, I want to be a teacher."

---

[22] "Report of the Hospital Economics Committee, 1908–1909," Department of Nursing Education Archives, Teachers College.

[23] Effie J. Taylor, "Isabel Maitland Stewart," National League of Nursing leaflet (n.d.), MAN Papers.

[24] Ethel Gordon Munson Fenwick, the wife of Dr. Bedford Fenwick, was formerly matron of St. Bartholomew's Hospital, London, and in 1888 was one of the founders of the British Nurses Association. In 1893 she became editor of an independent nurses' journal, *The Nursing Record*, later renamed *The British Journal of Nursing*. She proposed the International Council of Nurses in 1899 and became its first president. Stewart and Austin, *A History of Nursing*, pp. 166–70.

Although there was only one program in nursing, Adelaide quickly showed Isabel how the various courses could help her become the kind of teacher hospital training schools so desperately needed.[25]

The class entering in the fall of 1908 was memorable not only because it was the largest but also because of its members' qualifications. The course was beginning to attract nurses who were college graduates—for instance, Helen Wood, Helen Stewart, and Laura Logan. Among other members of the class were Bertha Erdman, Louise Powell, Bessie Simmons, Linette Parker, Harriet Bailey, and Effie Taylor, who had been in Adelaide's last class at Johns Hopkins.[26] Choko Suo, from Tokyo, Japan, was among the first of a long succession of foreign students who were to study nursing education at Teachers College.[27] Some of these students wanted to teach, others wanted to do philanthropic work, a few would study administration. Adelaide explored the resources of Columbia University and saw to it that graduate courses in social economy under Dr. Devine, Mrs. Simkovitch, and Dr. Lindsay were opened to her better-qualified students. Excursions to social centers were arranged and extra lectures were brought in. Isabel Stewart said she would never forget her field trip to Ellis Island and Henry Street, because of the way it was interpreted by Miss Nutting. That year Lillian Wald lectured on the "Visiting Nurse," and Irving Fisher spoke on "Hospital Accounts and Bookkeeping." Dr. Hurd seemed pleased to come up from Hopkins and lecture on "Hospital Administration."[28] Practice-teaching facilities were provided by one of the nearby hospital training schools.[29]

In addition to launching a new class, buying furniture, and settling into her apartment, Adelaide prepared a paper for the meeting of the American Hospital Association to be held in Toronto in late September. She had planned to go, but later decided she could afford neither the time nor the money, and so she sent the paper to be read. It was well received, but Adelaide wrote her sister she would never understand why. She promised to give a paper in Buffalo in October, and thought she would have ample time to write it after school started, but,

[25] Isabel M. Stewart, *Oral History*, 2 vols. (New York: Columbia University, Butler Library, 1958), 1: 75, 82, 104, 120.

[26] *Nursing Education Bulletin*, the special issue commemorating the fortieth anniversary of nursing education at Teachers College, October 13–14, 1939, p. 7.

[27] Adelaide Nutting (New York) to Armine N. Gosling (St. John's, Newfoundland), November 1, 1908, MAN Papers.

[28] "Speech by Dr. Henry M. Hurd at Teachers College, [1908–9]," *ibid.*

[29] "Report of the Hospital Economics Committee, 1908–1909," Department of Nursing Education Archives, Teachers College.

as the days went by, every minute had to go for other things . . . the day before the Buffalo meeting not a line of the work touched. So as not to break my promise, I took the train, traveled all night, gave an informal address the next day and traveled all night back again and was on duty in my office bright and early the next morning. I have an engagement to lecture two successive weeks in Patterson, New Jersey, and am going up to Providence to speak next week. You have no idea what an effort these things are. . . . I am not forced to go about lecturing. It is entirely a matter of choice, the result of I don't know what impulses— the desire to learn how to speak in public and the hope of helping in my work here at the bottom. By and by, when I become more accomplished I mean to make a charge now and then for lecturing and thus have a penny or two for the suffrage cause.[30]

New Year's Day, 1909, found Adelaide in Washington, D.C., attending a meeting of home economists for the purpose of organizing a national association, a plan which grew out of the Lake Placid conferences Melvil and Annie Dewey had first sponsored ten years before.

In 1906 a teachers section had been organized at Pratt Institute, Brooklyn, which held a meeting the following year at the University of Chicago. Dr. C. F. Langworthy of the U.S. Department of Agriculture was chairman of the committee for the Washington meeting. Other members were Isabel Bevier, University of Illinois; Mrs. Melvil Dewey; Alice P. Morton, assistant professor of Domestic Administration, University of Chicago; M. Adelaide Nutting, professor of Domestic Administration, Teachers College; Benjamin R. Andrews, secretary, Department of Domestic Economy, Teachers College; Ellen Richards, Massachusetts Institute of Technology; and Maurice LeBosquet, University of Chicago. One hundred forty-three persons attended the first session. Before the session closed, the conferees had voted to organize the American Home Economics Association and to draw up a constitution and by-laws. Adelaide was named to the by-laws committee. The association committed itself to "the improvement of living conditions in the home, institutional household and community."[31] It welcomed to membership all teachers of domestic economy, interested teachers in allied fields, managers of institutions, social and municipal workers, hygienists, and sanitary experts. Quickly its committees went into action. One month later, membership had risen to 830. In February, following the organization of the association, Volume I, number 1, of the *Journal of Home Economics*

[30] Adelaide Nutting (New York) to Armine N. Gosling (St. John's), November 1, 1908, MAN Papers.
[31] *Journal of Home Economics* 1 (1909): 93.

appeared.[32] Few professional organizations have gotten off to such an auspicious start.

A year later 150 delegates attended the annual meeting of the Home Economics Association at Simmons College, Boston. Adelaide spoke before the Dietitians' Section. Later she was named chairman of a committee to study children's nurses. At the Lake Placid Conference of the Administrative Section of the Home Economics Association (June 28–July 1, 1910), she spoke on the "Field of Administration," its history, the avenues ahead in institutional life, hospital and tubercular agency work, dietitians, and the need for trained women.[33]

Meanwhile, the Society of Superintendents, which had originally underwritten the hospital economics program at Teachers College, was concerned about the future, which only an endowment could secure. The amount it sought was only $50,000, but, generous as the superintendents and nurses were in comparison to their means, that amount was not forthcoming. By May 1, 1908, only $5,000 had been raised.[34] Two years later the total sum collected amounted to only $11,748.30.[35] This situation troubled nursing leaders.

Why should nursing education not be tax supported, as was education for the professions of medicine, law, and engineering? Why must nursing education always pay its way or be the object of private philanthropy? Why was the training school always the handmaiden of the hospital? When hospitals were maintained by the state for the few hours' weekly clinical experience required for the education of physicians, why were student nurses committed to an eight-to-twelve-hour-a-day internship?

When Isabel Robb was elected president of the Society of Superintendents in 1908, she decided to focus the society's attention on the collegiate school as one of the great needs of nursing education. Since 1901 several detached preparatory courses had been tried, at Drexel Institute in Philadelphia, Pratt Institute in Brooklyn, and a few other places, but most of them had been short-lived. The one at Simmons College, Boston, continued for many years, however, and eventually developed into a collegiate school with basic and graduate programs.[36]

[32] Adelaide Nutting is listed as an original member of the American Home Economics Association. Original life members were Mr. and Mrs. Melvil Dewey, Grace Dodge, and Fanny Merritt Farmer. *Ibid.*

[33] *Ibid.*, 2 (1910): 11.

[34] Adelaide Nutting (New York) to Annie W. Goodrich (New York), October 12, 1908, MAN Papers.

[35] "Report of the Hospital Economics Committee, 1910," Department of Nursing Education Archives, Teachers College.

[36] Stewart and Austin, *A History of Nursing*, pp. 207–8.

The Society of Superintendents' 1909 meeting was scheduled for St. Paul–Minneapolis in early June. Adelaide promised to read a paper there and planned to return by way of Cleveland in order to stop over for a few days with the Robbs. Isabel was proud of her boys— Hampton, aged thirteen, and Philip, seven—and devoted to their father. Later in the summer Isabel, Dr. Robb, and the boys would vacation in Germany, and Isabel would stop over in London for the Third Congress of the International Council of Nurses. Lavinia Dock, the council's secretary, Annie Goodrich, and a number of other friends would be there. Adelaide had been asked to present a paper on "Preparation for Institutional Work." She had agreed to write it and would ask Isabel to read it.[37]

The superintendents' meeting in St. Paul–Minneapolis was a success from every angle. The superintendents came in their best and the most enthusiastic convention mood. Isabel Robb presided with dignity and dispatch. Adelaide thought she had never looked so beautiful, standing there handsomely dressed as she had been since her marriage. Tall, large of frame, well proportioned, and only a trifle matronly, there was something regal about Isabel; with her sincere, pansy blue eyes, gracious smile, perfect teeth, and strong but well-modulated voice, she seemed born to command. No wonder Lavinia Dock's father called her "Juno."

The papers read at the meeting were timely, and a feeling of unity and harmony prevailed. Adelaide Nutting was elected president for the next year. Then the most thrilling moment came. Dr. Richard Olding Beard announced that the University of Minnesota had approved the establishment of a school of nursing. The audience rose to its feet, applauding the news. Mrs. Robb shed tears of joy. To Adelaide beside her, this was indeed a dramatic event in nursing history.

"I was not ashamed to have you see me cry," Isabel later told Dr. Beard. "My tears came from a deep well of gratitude." Dr. Beard smiled, for it had been Isabel Robb's enthusiasm that had led him to become an exponent of the university approach to nursing education.[38]

On her way home from the convention, Adelaide stopped over in Chicago and Cleveland to talk to small groups of nurses about the work at Teachers College. After four or five days of hard work in

[37] Margaret Breay and Ethel Gordon Fenwick, *History of the International Council of Nurses* (Geneva: International Council of Nurses, 1931), pp. 65–70.

[38] Richard Olding Beard, "The University Education of the Nurses" (Report made at the Fifteenth Annual Convention of the American Society of Superintendents of Training Schools for Nurses, 1909), pp. 111–25; *idem*, "The Social, Economic and Educational Status of the Nurse," *American Journal of Nursing*, August, 1920, pp. 877–78.

New York, she went to Baltimore "to get those troublesome tonsils out." The day before she left for Hopkins, she signed a contract with the U.S. Bureau of Education for a bulletin on nurse's training, for which she would receive $200.[39]

Back in New York Adelaide spent a week "pounding" out her paper for the Third Congress of the International Council of Nurses in London. She felt that it was the "very worst" she had ever written, and was almost ashamed to send it. Knowing that the matter of woman suffrage would be coming up at the meeting, she sent along a statement: "Although I have no opportunity of expressing it in an official way, I am glad to say, personally and heartily, I support the resolutions in favor of the enfranchisement of women." She learned later that, of the forty-three persons present, thirty-eight voted in favor, two voted against, and two abstained. To her dismay, the two who voted against were members of the American delegation.[40]

Many of Adelaide's friends were becoming deeply involved in the suffrage movement. Lillian Wald kept in close touch with Mrs. Pankhurst and her daughters in London as they battled for women's rights in Britain. Lavinia Dock had been an ardent feminist as long as Adelaide had known her, and the years had only heightened her enthusiasm. Dr. Florence Sabin sent clippings from the Baltimore papers and added a note.

> The suffrage cause moves on. No one talks of anything else. We have 380 members and the league grows each day. Of the full professors on the medical side, we have all but Drs. Hurd, Halsted, Abel, Thayer, Williams, and McCollum. Of these, I believe all are in favor except Dr. Williams. . . . He told Miss Hamilton the other day that he thought the study of Latin and mathematics for girls produced diseases of women. Did you ever hear anything so preposterous? . . . We want 5,000 members this year.[41]

Adelaide's sister, Armine Gosling, was interested in securing the enfranchisement of women in Newfoundland. From time to time they exchanged clippings and magazine articles relating to the suffrage cause, but Adelaide never felt she could spare the time or energy to enter actively into the movement.

While friends attended the International Council of Nurses congress and toured Europe, Adelaide vacationed in Waterloo, "the least

---

[39] Adelaide Nutting (Waterloo, Quebec) to Armine N. Gosling (St. John's), July 18, 1909, MAN Papers.

[40] Breay and Fenwick, *International Council of Nurses*, p. 55.

[41] Florence R. Sabin (Baltimore) to Adelaide Nutting (New York), March 15, 1909, MAN Papers.

expensive place to be had." Before leaving New York she rented some of the rooms in her apartment to three summer students at $25 a month for the six-week term. This, she wrote her sister, made her feel "quite jubilant . . . hating to pay such a large rent for a closed apartment."

New York was broiling hot when I left last Monday night but Montreal was comfortably cool. I had a whole day there spent walking about the streets in company with various ghosts, men and women, from poor old Russ Huntington down to Oliver Booth and two or three school friends who faded away it seems to me whole centuries ago. I know no one in the city now, and truly I go about as one who "treads alone some banquet hall deserted." It is much the same thing too, here in Waterloo except for the human ties which survive everything in the way of absence, change, etc. The moment I step off the train at the station and see Charlie, the old affection springs up warm and alive, making me feel that the family tie is after all the strongest, most enduring and vital thing we have.[42]

As usual Adelaide took along "quite a lot of work, among other things a report for the Bureau of Education at Washington for which," she wrote her sister, "I am to be paid! Thank heaven." She found Waterloo "sweet and quiet," although Jim's two older boys, Harold and Keith, were visiting there too: "This is the second Sunday that I have girded up my loins and propelled myself to church, and have been almost narcotized with the parson's droning flight of words, words, words. And all for what—because I dare not permit Keith to stay away. So much for the disciplinary power of the child over the adult."[43]

Adelaide was looking forward to the coming school year. The new Household Arts building[44] was ready for occupancy, and there were special accommodations, classrooms, and offices reserved for the Hospital Economics Division. A School of Household Arts had been set up in the reorganization of Teachers College, and Adelaide had been given more latitude in expanding the offerings for nurses. She would have as her assistant Isabel Stewart.

Isabel and her sister Helen's apartment was just across the street from Adelaide's. After the first term, when Isabel had thought she might have to withdraw and go to work, Adelaide had been able to

[42] Adelaide Nutting (Waterloo) to Armine N. Gosling (St. John's), July 18, 1909, *ibid.*

[43] Adelaide Nutting (Waterloo) to Armine N. Gosling (St. John's), August 1, 1909, *ibid.*

[44] The Household Arts building was later renamed Dodge Hall for its donor, Grace Hartley Dodge.

secure a scholarship of $500 and had divided it, half to Isabel Stewart and half to Louise Powell, another promising student.[45] During the summer, Isabel had worked at Bellevue Hospital. Now she was returning to Teachers College to work on her bachelor of science degree and to assist in nursing instruction at a stipend of $600 a year, of which $400 would come from department funds and $200 from the Society of Superintendents. Lydia Anderson would also be an assistant, with $300 of her salary coming from the department and $200 from the Society of Superintendents.[46]

Isabel Stewart's positive, practical approach to nursing education appealed to Adelaide, and she was quick to have Isabel apply her eager, inquiring mind to the field of graduate education for nurses. Isabel had been frank in saying that the course in hospital economics was weighted with too many courses in home economics.[47] The new School of Household Arts would open up a wider range of resources along scientific and technical lines. Drs. Henry Clapp Sherman and Mary Swartz Rose were to teach new courses in nutrition, Miss L. Ray Balderston would give courses in laundering and housewifery, and Dr. Josephine Kenyon would teach child care.[48]

So far the emphasis and direction of Adelaide's work had been toward hospital administration and the preparation of graduate nurses for teaching in training schools. She realized, however, that there were other nursing specialties that might be developed if funds and personnel were available. Lillian Wald, who had come to lecture at Teachers College and had volunteered the facilities of the Henry Street Nursing Service for observational purposes, was anxious that Miss Nutting provide courses that would better prepare the graduate nurse for the kind of health work her visiting nurses were doing. There were many things a graduate nurse needed to know about sanitation, legal aid, and mental hygiene before she ever went out on a case. Although the School of Social Work, then comparatively new in the city, offered some instruction of a suitable kind, Miss Wald spoke to Adelaide about the possibility of Teachers College and the Henry Street Nursing Service working out a joint program of instruction. Adelaide wrote of this in a memorandum:

> One of my hopes in coming to Teachers College was to open some opportunities for good instruction, and for supervised field work in this

[45] Stewart, *Oral History*, 1: 120–26.

[46] Adelaide Nutting (New York) to Dean James E. Russell (New York), March 3, 1909; and James E. Russell (New York) to Adelaide Nutting (New York), March 6, 1909; MAN Papers.

[47] Taylor, "Isabel Maitland Stewart."

[48] *Twenty-five Years of Nursing Education in Teachers College*, p. 9.

branch, etc. But money was needed to pay for suitable courses for nurses, in housing, tenement inspection, social conditions, sanitation and hygiene, the health problems in the public schools, tuberculosis, mental hygiene and other pertinent subjects.

Lacking further resources of our own, virtually none of the needed instruction could be obtained through the College. I thought of the C.O.S. [College of Surgeons] then the recipient of a gift of some millions as a possible source of aid, in that some such courses might, in part, be helpful to their students and Miss Wald. Miss Wald who was one of its directors agreed to go with me to see Dr. S. McCune Lindsay to look into the possibilities of such cooperation.[49]

Adelaide was unaware that Mrs. Helen Hartley Jenkins, a member of the Board of Trustees of Teachers College since 1907, was quietly observing from afar the work that was being done there in the field of nursing education. She discussed the program's possibilities with Dean Russell and with Mrs. Robb. Mrs. Jenkins took her work as a trustee seriously. Her family had long been identified with philanthropic enterprises in New York. Her father had founded Hartley House, a West Side settlement, and her grandfather had been one of the original members of the Association for Improving the Condition of the Poor. Mrs. Jenkins saw the significance of the new venture in nursing education at Teachers College and decided to provide the means for translating its possibilities into vigorous realities.[50]

Meanwhile, Adelaide Nutting and Lillian Wald went to see Dr. Lindsay at the College of Surgeons. Miss Wald "gave all the weight of her practical experience" in supporting Miss Nutting's presentation of the problem, and Dr. Lindsay promised to consider the question carefully.

Shortly afterward, Mrs. Jenkins, a friend and admirer of Miss Wald, called to see her about another gift, whereupon Miss Wald brought up the matter of training visiting nurses at Teachers College.[51] Mrs. Jenkins seemed interested and asked several questions. On the assumption that Mrs. Jenkins might have something in mind, Lillian Wald telephoned Adelaide and told her of the conversation with Mrs. Jenkins. Adelaide went at once to see Dean Russell and told him of the call which she and Miss Wald had made on Dr. Lindsay and of Miss Wald's subsequent conversation with Mrs. Jenkins.

[49] M. Adelaide Nutting, "Notes for Isabel Stewart regarding Mrs. Helen Hartley Jenkins' Endowment," Department of Nursing Education Archives, Teachers College.

[50] M. Adelaide Nutting (New York) to Dean William F. Russell (New York), December 14, 1935, MAN Papers.

[51] Adelaide Nutting, "Teachers College Endowment," (n.d.), MAN Papers.

The dean then arranged for Mrs. Jenkins to meet Miss Nutting. Later, when Mrs. Jenkins mentioned an endowment of $150,000 to Dean Russell, he thought the amount far larger than necessary to carry out the visiting nurse instruction. Hard-pressed as always for funds, he suggested that Mrs. Jenkins make her gift to the entire nursing education program, which would enable him to shift funds formerly allocated to nursing education to other needy departments. Mrs. Jenkins conferred with Isabel Robb, and, when the terms of the investiture of December 2, 1909, were announced, the endowment provided for the creation of a separate Department of Nursing and Health. Instruction would now be offered in three fields: administration, nursing education, and public health.

When the gift was finally turned over to Teachers College, Dean Russell went to Adelaide's office and made out a simple budget, which listed the members of her staff and their salaries; the total amount was slightly less than the 4.5 or 5 percent interest on the endowment.[52] This cut to a very small sum the amount available for the new work in health education in cooperation with the Henry Street Settlement.

Lillian Wald, who always thought she was responsible for Mrs. Jenkins' interest in nursing education, and Adelaide, who shared this impression, were astonished at the dean's action. Mrs. Jenkins apparently approved, and they could only hope that the withdrawal of college funds from the department was temporary, and that, with increased enrollments and more prosperous times, these would be restored.[53]

Lillian Wald recommended Ella Crandall, then at the Henry Street Settlement, as the person best prepared to take charge of the visiting nurse phase of the nursing education program, and she was appointed. Adelaide then turned to such persons as Dr. Josephine Baker, eminently qualified in the field of public school nursing; Dr. C. E. A. Winslow, associate professor of biology at the College of New York and curator of public health for the American Museum of Natural History, an authority on sanitation; and Dr. Herman Biggs of the New York Board of Health. She asked them to give single courses or a series of lectures for which not more than $200 could be paid.

Unaware of Dean Russell's action, the nursing profession hailed the endowment by Mrs. Jenkins as a great boon to nursing education. Dr. Richard Olding Beard, head of the Minnesota University School

[52] Adelaide Nutting, "Memorandum on the Helen Hartley Jenkins Endowment," for Isabel Stewart (n.d.), *ibid.*
[53] *Ibid.*

of Medicine, wrote enthusiastically: "Mrs. Helen Hartley Jenkins of New York has set a fine example of the noble use of wealth during the life time of its possessor or accumulator and at the same time has shown appreciation of one of the most effective means of meeting the needs of the social service agencies of the times."[54] Dr. Osler wrote Adelaide congratulating her on the benefaction: "delighted to hear of your good fortune which will enable you to carry out your plans and it should be a stimulating thing to the profession throughout the country."[55]

Adelaide was puzzled why Isabel Robb had not discussed Mrs. Jenkins's gift with her and why she had not been included in the original planning. Was this another manifestation of Isabel's child-like fondness for surprises? Adelaide believed it went much deeper. There had been a coolness between them since Isabel had published an article which Adelaide considered to be based on an idea that she had sketched. Adelaide was always scrupulous about giving credit where credit was due and was hurt to think that her friend was not equally meticulous.[56] Sometime she would talk the matter over with Isabel.

Adelaide had been busy throughout the school year and was far behind in her correspondence. In September she had published an article on the "New Developments in Hospital Economics" in *The Johns Hopkins Nurses Alumnae Magazine*,[57] and she had also inaugurated a preparatory course in connection with the Bellevue and Allied Hospital Training School. Students completing the preparatory course at Teachers College could go on to these hospitals and complete their work in two years. The course included general and applied psychology, applied bacteriology, first principles of chemistry, personal hygiene, elementary materia medica and therapeutics, food production, food preparation, cookery for invalids, housewifery, principles of nursing, and social economy. The preparatory course also provided practice teaching for graduate nurses planning careers in nursing education. Adelaide had written up the course in detail for the October issue of the *American Journal of Nursing*.[58]

[54] Richard Olding Beard, "Practical Endowments," *Bellevuan*, March 26, 1910; clipping in the MAN Papers.

[55] William Osler (Oxford) to Adelaide Nutting (New York), December 21, 1909, *ibid*.

[56] Isabel M. Stewart, "Notes" (made at Chalfonte-Haddon Hall, Atlantic City, N.J., n.d.), *ibid*.

[57] September, 1909, p. 3.

[58] Adelaide Nutting, "Hospital Economics," *American Journal of Nursing*, October, 1909, pp. 27–30.

From December 30, 1909, to January 1, 1910, Adelaide attended the annual meeting of the American Home Economics Association at Simmons College in Boston. Teachers College was represented by three other staff members, Helen Kinne, May B. Van Arsdale, and Mrs. Mary Woolman. Adelaide spoke before the Dietitians' Section.

In May, New York nurses and hospitals would join the Society of Superintendents and the Associated Alumnae in celebrating the fiftieth anniversary of the first Nightingale School of Nursing with a grand salute to Florence Nightingale. Adelaide was in charge of bringing together an exhibit of Nightingaliana for display at Teachers College, a large part of which would come from the personal collection she had been building since acquiring her first copy of Miss Nightingale's *Notes on Nursing*.

When Isabel Robb came to lecture at Teachers College in January, Adelaide was not of a mind to discuss the matter that was troubling her. Isabel had asked to give the lectures on the fiftieth anniversary of the founding of Florence Nightingale's first training school because the occasion afforded her an excellent opportunity to appeal to graduate nurses to affiliate with the American Red Cross for service in times of war or disaster.

Adelaide took a few days off in February to go to Baltimore to gather up some items for the Nightingale exhibit and to attend a meeting of the Teresians with her friend Samuel S. McClure, who spoke on the making of a magazine.

With teaching, writing letters, preparing lectures, attending faculty and staff meetings, and getting ready for the meetings of the Society of Superintendents and the Associated Alumnae in May, the days passed all too quickly. Almost before Adelaide realized it, the winter snows had melted and the sun rose earlier and set later. The trees in Morningside Park had turned a soft green, and here and there among the rocks one found a crocus.

Late in the afternoon of April 15, as Adelaide was gathering up her papers to go home, a messenger boy hurried in with a telegram. She quickly opened it. It was from Dr. Robb. Isabel had been killed in a streetcar accident that afternoon. Funeral services would be held on Monday. Adelaide was stunned. Stopping by to walk home with Miss Nutting, Isabel Stewart found her in tears.[59]

The morning papers carried the gruesome details. Mrs. Robb and a friend had been crossing a downtown street. Frightened by a speeding automobile, Isabel stepped back, was caught on the devilstrip

[59] Stewart, "Notes" (Chalfonte-Haddon Hall).

between the tracks, and was crushed between two streetcars coming from opposite directions. She died instantly.[60]

Adelaide, Anna Maxwell from Presbyterian Hospital, and Jane Delano, president of the Associated Alumnae and national director of the American Red Cross Nursing Service from Washington, went to Cleveland for the funeral. Dr. Henry Hurd and Dr. Lewellys Barker came from Baltimore. There was a private service for the family and friends at the Robb home, followed by services in Trinity Episcopal Cathedral.

That night, as the train sped back to New York, Adelaide could not sleep. There were things deep inside that hurt, and she did not want to talk. Isabel's portrait had not been painted. It had been one of the first things Dr. Osler asked about the year before, when he returned to Johns Hopkins for the dedication of the surgery building.[61] Isabel must have a memorial worthy of her, a chair of nursing education or scholarships. Isabel had been only fifty, and left so many plans, so much unfinished work! At least she had known about the Teachers College endowment.[62]

As Adelaide sat in the darkened coach, surrounded by sleeping passengers, her thoughts went back to that night at Hopkins when

[60] *Cleveland News*, April 16, 1910; *Cleveland Plain Dealer*, April 16, 1910; *Cleveland Leader*, April 16, 1910, clippings in the MAN Papers.

[61] *The Johns Hopkins Nurses Alumnae Magazine*, June, 1909, p. 52.

[62] Isabel Adams Hampton (1859–1910) was born in Welland, Ontario, on August 28, 1859. She taught in public schools prior to entering the Bellevue and Allied Hospital Training School for Nurses on August 24, 1881, from which she received her diploma in October, 1883. Isabel substituted for the superintendent of Womans Hospital, New York, from 1883 to 1885; worked out of St. Paul's House, Rome, in 1885 and 1886; was superintendent of the Illinois Training School for Nurses, Chicago, from 1886 to 1889; and served as superintendent of nurses and principal of The Johns Hopkins Hospital Training School for Nurses from 1889 to 1894. She helped organize the Association of Superintendents of Training Schools for Nurses in 1893 and 1894, and the Associated Alumnae in 1896, which became the American Nurses Association later in that year.

Isabel Hampton married Dr. Hunter Robb in London in 1894. In 1898, at the Society of Superintendents' meeting in Toronto, she read a paper relative to graduate study for nurses which resulted in the establishment of the hospital economics course at Teachers College in 1899. Isabel Robb helped establish the *American Journal of Nursing* in 1899. Her major publications were *Nursing: Its Principles and Practice* (1894); *Nursing Ethics* (1900); and *Educational Standards for Nurses* (1907). She served as president of the American Nurses Association from 1897 to 1901 and as president of the Society of Superintendents in 1908 and 1909.

The mother of three sons—Hampton (born in 1896), a son who died in infancy, and Philip (born in 1902)—Isabel Hampton Robb died in Cleveland, Ohio, on April 15, 1910. See Adelaide Nutting, "Notes on Mrs. Isabel Hampton Robb," MAN Papers; Mrs. Carolyn Scholfield (Port Colborne, Ontario) to Isabel Stewart (New York), July 14, 1939, IMS Papers; and *Cleveland Plain Dealer*, April 16, 1910.

she first met Isabel. Silently she retraced the highlights of their long friendship: the first lessons at Isabel's feet, the language classes at the Berlitz School, the plays and concerts they attended together, the day Isabel confided she was marrying Hunter Robb and wanted Adelaide to succeed her as superintendent and principal of the Hopkins Training School, shopping with Isabel in London, their long talks about nursing and the organization of the Society of Superintendent's, and the Associated Alumnae, the conventions, the hospital economics course at Teachers College, and now the Department of Nursing and Health.

She owed Isabel so much; that she had ever doubted her was the torment.

XVI

The Commission of Leadership, 1910–1912

On Tuesday, April 19, Adelaide checked her calendar. The superintendents' meeting was less than a month away. She was tired from
the long trip to Cleveland, but it was no time to give way to weariness. Isabel Robb's death necessitated some changes in the program.
She was to have given one of the principal addresses on Florence
Nightingale at the joint meeting of the Society of Superintendents
and the Associated Alumnae in commemoration of the fiftieth anniversary of the founding of St. Thomas's Hospital, the first Nightingale school of nursing. There were telephone calls to make and
letters to be written. This was the second time Miss Nutting had been
elected president of the Society of Superintendents, a distinction no
other member had been given; she was determined that the New
York meeting would not fall short of expectations.

Adelaide had no difficulty in obtaining the assistance of her friends
and colleagues, especially Isabel Stewart, who was proving to be a
most capable, imaginative, and enthusiastic assistant. Dean Russell,
Mrs. Jenkins, and the other trustees were pleased to have the nursing
profession take a firsthand look at Teachers College.

On Sunday, May 8, prior to the convention, memorial services for
Mrs. Robb were held in Baltimore in the Nurses' Home of The Johns
Hopkins Hospital, and Adelaide went down to speak on Isabel's educational work. After Dr. Hurd had spoken of Mrs. Robb's work as an
administrator and of her first days at Hopkins, Adelaide, in a clear
calm voice, spoke simply and affectionately of the woman who had
organized The Johns Hopkins Training School, established its standards, and placed it on the educational basis which had enabled it to
hold for nearly twenty years a leading place among the training
schools of the world. She told of Isabel Hampton's training at Bellevue, sketching the dour picture of nursing education in those days,
with its long hours, back-breaking toil, and limited instruction. She

175

described Isabel's work in Rome, the Illinois Training School in Chicago, and the great opportunity that had been hers at Johns Hopkins, how she had aroused an unshaking loyalty in her students and had emphasized the responsibilities of the nurse and pride in the profession. Isabel Robb had insisted on uniformity in standards and performance, and had eventually succeeded in filling every post in the hospital with persons she had trained, thereby achieving a uniformity of method in caring for Hopkins patients.

Adelaide emphasized Mrs. Robb's unique role in organizing the Society of Superintendents, the Associated Alumnae, and the graduate course in hospital economics at Teachers College. She told of the books Isabel had written and of her notes for the address on Florence Nightingale at the fiftieth anniversary of the first training school for nurses. She concluded: "Every year that passes will but add to our gratitude for her gifts and devotion to her memory."[1]

On the train returning to New York, Adelaide pondered the matter uppermost in the minds of Hopkins alumnae, a memorial to honor Mrs. Robb. Of course, her portrait must be painted, but the living memorial, should it be a professorship in nursing education or a scholarship fund that would enable deserving graduate nurses to undertake further study? Jane Delano would present the matter at the Associated Alumnae meeting and Adelaide herself would bring it before the superintendents.

One of the concerns of the Committee on Arrangements had been the matter of exhibits at Teachers College. A large amount of Nightingaliana was brought together. Dr. Alfred Worcester, of the Waltham Training School, and the New York Academy loaned autographed letters and articles written by Miss Nightingale. The matron of St. Thomas's Hospital in London sent a collection of photographs and copies of portraits, and the Surgeon General's Library loaned valuable documents. Adelaide was displaying her own collection of Miss Nightingale's writings and had prepared a bibliography as a souvenir. Also on exhibit would be the Parian marble statuette of the Lady of the Lamp, by Hilary Carter, sister of Sir Arthur Bonham-Carter, who had presented it to The Johns Hopkins Training School. In addition to the historical items, there would be exhibits of occupational therapy, featuring weaving, carving, painting, pottery, and rugs loaned by Dr. Hubert J. Hall of Marblehead, Massachusetts.[2]

---

[1] Adelaide Nutting, "Memorial Service for Isabel Hampton Robb, May 8, 1910," *The Johns Hopkins Hospital Bulletin*, August 1910, pp. 252–54.

[2] Adelaide Nutting (New York) to Dr. Hubert J. Hall (Marblehead, Mass.), February 10, 1910, MAN Papers.

On the morning of May 17, the Society of Superintendents held its opening session at the Academy of Medicine. After the invocation, Adelaide introduced Dr. John Finley, president of the College of the City of New York, who welcomed the nurses and paid tribute to Florence Nightingale. After Georgia Nevins' response, Adelaide began her presidential address with a brief tribute to Isabel Hampton Robb, "to whose broad vision we owe so much, as a friend and comrade, at the same time tribute is being paid to Florence Nightingale."[3]

In the course of the morning Adelaide introduced Mrs. Helen Hartley Jenkins, who had recently given an endowment of $150,000 to carry on the work in nursing education at Teachers College. Mrs. Jenkins was greeted with a standing ovation. When the applause died down and the audience was seated, Adelaide announced that Mrs. Jenkins favored a memorial to Mrs. Robb and in her honor was presenting a scholarship of $250 in nursing education at Teachers College for the academic year 1910–11. Before the meeting adjourned for lunch, a cablegram was dispatched to Miss Nightingale, now in her ninetieth year.

The meeting moved to Teachers College on Wednesday afternoon, and the Associated Alumnae, who were to convene the next day, were invited to join the superintendents for the lectures, exhibits, and reception. In welcoming the nursing organizations, Dean Russell spoke enthusiastically of the hospital economics course, which the superintendents had underwritten, and predicted a glowing future for nursing education under the new endowment. At the conclusion of the addresses a reception was held and the visitors were invited to inspect the new household arts building and the exhibits.[4]

The grand climax of the conventions came with an evening of tribute to Florence Nightingale. So much interest was manifested that it was necessary to rent Carnegie Hall for the event. The stage was decorated with American and German flags and palms. Honoring Miss Nightingale, a Union Jack with a wide black band in memory of the late King Edward VII hung in the center. The main floor was reserved for the nursing organizations and the balconies and boxes for distinguished guests. On the platform were officers of the societies, boards of trustees of various hospitals, the speakers, and prominent friends of nursing. At the back sat the surpliced choirs of St. George's and St. John the Divine. Joseph Choate, the great jurist and until recently ambassador to the Court of St. James, spoke on "What Florence Nightingale did for Mankind." Colonel John Van R.

[3] Nutting, "Memorial Service for Isabel Hampton Robb."
[4] American Journal of Nursing, July, 1910, pp. 760–72.

Hoff's speech was entitled "The Soldier Nurse." Then the cablegram dispatched to Miss Nightingale earlier in the day was read:

> Representatives of 1,000 training schools and 26,000 nurses in the United States assembled in your honor on the Fiftieth Anniversary of your founding the first school for nurses, desire to send you a message of admiration, gratitude and affection. They cherish your name and example as a guiding star in their profession.[5]

The choirs sang, and the conventioners went home pleased with the beauty and dignity of the service.

Early the next morning Adelaide was on her way to address the Associated Alumnae on the work of Mrs. Robb. Again she outlined Isabel's strengths and character, her pleas for uniformity and standards in training, her gift for planning and organization, her accomplishments, the dreams she left to be fulfilled by others, and the great debt of the nursing profession to a great leader. She reported the new departmental organization in nursing education following the gift of Mrs. Jenkins and repeated Mrs. Jenkins's offer of a scholarship to a nurse for the year 1910–11 in honor of Mrs. Robb.

Before the nurses adjourned they approved setting up $50,000 as a memorial to Isabel Robb. Adelaide, who had first thought of an endowed chair of nursing education, agreed that scholarships from $150 to $500 would bring greater benefits to the profession. Before adjournment, $2,136 was pledged.

The gavel of adjournment had barely sounded when Adelaide summoned Isabel Stewart to her office to begin the routine post-convention task of writing letters of appreciation to all who had helped with the convention, the program, the exhibits, the reception, and the meeting in Carnegie Hall. The entire May issue of the *Teachers College Record* was given over to "The Education of Nurses and the Function of the Hospital." For it Adelaide had written "A Brief Account of the Course in Hospital Economics," and Isabel Stewart had submitted an article on the "Problems of Nursing Education." Dr. Richard Olding Beard's address on "The University Education of the Nurse" at the convention in Minneapolis was reprinted. Anna Alline wrote an article on "The State Supervision of Training Schools for Nurses," and Dr. Henry Hurd of The Johns Hopkins Hospital contributed one on "The Relation of the Hospital to the Community."[6]

---

[5] *Ibid.*, February, 1911, pp. 331–57.
[6] *Teachers College Record*, May, 1910, pp. 1–57.

Adelaide was proud of the record of nursing education at Teachers College. In the twelve years since the first two graduate nurses had enrolled in the hospital economics course, ninety-one had entered, of whom ten had dropped out for various reasons. Seventy-two had received the certificate at the end of a year; eleven had received the diploma for two years of study; three had remained for a third year to pursue some special study; two had received the bachelor of science degree; and one was working toward her master of arts degree.

Students in the nursing program had come from twenty states and five foreign countries; thirteen had come from Canada and five from England. They were graduates of fifty-three training schools, ranging from New York hospitals and Johns Hopkins as far west as the schools in Chicago and Winnipeg. Graduates of the hospital economics course were in constant demand. One was serving as a state inspector of training schools, ten were now hospital superintendents, twelve were training school superintendents, and eight were doing social service and school nursing. During a period of two and a half years Adelaide received 208 requests to recommend graduates for positions as hospital superintendents, training school superintendents, instructors for probationers, supervisors of district nursing, social service nurses, visiting nurse teachers, instructors or teachers for mothers, dietitians, matrons, and housekeepers, most of which represented important areas where women of training and ability were needed.[7]

Meanwhile, Adelaide was working on the report for the U.S. Office of Education. The more she worked on the project, the more intriguing its ramifications became, and she asked for an extension of time. The report offered her a great opportunity to focus attention on the status of training schools for nurses. She wanted to go into the subject deeper and to make recommendations as thorough and provocative as Abraham Flexner's report on medical education in the United States and Canada had been for the Carnegie Foundation for the Advancement of Teaching.[8] Adelaide's funds were limited, however, and she was forced to rely on the questionnaire and to draw her conclusions from them rather than from on-the-spot observations. She hoped that some foundation, perhaps Carnegie, might advance funds for a more exhaustive study.

While preparing an article, "Isabel Hampton Robb: Her Work in Organizations and Education," for the October issue of the *American*

[7] *Ibid.*, pp. 1–7.

[8] Abraham Flexner, *Medical Education in the United States and Canada*, Bulletin no. 4 (New York: Carnegie Foundation for the Advancement of Science, 1910).

Journal of Nursing, word came that Miss Nightingale had died on August 13 in London. Adelaide's thoughts again turned to a memorial, a question which would undoubtedly be taken up at the International Council of Nurses' congress in Cologne in 1912.[9] She wanted very much to attend this convention because Sister Agnes Karll, who was translating the Nutting and Dock *History of Nursing* into German, had been elected president.

Sister Agnes' vision for nursing was as broad and far-reaching as that of Isabel Robb. In 1903 she and thirty trained German nurses had founded a nursing organization; four years later it had a membership of 1,400 nurses.[10] Sister Agnes was now in Switzerland working on the translation. Through Sister Elizabeth Kollman, Sister Agnes had met Herr Consul Vohsen, of the Dietrich Reimer Press, who agreed to publish the book at cost. A literary critic from the firm would go over the translation. The profits from the book would be turned over to the sick and pension funds of the German Nurses Association.[11]

When the September *Journal of Nursing* announced that Isabel Robb's text on nursing was being translated into Chinese, Adelaide remarked, "How far this little candle sheds its light!" Three months later a postcard from Lavinia Dock brought word that Volume I of the German translation of *History of Nursing* was off the press. "Have you received a copy? It is bewitching!"[12]

Since coming to Teachers College Adelaide had been writing articles on nursing education, but it was not until the Dean's Office requested a list of faculty publications from January 1, 1910, to January 1, 1911, that she realized how many articles she had written in a single year. Listing them, she found there were nine, which compared favorably with the most prolific of her colleagues.[13]

[9] Adelaide Nutting, "Isabel Hampton Robb: Her Work in Organizations and Education," *American Journal of Nursing*, October, 1910, p. 19. In 1909 the International Council of Nurses voted to hold meetings every three years instead of every five.

[10] Editorial, "Sister Agnes Karll," *British Journal of Nursing*, July 13, 1907, p. 30; clipping in the Department of Nursing Education Archives, Teachers College.

[11] *American Journal of Nursing*, February, 1911, p. 381.

[12] Lavinia Dock (New York) to M. A. Nutting (New York), December 27, 1910, MAN Papers.

[13] "List of Publications by Adelaide Nutting, January 1, 1910, to January 1, 1911" (prepared for W. Dawson, Columbia University), *ibid.*:

    1. Review of Waters, "Visiting Nurse in the United States," *Survey* XXIII (February 2, 1910), 725–6.
    2. "Social Services of the District Nurse," *Household Arts Review* II (April, 1910), 8–15.

The extent to which she was involved in committee work was almost as startling to Adelaide as it was to Dean Russell when in December, 1911, he asked for a list of current committee activities, both on and off campus. She listed: chairman, Committee on Education, American Society of Superintendents of Training Schools for Nurses; chairman of the Society of Superintendents' Committee on Nursing and Society Work and a member of its Committee for Prevention of Infant Mortality; member, Committee for Prevention of Blindness, New York Association for the Blind; member, Committee on School Lunches, New York Public Education Association; member, Executive Committee, Nurses Associated Alumnae; member, Council, American Society of Superintendents of Training Schools for Nurses; member, Advisory Council on Nurses Training Schools, New York Education Department; chairman, Education Committee, International Council of Nurses. Under current publications she listed "Educational Status of Nurses," her study for the U.S. Office of Education.[14]

The Jenkins endowment made it possible to employ Ella Phillips Crandall, a graduate of "Old Blockley" (Philadelphia General Hospital) and a member of Lillian Wald's Henry Street staff, to develop courses in district nursing and health protection.[15] With two regular staff members, two assistants, and special lectures, Adelaide began to plan more ways in which Teachers College could be of service to nursing. For instance, occupational therapy could be easily developed by utilizing the resources of the manual arts and crafts center.

As for lightening her own load of responsibilities, Adelaide saw slight prospect. In 1910, when Helen Scott Hay resigned as chairman

3. "Nursing and Health," *Cleveland Visiting Nurses Quarterly* II (April, 1910), 10–13.
4. "Nursing Conventions and Nightingale Anniversary," Guest Editorial, *Survey* XXIV (June 4, 1910), 263–4.
5. *Bibliography of Florence Nightingale's Writings.* (Privately printed, May, 1910.)
6. "Florence Nightingale, O.M.: In Memoriam," *The Johns Hopkins Hospital Nurses Alumnae Magazine* (June, 1910).
7. "Isabel Hampton Robb," *The Johns Hopkins Hospital Bulletin*, August 21, 1910.
8. "Isabel Hampton Robb: Her Work on Organizations," *American Journal of Nursing* XI (October, 1910), 9–25.
9. "Problems of Nursing Education" (with Isabel M. Stewart), *Teachers College Record* XI (October, 1910), 7–26.
10. *Geschiste der Krankenflege* (in collaboration with L. L. Dock), tr. Agnes Karll, vol. I (Berlin: Dietrich Reimer, 1910).
14 Adelaide Nutting (New York) to Dean James H. Russell (New York), December 31, 1911, Department of Nursing Education Archives, Teachers College.
15 Mary M. Roberts, *American Nursing: History and Interpretation* (New York: Macmillan, 1954), p. 67.

of the Society of Superintendents' Committee on Education, Adelaide agreed to serve and to investigate the matter of preliminary instruction in nursing schools. She sent questionnaires to 230 hospitals having training schools, but when only 125 replied she did not feel conclusions would be warranted. She did learn, however, that eighty-four schools with preparatory courses in 1910 had not had them in 1905, and that the length of the preparatory period was usually three months. The curriculum uniformly consisted of anatomy and physiology, bacteriology, hygiene, materia medica, dietetics and cookery, and practical nursing. Only three schools offered courses in chemistry. Only five charged tuition.[16] It was quite evident that much work lay ahead for nursing's leaders.

Adelaide was by now quite accustomed to academic procedures. She could hold her own in a discussion, making logical and worthwhile contributions, and had become known as a person who got things done. Dr. Maurice A. Bigelow, director of the School of Practical Arts, referred to her as "General Nutting." Years later Dr. Thomas Briggs, professor of secondary education, wrote a vivid description of her.

> [Miss Nutting was] in a sense unique, since she had made respectable a non-academic department. She first made an impression on me when in faculty meeting she uttered convincing common sense, which contrasted pleasingly with the commonplaces and the echolalia so often heard.
>
> After a professional relationship had been established, I ventured to ask if my wife and I might make a social call. Permission was granted so graciously that we felt we were already going to see an established friend. She was such a *grande dame* that instead of shaking her hand at greeting and leaving I always kissed it and felt honored at being permitted to do so.
>
> . . . She had dignity that did not conceal charm. Although full of ideas on a wide variety of topics, she drew out her friends to express what they themselves thought and felt. . . . When a caller left Miss Nutting's apartment, his mind was excited not only by what she had said but what she had inspired him to say.[17]

Adelaide's friendship with Lillian Wald and her interest in cultural and civic affairs brought, in the fall of 1910, an invitation to join the Cosmopolitan Club, a membership she maintained proudly for nearly twenty-five years. The Cosmopolitan Club included women who were prominent in the arts, law, medicine, theater, and finance, and pro-

16 Adelaide Nutting, "Report of Committee on Education, American Society of Superintendents," MAN Papers.

17 Thomas H. Briggs, "Notes on Miss Adelaide Nutting, for Helen Marshall," 1964, Marshall Papers.

vided a pleasant place to dine with friends or entertain guests. Adelaide enjoyed the companionship of stimulating persons, and the Cosmopolitan, as well as the Arundel Club in Baltimore, provided some of her happiest associations.

At Teachers College Adelaide missed the full community life that had been hers in Baltimore. She had lived and worked within the walls of a great and famous hospital and had shared to the utmost its sleepless energy, its physicians, nurses, medical students, student nurses, and patients working as one great family.

> The college seemed just a little empty and the members a bit remote, aloof. This was more noticeable among the women than among the men, and it finally seemed to me to be due, among other things, to the fact that no place was provided either in the college or out of it where the women of the faculty could get together. It was difficult to make friendships or to build up much real companionship . . . when the only place one could meet one's fellows was in the corridors.[18]

Thus, she invited Patty Hill, Willystine Goodsell, Mary Woolman, Helen Kinne, and a few other women teachers to her apartment to discuss the possibility of forming a faculty women's club. A winter was spent trying to work out a plan, and a series of dinners was held to interest others. Counting the women teachers at Barnard, Teachers College, Horace Mann and Speyer School, and the women in administration, there was a potential membership of 130.

It was the custom of the trustees to entertain the faculty at an annual dinner prepared and served by the students of the Department of Foods in the School of Practical Arts and to make this an occasion to discuss college matters. At one of these annual dinners Dean Russell brought up the matter of quarters for a faculty women's club. Subsequently, Mrs. Jenkins offered rent free some rooms in a first-floor apartment at 50 Morningside Drive, and the women then got together the funds needed for furnishings. When the formal organization of the Faculty Women's Club was effected in 1912, Adelaide was elected president, and Virginia Gildersleeve, of Barnard, was elected vice-president. In appreciation of her contribution, Mrs. Jenkins was made honorary president.[19]

Believing that her students should cultivate social and professional interests, Adelaide invited her staff and the twenty students currently

[18] M. Adelaide Nutting, "Address at the Lighting of the Fireplace at the Faculty Women's Club House, Columbia University, February 9, 1925," MAN Papers.
[19] Ibid.; see also unidentified clippings, ibid.

enrolled to meet with her in Whittier Hall on Wednesday, November 2, 1910, to consider the formation of a departmental club. The idea appealed to the students and they decided to meet monthly, to pay dues of twenty-five cents, and, instead of organizing formal programs, to submit topics they would like to have discussed. The name, Isabel Hampton Robb Club, proved cumbersome and was soon changed to the Nurses' Club.[20] The topics first submitted for discussion were "Military Discipline in Training Schools" and "Woman Suffrage."

Adelaide always found a haven of peace and friendliness at the Henry Street Settlement House, where on Sunday evenings she ate with Lillian Wald, Lavinia Dock, and one or two other friends. The conversation often ran the gamut from public service to grand opera and back again. Adelaide would plead for improvements in hospitals and training schools, while Lillian pleaded for more and better-trained public health nurses.

The training of the visiting nurse or public health nurse was of great concern to Adelaide. Although the visiting nurse primarily ministered to the sick, she was concomitantly a teacher of health, advising families how to prevent the spread of disease and demonstrating the need for fresh air, cleanliness, proper feeding, and sanitation. Adelaide often paraphrased Ellen Richards: "Our laboratory wisdom must reach the street, the visiting nurse must become the middleman of science."[21] She foresaw the day of greater specialization and believed that training schools must be prepared to meet the challenge. For her own department at Teachers College, the changing pattern of nursing services had special meaning. Lillian Wald began to agitate for a national public health organization, a group apart from the two existing nursing organizations. By 1911 approximately three thousand nurses were engaged in public health work under state, municipal, county, or private agencies such as that organized in 1909 by the Metropolitan Life Insurance Company, which now employs more than four hundred nurses in the United States and Canada.[22]

The late winter and spring of 1911 raced by. Lillian Wald, home from her trip around the world with Ysabella Waters, had given seven lectures to the students: "The Development of District Nursing: Relation to Public Welfare"; "Infant Mortality"; "Home Care Ad-

[20] Record book given by Adelaide Nutting to the Isabel Hampton Robb Club, Department of Nursing Education Archives, Teachers College.
[21] Adelaide Nutting, "Training of Visiting Nurses," Transactions of the Fifteenth International Congress on Hygiene and Demography (Washington, D.C.: Government Printing Office, 1913), pp. 1–7.
[22] Roberts, American Nursing, pp. 86–88.

vantages vs. Institutional Care"; "Methods of Organizing Visiting Nurse Associations: Expansion and Extension"; "Duties of Officers and the Financing of District Associations"; "Milk Stations"; and "Care of Convalescents." These lectures provided a fine orientation to public health nursing.[23]

The terrible fire in the Triangle Waist Factory, in which 143 girls died, heightened Lillian Wald's and Adelaide Nutting's conviction that not enough was being done to protect the lives of workers. Adelaide promptly started a campaign at Teachers College to raise funds to help the victims' families, while Miss Wald sought more stringent regulations to protect the city's workers.

In late May, 1911, Adelaide went to Hopkins to attend commencement exercises, the alumnae reunion, and to pay tribute to Dr. Henry Hurd, who was retiring after twenty-two years of service as superintendent of The Johns Hopkins Hospital.[24] She had already written an editorial on Dr. Hurd's work for the March issue of *The Johns Hopkins Nurses Alumnae Magazine*.

Adelaide was always happy to return to Hopkins, where she had "found herself" and spent sixteen congenial, work-laden years. In retrospect, only the joyous incidents stood out. Baltimore was warm and hospitable with its newly emerging summer beauty of green grass, bright flowers, and heavily leafed and shady trees. Some members of the class of 1891 always returned: Evelyn Pope Lord, Marion Turner Brockaway, and Susan Read Thayer, who lived in Baltimore, and Georgia Nevins from Washington. In addition, many of Adelaide's students attended. One of them, Elsie Lawler, class of 1899, was now superintendent of nurses and principal of the training school at Hopkins. Miss Lawler was a strong, friendly, conscientious person who got along well with the doctors, patients, nurses, and students, and whose first thought was the care and comfort of the patients.[25]

Adelaide promised Georgia Nevins she would spend a few weeks of her vacation with her at a resort in Maine before making a visit to her brother's home in Waterloo. This year Adelaide had to choose

[23] Lillian Wald (New York) to Adelaide Nutting (New York), February 8, 1911, New York Public Library.

[24] *The Johns Hopkins Nurses Alumnae Magazine*, June, 1911, p. 57.

[25] Elsie Mildred Lawler (1873–1962) entered The Johns Hopkins Hospital Training School in 1896 and graduated in 1899; from 1899 to 1906 she served as head nurse, night superintendent, and assistant superintendent. On March 10, 1910, Miss Lawler became superintendent of nurses and principal of the training school at Hopkins. During her superintendency, 1,796 nurses were graduated. She retired in 1940. Ethel Johns and Blanche Pfefferkorn, *The Johns Hopkins Hospital School of Nursing* (Baltimore: The Johns Hopkins Press, 1954), pp. 180–238.

between the Fourteenth Annual Convention of the Associated Alumnae in Boston and the Society of Superintendents' meeting in Chicago because the two were being held at the same time. As a member of the Alumnae Council she felt it was her duty to go to Boston. Both societies were considering reorganization and a change of name, but more important was the Associated Alumnae's plan to buy up the stock of the original shareholders of the *American Journal of Nursing,* a proposition which had been under consideration for several years. In 1904 Lavinia Dock had donated a share to the Associated Alumnae in the hope that the other shareholders would do the same, but not all of them were willing to give away the shares for which they had denied themselves necessities, and it soon became apparent that most of the shares would have to be purchased.

The Associated Alumnae convened in the famous Park Street Church on June 3 and 4, 1911, and it proved to be a historic gathering. The articles of incorporation were affixed to the constitution, and the organization emerged with the name the American Nurses Association (ANA). Helen Hartley Jenkins, who had contributed so generously to Teachers College, nursing education, and public health, was made an honorary member. Adelaide was named to the Program Committee for 1912.[26]

Between the nurses' meeting in Boston and the home economics meeting at Lake Placid, Adelaide returned to New York to work on her survey of the status of nursing, for which she had been under contract to the U.S. Office of Education since 1909. Originally, Adelaide was to have completed the work in ninety days and been paid $200 for her labors.[27] The longer she worked on the survey, however, the more facets she wished to explore. In February, 1910, she wrote Ellsworth Brown, U.S. Commissioner of Education, that she would try to complete the survey by July. On July 15, 1910, she wrote him that she was so dissatisfied with what she had written that she was not willing to have it published.[28] Again an extension of time was granted, with the stipulation that the money would lapse if the manuscript were not submitted by July 1, 1911. Response to the final questionnaire had been slow, but as a result of follow-up letters,

[26] *The Johns Hopkins Nurses Alumnae Magazine,* June, 1911, pp. 80–85; Blanche Pfefferkorn, "Nursing Organizations in the United States: Their Origin, Purpose, and Some of Their Results," *Modern Hospital,* February, 1917, p. 2.

[27] "Contract between Adelaide Nutting and Elmer Ellsworth Brown, representing Bureau of Education, Department of Interior, Washington, D.C., June 19, 1909," MAN Papers.

[28] Adelaide Nutting (New York) to Elmer Ellsworth Brown (Washington, D.C.), July 15, 1910, *ibid.*

a large percentage of the schools agreed to fill out the questionnaire. Since more than 1,100 schools were participating, organizing and interpreting the answers to several hundred questions was a grilling task.

On June 24, 1911, Adelaide mailed the manuscript, but requested that it be sent back later so that additional information might be added. Isabel Stewart breathed a sigh of relief at the prospect of clearing the office of those unsightly baskets of questionnaires, letters, and tabulation sheets. Nothing would be thrown away, just put out of sight, Adelaide was assured, as she prepared to leave for Lake Placid.

Meanwhile, exciting news had come from England. Dr. Osler had been invested with the title of baronet on the occasion of the coronation of George V. Canada had only one other baronet. How strange yet delightful to say "Sir William and Lady Osler." Adelaide joined with other Canadians in congratulations.[29]

Prior to the Lake Placid Conference on Home Economics, Adelaide read student papers and examinations at the college and held the traditional convocation of her nursing education students, in which she talked intimately of the problems and responsibilities of nursing and charged her students "to live up to the high calling of their profession."

Adelaide always looked forward to the Lake Placid conferences, where there were seldom more than forty or fifty persons in attendance. The cool, fresh air of the Adirondaks was invigorating, the papers read were pertinent, and the discussion was stimulating. Adelaide's topic was "General Problems in Administrative Work." She decided to present first the field of administration, then the new avenues, and finally the growing tendency toward specialization, especially in nursing. In 1885 perhaps 100 institutions in America could rightfully be called hospitals; by 1910 the number was well above 6,000. With hospitals, college dormitories, clubs, settlements, hotels, apartment houses, and lunchrooms shared the need for organization and skillful housekeeping, which in turn called for an educated administration.

To Adelaide the hospital was a center for study, experiment, and the application of new discoveries in food and nutrition, theories and methods. The dietitian in a hospital often had to plan as many as five menus: one for non-paying patients; one for paying patients in the wards where the per capita allowance might be from eleven cents

[29] Harvey Cushing, *Sir William Osler*, 2 vols. (Oxford: Clarendon Press, 1925), 2: 275–83.

to forty or fifty cents a day; one for the private patients, where choice and combination had to "satisfy people accustomed to such standards in their own homes"; a simple, well-cooked, well-balanced, and tasty menu for student nurses; and a fifth menu, hearty and generous, for the hospital helpers, groundsmen, and janitors. Adelaide appealed for trained dietitians who not only understood cooking and nutritive properties of food and were not content to order by telephone, but who studied market conditions, prices, and quality, and had a knowledge of sanitary precautions in storing and preparing foods.[30]

There was something very sociable about the Lake Placid meetings, relaxed yet stimulating. After the formal sessions the discussions continued in groups of five or six in a corner of the porch, under a tree, or in a protected spot overlooking the lake. Adelaide felt she came to know her colleagues better in this quiet give-and-take atmosphere. Professor Benjamin Andrews and his wife seldom missed a meeting. Among the new people who came from time to time was Katharine Fisher, a teacher of home economy at McDonald College, Ste. Anne de Bellevue, Quebec, who so impressed Adelaide that she hoped she would sometime join the Columbia staff. This year Adelaide missed Ellen Richards, who had died the past March. They had first met when Adelaide was struggling to inaugurate a diet kitchen with student help at Hopkins, and the past January Mrs. Richards had lectured to the nursing education students at Teachers College. Adelaide had no responsibilities for this conference, but at the conclusion of the deliberations she was named chairman for the next year. She had some misgivings about taking on the responsibility, but, when the Deweys assured her they would help, she could not refuse.[31]

It was August before Adelaide and Georgia Nevins left for Ogonquit on the first of many vacations they were to spend at this lovely resort, reading, walking along the beach, sky and water gazing, meeting other vacationers, and occasionally joining them for a game of whist or bridge.

At Waterloo things were little changed. Charlie and Lizzie were beginning to show their age, but on the whole their health was good. Lizzie still kept up with her church and temperance work, and taught a Sunday school class; Charlie was busy with his law practice and in the evenings read or played cards with his old cronies. On pleasant afternoons Adelaide and Lizzie went for long drives in the country,

[30] Adelaide Nutting, "General Problems in Administrative Work" (Paper given at the Lake Placid Conference, Essex County, N.Y., June 28–29, 1910), printed in the *Journal of Home Economics*, November, 1910, pp. 477–83.

[31] *Journal of Home Economics*, October, 1911, p. 408.

north toward the Shefford hills or south to Frost Village. Sometimes Lizzie's friends came for tea, but, as always, Adelaide soon found Waterloo "unbearably dull" and was glad for an excuse to leave. This time she took refuge behind the unfinished manuscript of an address on "Nursing and Social Work" which she was to give in the early fall at the second annual meeting of the American Association for the Study and Prevention of Infant Mortality. She also wanted to do further work on the "Status of Nursing" manuscript. She explained further to Lizzie and Charlie that Armine, who had been in England since January putting her daughter Frances in school and seeing her husband's *Life of Sir Humphrey Gilbert*[32] through the press, was returning by way of New York and that she wanted to clear her desk of as much work as possible. It would be Armine's first visit of any length to New York, and Adelaide wanted it to be a memorable one.

Armine Gosling was a clever and brilliant woman, and Adelaide was proud to introduce her to friends at the Cosmopolitan Club and to members of the Teachers College faculty, especially those residents of Lowell and Emerson Halls who took so many of their meals in the faculty dining room. Adelaide and Armine attended concerts and plays, and in the evenings when they were at home they read and sewed together.

As soon as Armine sailed for Newfoundland, Adelaide plunged into a final revision of the "Status of Nursing" manuscript, working day and night until she became quite ill. The first week in November she went to an old familiar hotel in Atlantic City to sleep off a cold and generally recuperate. After a few days she returned home somewhat improved but then had a relapse and was confined to her apartment "with all miserable paraphernalia, inhalation, plasters, hot water bottles, shawls and sofas. . . ." No amount of exposure to medical science would ever alter her belief in the efficacy of a mustard plaster when beset by pains of pleurisy and congestion.

It was December 5 before Adelaide finally mailed the manuscript *"Educational Status of Nursing"* to the Hon. Philander P. Claxton, who then represented the U.S. Office of Education.[33] The study in its final form presented a graphic picture of nursing education, recent progress, and suggested standards and goals to be achieved. It dealt with the troublesome problems of the relation of training schools to hospitals, the requisite hospital capacity for training school mainte-

[32] William Gilbert Gosling, *Life of Sir Humphrey Gilbert* (London: Constable & Co., 1911).
[33] Adelaide Nutting (New York) to the Hon. Philander P. Claxton (Washington, D.C.), December 5, 1911, MAN Papers.

nance, special hospitals, hospital finance, education and age requirements, hours of work, length of academic work, curriculum, preparatory courses, instructors, libraries, tuition, payment of students,
state registration, and examining boards.

Adelaide documented her facts. In neat tables the reader could see
for himself the statistical record of 1,028 training schools in the
United States and Puerto Rico. The data were presented and included
the name and location of the school, the name of the current superintendent, the length of the course, the number of graduates in 1911,
the capacity of beds in the hospital, the average number of patients,
whether or not students were sent out to families, daily hours on
duty, and requirements for admission. There was a similar chart for
mental hospitals providing training. Another table listed training
schools where preparatory courses were given, the size of these
hospitals, the number of students enrolled, when the schools had
been established, the subjects taught, the daily hours given to theory
and practical work, the type of work—that is, in wards, diet kitchen,
or laundry—tuition if charged, whether or not textbooks and uniforms were furnished, and affiliation, if any, with a college or technical school.[34]

Status of Nursing was the first comprehensive study made of the
education of nurses in the United States, perhaps the first anywhere
in the world, and Adelaide tried to overlook nothing. She hoped that
some foundation would see it and be sufficiently impressed to underwrite a full-scale investigation and that administrators of training
schools would awaken to the need for standards. She little dreamed
that in less than two years the government's entire printing would be
disposed of (at ten cents each), that the study would be reviewed
widely, and that newspapers would be led to comment editorially.
Nothing more in the nature of such a study was published until the
Rockefeller report was issued in 1923.[35]

At the same time Adelaide was supplementing the *Educational
Status of Nursing*, she was preparing a study of training school committees by writing to principals of the schools of leading hospitals.
Most of the principals replied in favor of a five-member committee,
and some suggested that an educationalist and a doctor attend the
monthly meetings in an advisory capacity. Adelaide learned that

[34] M. Adelaide Nutting, *Educational Status of Nursing* (Washington, D.C.:
Government Printing Office, 1912).

[35] Isabel M. Stewart, "Notes on the *Educational Status of Nursing*," IMS
Papers; see also Joseph H. Brinker (Washington, D.C.) to Isabel Stewart (New
York), n.d., *ibid.*

Massachusetts General had a special advisory committee and that Presbyterian of Chicago had a very large committee which seldom met.[36]

Between Christmas and the middle of January, 1912, Adelaide reworked her paper on "Nursing and Public Health" for an address to be given at the graduation exercises of the Massachusetts General Hospital Training School for Nurses on January 18. She was always glad to give commencement talks and share with young nurses some of the things she had learned over the years so that they might go forward with a greater understanding and awareness of the opportunities and obligations inherent in the profession. More and more as she spoke to young graduates she emphasized the teaching function of the nurse, whether she be employed in the home, the school, industry, or as a visiting health worker. The nurse's responsibility was to prevent disease as well as to alleviate its miseries.

Adelaide invariably injected into these addresses some thought for the administrators and trustees present.

> Do we seriously believe that we can develop in our students any real mental power in their work, or expect them to maintain high ideals in it while we require of them as students ten hours of work a day of hospital work (yet these hours exist) . . . nearly fifty percent of the entire number in this country, even longer, or while . . . nearly twenty-five percent still send their pupils out into families to act as nurses, and that remuneration goes in almost all instances directly into hospital funds, and that the majority of training schools, probably not less than ninety percent, have not on their staffs one single paid instructor whose whole time is devoted to teaching students, while a pathetically large number do not own to having anything whatever in the way of a library for their students.[37]

Adelaide's survey of records from more than 800 schools showed how discouraging the situation was; 229 schools either stated they had no library or ignored the question.

Adelaide asked the new nurses to measure their strength against the obstacles to progress in nursing education and to set high standards and maintain them. "In the last analysis the great improvements in nursing must come from within. They must be brought about by nurses for nurses. . . . If we honestly believe in our work and its value to our neighbors, we will count no sacrifice too great to make that it may be strengthened."[38]

[36] Adelaide Nutting, "Training School Committee Survey Data," MAN Papers.
[37] Adelaide Nutting, "Nursing and Public Health," *Boston Medical and Surgical Journal*, March 14, 1912, pp. 401–5.
[38] *Ibid.*

Notice that she had been named official delegate to the International Council of Nurses in Cologne in August was a factor in reshaping Adelaide's plans for the summer of 1912. She had wanted to attend this particular congress ever since she had heard that Sister Agnes Karll had been elected president, but she did not see how she could get away; for the first time, a summer session for nurses was to be held at Teachers College. Isabel Stewart, however, assured Adelaide that she could take over the responsibility of channeling the students into the proper courses and of providing professional lectures and field trips. Melvil Dewey volunteered to preside at the Lake Placid conference. In February, Adelaide went to Baltimore to consult Dr. Thayer about her health. He thought she was quite equal to the European jaunt and that the trip would do her much good, so she decided to go.

Before leaving for the summer, Adelaide hoped to interest the Carnegie Foundation in underwriting a comprehensive investigation of nursing schools. Prior to making a proposal for funds she had written to thirteen outstanding medical men about the province of the nurse. "What is necessary beyond strict obedience to doctor's orders so that we may better train them?" Their opinions, she wrote, would carry much weight in shaping future training programs.

Dr. Henry Baird Favill, Chicago, replied that nurses should be trained in observation so that they could interpret the patient's condition. Dr. Theodore Janeway asked that not all nurses be trained to do the same things. Dr. George Goler, Rochester, insisted on new skills, knowledge of other therapy, since less medicine was being used; he urged that nurses be trained in the therapeutics of air, water, food, rest, recreation, pathology, and observation and asked that they be intelligent assistants to the physician. Richard Cabot of Boston wrote: "I think the nurse in relation to the doctor should be parallel to the province which in my opinion women have largely occupied in this relation to men in the more civilized countries during the Christian era. Men discover and bring home what is new; women make it useful, preserve it and criticise it. . . . Physical treatment falls more and more on the nurse." Dr. Herman Vickery of Boston concluded, "the better the intellectual training of the nurse, the better the nurse."[39]

[39] The physicians from whom Adelaide solicited opinions on the role of the nurse were: Dr. Henry B. Favill, Chicago; Dr. George W. Goler, Rochester, N.Y.; Prof. C. E. A. Winslow, New York; Dr. H. J. Gerstenberger, Cleveland; Dr. John S. Fulton, Washington, D.C.; Dr. J. F. Edwards, Pittsburgh, Pa.; Dr. Herman Vickery, Boston; Dr. William H. Welch and Dr. Lewellys S. Barker, The Johns Hopkins Hospital; the Hon. Ernest Lederle, commissioner of health, New York; Dr. Richard Cabot, Massachusetts General Hospital, Boston; Dr. Alexander Miller and Dr. Theodore Janeway, New York. MAN Papers.

In her appeal to the Carnegie Foundation, Adelaide declared that an intensive study of the system of training was imperative. The public was suffering from incompetent nursing, the nurses themselves were not satisfied with it, teaching in hospitals was outmoded and did not conform to standards in other fields of education, the relation between hospital and school was confused, there was too much turn-over in training school administration, and there was too much exploitation of student nurses by the hospitals. She cited the investigation that had already been made on the educational status of nursing and listed the areas yet to be surveyed: the fields in which nurses were currently engaged; the teaching given students whether it was by graduate nurses, paid or unpaid; lectures by doctors, paid or unpaid; the physical condition of the schools; dormitory or other housing; type of board, laundry; the financial condition of the schools—tuition paid by students, payment to students, cost per student for maintenance and teaching—and the cost of teaching students outside hospitals. The practical results of such an inquiry, she said, would provide exact knowledge of the wide variation in curriculums and practical work, as well as definite knowledge of the cost of educating nurses and the amount saved by hospitals that used student nurses. To accompany the proposal she worked out a modest budget.

Social investigator for a year	$4,000
Secretary-stenographer, postage, travel	2,000
Printing and distribution of report	1,000
Follow-up	500
	$7,500[40]

In a short time Dr. Henry Pritchett replied that the Carnegie Foundation was interested in nursing education but was not presently ready to undertake the study. It was disappointing, but Adelaide took heart that the U.S. Office of Education bulletin *Educational Status of Nursing* had not fallen on deaf ears. She received a letter from E. H. Lewinski-Corwin, executive secretary of the Academy of Medicine, inviting her to serve on a committee to investigate the nursing problem in New York. This was the same Academy of Medicine that six years before had expressed concern about the "over-trained nurse."[41]

[40] Adelaide Nutting, "Plan for Investigation of Nursing Education," *ibid.*
[41] E. H. Lewinski-Corwin (New York) to Adelaide Nutting (New York), April 12, 1912, *ibid.*

Instead of going to Chicago for the concurrent conventions of the Society of Superintendents and the Nurses Associated Alumnae, which in 1911 had taken the name American Nurses Association, Adelaide sent letters to be read by Isabel Stewart and assumed that Annie Goodrich, Lillian Wald, Mary Gardner, and Miss Crandall would be present to interpret the public health aspect of nursing. After writing two professional papers and registering nineteen nursing students for the summer school, Adelaide would go to her sister's home in Newfoundland for a rest en route to the International Council of Nurses congress in Cologne.

By 1912, there were 3,000 nurses engaged in various phases of public health nursing and it seemed that the time had come for a national organization of public health workers. Since 1908 the *American Journal of Nursing* had provided space for a department of visiting nursing, but this did not seem adequate to the public health nurses' needs. Since January, 1912, a joint committee from the Society of Superintendents and the American Nurses Association, representing 20,000 nurses, had been working on a study of health nurses. On the strength of the committee's findings, summaries were sent to 1,000 health agencies employing visiting nurses, inviting them to send representatives to a meeting to be held in Chicago in connection with the two other nursing organizations.[42]

Adelaide had no doubt that an organization of public health nurses would be effected in Chicago. It was also probable that the Society of Superintendents would be reorganized, delineate new functions, and change its name. For what actually transpired she would have to wait until she saw the newspapers, had a letter from Isabel Stewart, or talked with Lillian Wald in Cologne. That her wisdom and counsel were missed was noted in a telegram from the superintendents.

After a month in St. John's, Adelaide went on to London and then to Cologne, where the meeting of the International Council of Nurses began on August 14.

From the opening reception in the elaborate banquet hall of the fifteenth-century Gurzenich to the concluding banquet at the Hotel Disch, Adelaide was impressed with the drama of the settings, the proud hospitality of the Germans and the efforts of Sister Agnes Karll to make the congress a memorable experience. The ceremonies, the induction of the national nursing associations of India and New Zealand, the presentation of flowers, and the memorials to the great

42 Roberts, *American Nursing*, p. 87.

nursing leaders Florence Nightingale, Isla Stewart, and Isabel Hampton Robb, all of whom had died since the last congress in London, were dignified and impressive.[43]

Adelaide presided at a session on the "Overstrain of Nurses," and appeared on the program at a section on "The Social Service of the Nurse." Great responsibilities, she said, rested upon the directors of training schools.

> Against the confusions and contradictions into which nursing has been thrown by various institutions and individuals controlling or utilizing the educational system, one fact stands out sharply, there is an imperative increasing demand in every branch of nursing for better educated and more liberally trained women. If we can not under the present system find strength to pull ourselves up to a higher plane of mental power and effort, and cease to look upon nursing as a purely practical work requiring hard apprenticeship, heroic devotion, and little or no foundation in science or principles then our system must pass and a freer, more worthy one must replace it. . . . Into the hands of the teachers and superintendents of our training schools is largely committed the making of future thinkers and leaders upon whom our countries are coming to lean so heavily.[44]

Lavinia Dock introduced two resolutions which received unanimous approval: endorsement of the state registration of nurses, and adherence to the principle of woman suffrage. Adelaide promptly seconded the latter, noting that the American Nurses Association had voted solidly for it at its recent meeting in Chicago.

Adelaide found the late hours, the heavy diet, and the long meetings, with their tedious translation of papers, wearisome and exhausting, and she was glad when the conference ended. She went on an excursion down the Rhine to Dusseldorf and by train to Kaiserwerth to visit the Deaconess Mother House, where Elizabeth Fry and Florence Nightingale had studied under Pastor Theodor Fliedner. It was a journey she had wanted to take ever since Lavinia Dock had described her visit there. Now she would tread the sacred paths. Rain spattered down as the 300 delegates wandered through the peaceful little cemetery, past the graves of the pastor, his first wife, Friedreke, and his second wife, Karoline. The English nurses placed laurel wreaths on these graves, then continued on past the grave of Gertrud Reinhardt, the first deaconess, and the rows of small stones bearing the names of sisters who had toiled and died at Kaiserwerth. At the

[43] Margaret Breay and Ethel Gordon Fenwick, *History of the International Council of Nurses* (Geneva: International Council of Nurses, 1931), pp. 77–83.
[44] M. Adelaide Nutting, "Address at Cologne, ICN, 1912," MAN Papers.

Mother House the window of Florence Nightingale's room was draped with the British colors and its sill was bright with flowers. One by one the visitors ascended the narrow stairs to the small, simple room that had become a shrine, after which the guides took them on a conducted tour of the twenty-four buildings, the school for domestic training of young girls, the penitentiary, the School for Teachers, Hospital for the Sick, School for Deaconesses, the farm, and other departments.[45] Adelaide was content to walk quietly back to the tram, musing on the strides that had been made in nursing, and outlining the things she would write her sister. She had not missed a single session, and since her arrival in London had taken time to write only post cards.[46]

After the congress Adelaide and her friend Alice Boughton from Philadelphia traveled up the Rhine to Wiesbaden, where people flocked from far and near to bathe and drink waters from the healing springs, "for maladies which might not even exist." The place was gay with flowers and gardens, and Adelaide wrote that she was glad to have seen it. She looked forward to returning to America, however, to more fruit and vegetables and less meat. "I am impressed with the terrible vigor of the Germans. They are consciously or unconsciously building first rate fighting material and from superficial impressions England will need all the help her colonies can give her if she gets into a real conflict here, which Heaven forbid."[47] They spent a day in Heidelberg before going on to The Hague, Brussells, Bruges, and Antwerp, where Adelaide would board the S.S. *Finland* on August 31. Rain interfered with many of their plans for sightseeing. She wrote Armine:

> I had to leave the blessed Hague with very little of it seen owing to the incessant and heavy rains. You cannot imagine how depressing and exasperating it is to be in a city of great beauty architecturally and otherwise and full of beautiful things, and to have such drenching weather one can see nothing. . . . We left The Hague in the rain last Saturday and got to Brussells, also in the rain, but yesterday for the first time in nearly a month we had a beautiful day and we spent it in Bruges. Wonderful old peaceful canals, with their slow old barges,—these brown old churches, with their exquisite belfries and soft-toned bells—fine old squares and market places—with their magnificent old buildings, how impressive they are. I am just getting into the spirit of the thing, and off goes my steamer day after tomorrow.

[45] Breay and Fenwick, *International Council of Nurses*, p. 103.
[46] Adelaide Nutting (The Hague) to Armine N. Gosling (St. John's, Newfoundland), August 23, 1912, MAN Papers.
[47] Adelaide Nutting (Cologne) to Armine N. Gosling (St. John's), August 18, 1912, *ibid.*

Well, Brussells is a delightful city, gay, cheery, full of splendid wide
streets and boulevards—beautifully planned parks, squares, gardens,
fountains, statues, really I have grown very fond of Brussells and would
love to go back there again.[48]

Despite the incessant rain, Adelaide enjoyed Antwerp and the
beauties of the cathedral and marketplace. She liked the museum,
with its wealth of Reubens. Most of all she delighted in the Plantin
Museum, "the splendid old patrician home of the printer Plantin."
She thought how much Armine and Gilbert would have enjoyed it.
"There are the old presses with the type just as it stood, his office,
his account books, his very fine collection of other early printers—a
magnificent Gutenberg Bible."[49]

Early on the morning of September 8, the S.S. *Finland* steamed
past the Statue of Liberty. An hour later Adelaide had gone through
customs and was on the way to her apartment. The great news from
the international congress had preceded her on a post card to Isabel
Stewart: "We made Annie Goodrich president."[50]

[48] Adelaide Nutting (Antwerp) to Armine N. Gosling (St. John's), August 29,
1912, *ibid.*
[49] Adelaide Nutting (Antwerp) to Armine N. Gosling (St. John's), August 31,
1912, *ibid.*
[50] Adelaide Nutting (Cologne) to Isabel M. Stewart (New York), [August,
1912], IMS Papers.

XVII

The Portent of War, 1912–1917

By the time Adelaide had settled in her apartment, classes began. Thirty-four graduate nurses were enrolled that fall. The year before there had been twenty-three students. The announcement Isabel Stewart had helped to prepare the previous spring had grown from a two-page leaflet to a twenty-four-page pamphlet. Courses were now being offered in six major branches: hospital administration, administration in schools of nursing, teaching in schools of nursing, public health nursing, teaching and administration in public health nursing, and the preparatory course. The term "public health" nurse would replace the older term "visiting instructive" nurse, largely at the insistence of Lillian Wald, who thought the term "public health" more inclusive.[1]

Over a cup of good English tea Adelaide heard Isabel Stewart's spirited version of the superintendents' and nurses' meetings, and of the special conference on public health in Chicago. The Society of Superintendents had emerged with a revised constitution and a new name, the National League of Nursing Education (NLNE). Adelaide's letter had been read at the opening session on June 3. Isabel Stewart had presented her report on efforts to enlist aid from the Carnegie Foundation in conducting a study of training schools and had read the letter from Dr. Henry Pritchett expressing regret that for the time being the foundation could not undertake the study.

The ANA had bought up the last shares of *American Journal of Nursing* stock and was now the journal's sole owner. A board of directors elected by the association would manage the *Journal*, but Sophia Palmer would continue as editor.

[1] Isabel M. Stewart, *Twenty-five Years of Nursing Education in Teachers College, 1899–1925* (*Teachers College Bulletin*, 17th ser., February 1926), p. 8; idem, "An Outline of the History of the Department of Nursing Education," *ibid.*, February, 1920, pp. 10–11.

The NLNE would enlarge its membership to include teachers and supervisors of nurses, directors of public health nursing, members of state boards of nurse examiners, and all nurses whose work was directly concerned with education. State and local branches would be free to develop standards for training schools within the framework of state registration requirements, and the National League's function would be to help schools of nursing move forward toward a professional status comparable to that of school teachers, social workers, and similar groups.[2]

With the blessing of the NLNE and the ANA and an enthusiasm that almost astounded Lillian Wald, the National Organization for Public Health Nursing (NOPHN) was created with three classes of membership: agency; active public health nurses; and associate, composed of non–public health nurses and lay persons who would participate in discussions but would not vote. The organization followed much the same pattern that Lillian Wald had discussed with Adelaide Nutting.[3] For its first president the new organization chose Miss Wald, who had done yeoman's service in establishing the Henry Street Visiting Nurse Service, in arousing the citizens of New York to the need for school nurses, in promoting the Metropolitan Life Insurance Nursing and the Town and Country Nursing services of the American Red Cross, and in sponsoring the U.S. Children's Bureau signed into law by President Taft on April 9, 1912.[4]

The Cleveland Visiting Nurse Association promptly offered to transfer the ownership of its *Visiting Nurse Quarterly* to the new organization and to provide for its maintenance until the NOPHN could assume the financial responsibility.

Although Ella Crandall would be leaving the department to become full-time executive secretary for the new NOPHN, Mrs. Jenkins' gift would enable the department to emphasize all phases of nursing rather than just hospital and home nursing. As the department's enrollment justified, new staff would be added.

Interest in public health was growing. The International Congress on Hygiene and Demography was holding its fifteenth annual meeting in Washington from September 23 to September 28 and Adelaide had been asked to give a paper on "The Field of the Instructive Visiting Nurse in Public Hygiene." The organization's membership was inter-

[2] Isabel M. Stewart and Anne L. Austin, *A History of Nursing from Ancient to Modern Times: A World View* (New York: G. P. Putnam's Sons, 1926), p. 209.

[3] Lillian Wald (New York) to Adelaide Nutting (New York), January 16, 1912, MAN Papers.

[4] Mary M. Roberts, *American Nursing: History and Interpretation* (New York: Macmillan, 1954), p. 88.

national and was composed of various persons interested in the prevention of disease. Adelaide had heard something of its work through her old friend Dr. Welch of Johns Hopkins. Papers were to be read by scientists, statesmen, statisticians, health officers, town planning experts, and social workers. Lillian Wald had suggested that nurses be included among the speakers because of their vital role in the prevention of disease as well as in the care of the sick.[5] As a result Adelaide Nutting and Clara Noyes, superintendent of the Bellevue Hospital Nurses Training School, were invited to present papers. Miss Noyes's topic was "Trained Midwives."[6] Clara Noyes had graduated from Johns Hopkins in 1896 and was rated one of its most promising graduates. She was beautiful, charming, intelligent, and one of the "anointed"—students whom Miss Nutting had thought had much to offer, and whom she had advanced at every opportunity by recommending them for a position, a paper at a professional meeting, or a committee on which they might show their mettle.

In the five years since Adelaide had come to New York she had made many friends. The Faculty Women's Club, of which she was elected president for the year 1912–13, extended its membership to the wives of staff members, and, with the wise and generous financial backing of Mrs. Jenkins, the organization sponsored some delightful teas and lectures in the clubrooms at 50 Morningside Drive. The range of Adelaide's friendships widened. At the Cosmopolitan Club she met women who were outstanding in other professions, such as law, medicine, the arts, the theater, and philanthropic institutions. The Hopkins Alumnae held luncheon meetings from time to time, and at Teachers College there were the monthly meetings of the Nurses Club and an occasional supper with friends and an evening at the theater.

Through Lillian Wald and the little coterie on Henry Street, Adelaide's sympathy for the needy and unfortunate deepened. She learned much about practical philanthropy and local politics. The matters discussed at Henry Street were often disturbing, but one always left in an optimistic frame of mind. Lillian Wald knew who could help, and she never hesitated to ask people of wealth to share.

Lavinia Dock had not returned to Henry Street after the congress in Cologne but had gone straight to London to join Emmaline Pankhurst and her daughters, Christabel and Sylvia, in the crusade for woman suffrage. Lavinia, honorable secretary of the International Council of Nurses, soon took her place in Piccadilly, armed with an

[5] *The Johns Hopkins Nurses Alumnae Magazine*, June, 1912, p. 52.
[6] *Ibid.*, September, 1912, p. 100.

advertising board and a green bag on which "Votes for Women" was lettered in purple and white and in which she kept copies of the suffragist paper. "Votes for Women," she shouted in loud and piercing tones. "Votes for women, only a penny." Surprised by her American accent, people often stopped to stare and then, embarrassed, would buy a copy.[7] "How long will it be before Lavinia Dock has New York nurses marching down Fifth Avenue in a suffragist parade?" someone would invariably ask.

Adelaide's enthusiasm frequently involved her in far more than she realized. She committed herself to the writing of papers, articles, and lectures from one to two years in advance, and at times had to work frantically to keep her schedule, much to the detriment of her health. By the same token, and partly to compensate for this rugged schedule, she promised herself long vacations, free of work and worry. Already she was talking of another trip abroad, this time with Georgia Nevins, who had never been abroad and was anxious to go.

Again in 1912 Adelaide spent her Thanksgiving holiday with Miss Lawler at The Johns Hopkins Nurses' Home in Baltimore. It was the first time she had seen Isabel Robb's portrait since Sargeant Kendall had finished it and it had been hung in the foyer opposite her own by Cecelia Beaux. From photographs the artist had captured Isabel's youthful beauty, dignity, and charm, her lovely coloring and kind blue eyes, her full, almost smiling lips and soft, light-brown hair gently brushed back under a stiff, round cap, the familiar black uniform, with its high, narrow collar and a large pin in front, its mutton-leg sleeves, and its tight basque and girdle. Captured too were Isabel's strong, firm hands. The portrait looked just as she had looked that night so many years ago when, weary and hungry after the long journey to Hopkins, Adelaide had first seen her.

Each year Adelaide had new responsibilities thrust upon her. When William Sulzer was elected governor of New York in 1912, he was urged to apply up-state the principles of preventive medicine which had proved so successful in New York City. When this was found to be impossible under the law, the governor declared that the law must be changed so that the 1,438 local boards of health could be brought under state supervision. On January 10 Governor Sulzer summoned a committee of experts to begin at once the task of framing a new law. To this committee he named Adelaide Nutting. The committee's chairman was Dr. Herman Biggs; its secretary was Homer Folks; other

---

[7] Lavinia Dock, "On the Pavement," *British Journal of Nursing*, September 21, 1912; clipping in the MAN Papers.

members were Dr. E. R. Baldwin, John A. Kingsbury, Dr. W. E. Milbank, Dr. J. C. Otis, and Ainsley Wilcox.[8]

In one month the committee held ten public hearings, which, when typed, tallied 836 pages of testimony. Letters were sent to 1,033 local health officers, from whom 652 answers were received. Detailed investigations were made in three counties. On February 15 the committee's report was filed. Acting on the findings of the committee, the legislature reorganized the State Health Department, expanded public health services from six divisions to nine, in order to include child hygiene, tuberculosis, and public health nursing. The state commissioner of health was given power to enforce public health laws and to supervise local authorities. The legislature also created an advisory council to be composed of the state health commissioner and six members appointed by the governor; three were to be doctors with a knowledge of sanitary science, and another was to be a sanitary engineer. Although it had no legislative or political backing, no powers to enforce, could recommend but could not demand, had no staff, no operating budget, and no executive or administrative powers, the bill signed by Governor Sulzer on May 17, 1913, was hailed the greatest landmark in the history of public health since the creation of the first state health department in Massachusetts in 1869.[9]

Governor Sulzer had been impressed by the alert, imaginative woman he had appointed to the committee to frame the public health organization measure, and on March 26 he asked Adelaide Nutting to represent the state of New York at the Fourth International Congress on School Hygiene, to be held in Buffalo, New York, August 25–30, 1913.[10]

Meanwhile, as chairman of the Education Committee of the NLNE, Adelaide, with the help of Isabel Stewart, turned to the findings published in the *Educational Status of Nursing*. Of the 1,100 schools that had responded to Adelaide's questionnaire, the great majority ranked from poor to mediocre educationally and were geared to the nursing needs of the hospital rather than to the instruction of nurses. Adelaide and her committee began to concentrate on the development of a cur-

[8] William Sulzer, governor of New York (Albany, N.Y.) to Adelaide Nutting (New York), January 10, 1913, MAN Papers: "Special Commissioner to serve without pay or other compensation for purpose of collating facts relative to administration of public health. . . ."

[9] Larimore Granville, "The Public Health Council: New York's Giant Stride in Public Health," *Health News*, May, 1963.

[10] William Sulzer, governor of New York (Albany, N.Y.), to Mary Adelaide Nutting, R.N. (New York), March 26, 1913, "Commission to Represent State of New York at the International Congress on School Hygiene, Buffalo, N.Y., August 25–30, 1913," MAN Papers.

riculum which would equip nurses to meet such conditions as they might find in any type of community. Although she dreamed of autonomous nursing schools, Adelaide realized that for quite some time training schools would be controlled by hospitals. The committee thus set itself the task of defining the type of hospital which constituted a desirable teaching field.

Always Adelaide pleaded for the better-educated and better-trained nurse. In answer to a letter from Dr. John A. Hornsby, editor of *Modern Hospital*, inquiring if she favored a college education as a prerequisite to nurses' training, she wrote frankly:

> I am so far from favoring such a thing [a college education prerequisite for nurses] that I would be strongly opposed to it, as neither necessary, advisable nor practicable. Of course we need a good many well educated women in certain branches of our work, as superintendents of training schools and as assistants and teachers in such schools, educated women are necessary. Equally are they required as supervisors, and we must have training schools of such character and of standards of work as will attract these educated women and hold them through demands upon their intelligence, as well as upon their physical powers.

In her opinion, a high-school education should be the entrance requirement for training schools.[11]

Adelaide kept in close touch with Red Cross activities in Washington. After the American Red Cross was reorganized in 1910 and the new National Committee on Red Cross Nursing came under the capable direction of Jane Delano, also president of the ANA, many nurses took a new interest in the Red Cross and enrolled. To keep popular interest in the Red Cross alive and to maintain readiness for service in times of disaster, courses in home nursing and first aid would be given on a national scale. These would include ten lessons in first aid, fifteen in hygiene and home nursing, and fifteen in dietetics and household economy. Jane Delano and Isabel McIsaac, now superintendent of the Army Nurse Corps, planned to write a textbook, and Miss Marian Oliver would develop the first aid work.

Miss Oliver envisaged teams modeled after the Volunteer Aid Detachments in England. American nurses traveling abroad looked askance at units dominated by socialites who had little knowledge of real nursing. "The hope of glory, the fascination of the brassard

---

[11] *Modern Hospital*, was established in 1913; see M. Adelaide Nutting (New York) to Dr. John A. Hornsby (Chicago), November 8, 1913, *ibid.*

attract the moths and butterflies," commented Miss Dock.[12] Nevertheless, the plan received Red Cross approval and a prospectus was issued describing a two-year series of lectures on first aid, home nursing, and dietetics and a third year devoted to sanitation and hygiene. Uniformed corps were to be organized throughout the United States.

When Adelaide received a copy of the Red Cross circular she became alarmed that women completing these courses might offer their services to an ignorant and unsuspecting public. It had been to circumvent the evils of short courses and correspondence schools that the ANA and the NLNE had affiliated with the Red Cross. Other nursing leaders shared Adelaide's apprehension, and they too protested. The National Committee of the Red Cross promptly withdrew its plan for Women's First Aid Detachments, announcing in the January, 1913, issue of the *American Journal of Nursing* that all classes for women except first aid would be directed by the Nursing Service and that no uniforms for women other than nurses would be authorized by the Red Cross. If in times of calamity or war, volunteer women were needed in rest stations, to distribute supplies, or in relief work, they would be directed by the Red Cross Nursing Service.[13]

Jane Delano quickly supported her nursing colleagues. "I told the Red Cross that if this plan were put through I should sever my connections with the Red Cross, that I believe every member of the National Committee and every member of the state and local committees would go out with me." Miss Delano's stand was reassuring, and Adelaide and the other nursing leaders breathed sighs of relief. Five classes in home nursing were organized in 1912, ten in 1913, and, by the outbreak of World War I, 21,662 women had completed the course.[14]

Another peacetime Red Cross activity to which Adelaide and the nursing organizations gave full support was rural nursing. Suggested by Lillian Wald, and in large measure financed by Jacob H. Schiff, a New York businessman and philanthropist, and the Metropolitan Life Insurance Company, an experiment in rural nursing was undertaken. Nurses engaged in this work had to meet Red Cross registration requirements and had to have had at least four months experience under the supervision of a recognized visiting nurse association, such as the Henry Street Settlement or the visiting nurse associations of Chicago and Detroit. Since few nurses with sufficient training were available,

[12] Portia B. Kernodle, *The Red Cross Nurse in Action, 1882–1948* (New York: Harper & Bros., 1949), p. 62.
[13] *Ibid.*, p. 65.
[14] *Ibid.*, p. 308.

scholarships and loans were set up to attract others. The program got under way in 1913 with sixteen nurses, three of whom were preparing under scholarships, four under loans.[15]

Alert to the need, in 1913 Adelaide inaugurated a four-month post-graduate course in rural nursing at Teachers College. When the Red Cross expanded the service to include towns under 25,000 and changed the name to Town and Country Nursing Service, the course was altered accordingly. As scheduled from October 1, 1913, to January 30, 1914, this four-month course consisted of an "Introduction to Social Work," "Principles of Public Health Nursing and Industrial Hygiene," a series of lectures, conferences, and fieldwork from four to six hours weekly. Two months were allocated to work at the Henry Street Settlement, one month went to public schools and infant milk stations, and one month was spent with the Westchester District Nurses Association, where the students gained experience in village nursing. Lectures were given on such pertinent subjects as sanitation, contagious diseases, and sex education.[16] Three students enrolled in the Red Cross course; fifty-four registered for the regular course in nursing and health. The courses had barely been launched when Adelaide was asked to serve on the Red Cross Rural Nursing Service Committee. It was not unusual for one person to serve on several Red Cross committees at the same time, and Adelaide hastened to accept.[17]

In 1913 Mrs. Jenkins offered $2,000 annually to cover the salary of an assistant professor, and in 1914 Annie W. Goodrich, former superintendent of the Bellevue and Allied Training Schools and successor to Anna Alline as inspector of New York training schools for nurses, was appointed to the position. Miss Goodrich, currently president of the International Council of Nurses, was a valuable addition to the department at Teachers College. Her particular field was the administration of nursing schools. Three years in and out of Albany inspecting nursing schools, as well as experience as a postgraduate at St. Luke's, New York, and Bellevue hospitals, had given her an excellent background in her field. She was an outstanding authority on laws governing hospitals and nursing practices throughout the United States. She was brilliant, energetic, and forward-looking, quick at repartee, and had a "flashing rapier-like wit" that could be sarcastic at times. In many ways there was a marked contrast between Annie

[15] *Ibid.*, p. 77.

[16] "Rural Nursing—Red Cross Public Health Nursing," course outlines, 1914, Department of Nursing Education Archives, Teachers College.

[17] Sara Parsons (Boston) to Adelaide Nutting (New York), November 17, 1913; Adelaide Nutting (New York) to Sara Parsons (Boston), November 26, 1913; MAN Papers.

Goodrich and Adelaide Nutting, who was always remembered for her reserve, her scholarly and logical approach, firm will, and quiet charm.[18] Although their opinions sometimes clashed, they were intensely loyal and worked together for the advancement of nursing and nursing education. Annie Goodrich had been influential in Adelaide's coming to New York, and Adelaide had helped to have Miss Goodrich elected president of the International Council of Nurses.

After the Infant Mortality Conference in Washington on November 15, 1913, Adelaide talked with her old friend Georgia Nevins, and they began plans for a trip to Europe together. Coming toward the end of Adelaide's "long looked forward to and cherished sabbatical year," their trip would retrace part of a journey taken twelve years before, when Adelaide had become ill from economizing on food.[19] Although she promised herself she would make no such mistake this time, her salary of $3,000 would not permit indulgences. She wanted to see Greece and to have a feast of music in Vienna and Salzburg. Georgia, who had little experience in travel, entered enthusiastically into the plans. When Miss Goodrich found that she would have considerable time between the conclusion of her work in Albany and the beginning of classes at Teachers College, she asked to join the party. She offered to assume responsibility for the luggage on the trip, and Georgia agreed to serve as cashier, pay for excursions, lodgings, and other fees and keep financial records for the trio, if Adelaide would handle the itinerary.

On May 23, 1914, the three women departed on the North German Lloyd S.S. *König Albert* bound for the Mediterranean. The voyage was smooth and the weather pleasant. Although small, the ship was comfortable and the food was excellent. Adelaide did not find the passengers quite as interesting as those on her four previous trips. They included a number of Roman Catholic priests and bishops en route to a religious conclave; a Metropolitan tenor, with his wife and daughter, who was "carrying on a flirtation with a red-haired young siren"; a small party of tourists from California directed by a woman who did not know how to read her Baedecker maps and who mispronounced names of well-known places and persons; "a sweet-faced old lady entirely deaf and dressed like the last rose of summer, on her

[18] Esther A. Werminghaus, *Annie W. Goodrich: Her Journey to Yale* (New York: Macmillan, 1950), pp. 12–39.

[19] M. Adelaide Nutting, "Notes on Trip: Baths of Bornio, Italy," July 10, [1914], MAN Papers.

way to study the Montessori method"; and some other women from the Midwest.

> In a staid middle-aged way I am enjoying it and the anticipations of the next few months, but ah me! where is that high sense of adventure with which I embarked on anything in the days of my youth. Some beautiful and lovely thing that was always going to happen—and somehow never, never did. And yet I suppose I have had a share of life to be grateful for—the chance to work, and to grow, and as much freedom and power as I have had the sense to use.[20]

Miss Goodrich had qualms about seasickness, so Adelaide asked the steward to place her party at a table near the door. The precaution proved quite unnecessary, and too late they learned that they were to have been seated at the captain's table.[21]

An excursion ashore at Gibraltar proved hot, dusty, fatiguing, expensive, and disappointing. After walking through what seemed to be miles of tunnels they were permitted to look through a small aperture at the strait; it was so different from the pleasant drive through the Spanish countryside to the top of the rock which Adelaide had taken before. They "left Gibraltar in a blaze of sunshine" on Monday afternoon, June 1, and three days later steamed into the harbor at Naples at 4:00 A.M. Adelaide was on deck to enjoy the "blue sky, blue water, lovely little islands, a fairy like scene," which she had missed on her trip in 1902.

It was Adelaide's plan to leave Naples after spending a couple of days there and to go on to Palermo and Siracusa in Sicily, then over to Greece, to Athens and Corinth, and back to Naples by way of Corfu and Brindisi. "How shall I feel standing on Mars Hill?" Adelaide wrote, "Mars Hill, where St. Paul had preached to the Athenians on the unknown God. What of Mt. Olympus, Home of the Gods, and Delphi where their wisdom was dispersed?"[22]

In Naples they joined two "nice quiet" women from Boston on a motor trip to Pompeii, and thence to Sorrento and Amalfi. Much of this was old ground for Adelaide, but she found tea at the Cappucini Hotel and a climb to the top of a small mountain, Ravello, quite as delightful as before. They spent the night at the hotel and the next day went on to Salerno and thence to Paestum, a place Adelaide had long wanted to see.

[20] Adelaide Nutting (aboard the S.S. *König Albert*, approaching Gibraltar) to Armine N. Gosling (St. John's, Newfoundland), May 30, [1914], *ibid.*
[21] Nutting, "Notes: Baths of Bornio."
[22] Adelaide Nutting (nearing Gibraltar) to Armine N. Gosling (St. John's), May 30, [1914], MAN Papers.

Those great Greek temples deserted on a lonely waste of Italian coast, a great grim mountain behind and sea in front—no cities or villages in sight except one way up on a mountain side. No words can give any idea of the solemn beauty and charm of the scene. We spent hours there, had our luncheon at the foot of one of the pillars of the Temple of Neptune, gazing on sea and mountain, and trying as ever to think myself in the spirit of the men who made such a place for worship.[23]

By this time the three had decided to give up the trip to Greece because of the approaching very hot weather, the necessity of traveling over a great distance in an unduly short time at a great expense, and the conviction that so important a country should not be visited hastily. Adelaide resolved she would spend her next long vacation in Greece if she lived to have one.[24]

Naples had changed little since Adelaide's visit twelve years before, but it seemed less romantic. It was still lovely to look at, noisy, crowded, dirty, and colorful. She wondered if Naples seemed less exciting because she had grown older. The streets were certainly better kept, and the horses pulling wagons and carriages were better fed and more humanely treated, a result, she learned, of the persistent work of the Society for the Prevention of Cruelty to Animals. She was pleased by this and wrote a letter to the local society, enclosing a small donation. Although traveling was more expensive, Adelaide said she did not begrudge the increase, if a little more money was thereby getting into the hands of the poor.

Just as they were leaving Naples for Rome they were given an opportunity to travel by car to the great old Benedictine monastery Monte Cassino, high on the mountain top.

In Rome they found a clean, convenient pension—a beautiful room and three meals, at off-season rates, for only $1.80 a day—and they stayed for nearly ten days. From Rome they planned to go to Assisi, Perugia, Florence, Stresa, and Lake Maggiore. Adelaide was too weary to do many of the things one should do on returning to Rome, and she saw but 4 of its 400 churches. While Georgia and Annie went sightseeing, Adelaide took pleasant drives in the Borghese Gardens and in the Foria Pamphilia.

For the first few days in Rome a transportation strike hampered sightseeing. There were no street cars, no cabs, and only occasionally private carriages and taxis. The strike was soon settled, but the spirit of revolt was abroad in northern Italy, and visitors were advised to

[23] Adelaide Nutting (Palazza Moroni, Rome) to Armine N. Gosling (St. John's), July 18, [1914], *ibid.*
[24] *Ibid.*

hurry along, lest they become tied up in a railway strike. Adelaide and her companions hastened to the Tyrol and the Baths of Bornio, and from there to Stelvio Pass in an open diligence drawn by four horses.

It was a five-hour journey from Bornio up the steep mountain roads to the top. The driver stopped to rest his horses, and his passengers picked delicate Alpine flowers. At noon they reached the top of the pass and found themselves surrounded by great snow drifts through which the road had been cut. As they approached the summit a bugler in another diligence announced their arrival with "lovely silvery carolling of Tyrolese airs. It seemed as if we were arriving at some great gate in the upper world and so we were for there was the majestic Oeter just before us as we turned the corner, the highest peak in Austria, but not as high as Mont Blanc or the Matterhorn."[25] They drove down the mountain with five horses, very much in the manner Adelaide had become accustomed to in the Swiss passes. After tea at Neuspondinig they left by train for Meran and Bozen. These were typical towns of the Tyrol, "in lovely little valleys girt about by mountains," with the ruins of many old feudal castles on the lower peaks and hills. Adelaide was especially impressed by the number of chauffeur-driven cars that passed them. Later she described as quite the most wonderful and interesting thing in her experience a ninety-mile trip from Bozen to Cortina in a Royal Austrian Post motor diligence which held fifteen people.

From Cortina Adelaide and her party were going to Innsbruck and then to Salzburg for the Mozart anniversary festival, which would last ten days and was attracting the great conductors of the world. From Salzburg they planned to go to Lenz and travel via the Danube to Vienna and, after four or five days there, on to Prague and then to England and home. Adelaide was pleased to make the entire trip, exclusive of tickets over and back, for $500. She did very little shopping, unlike Miss Goodrich and Miss Nevins, who bought gifts for relatives and friends.[26]

While in Italy they learned that Archduke Franz Ferdinand of Austria had been assassinated on a visit to Sarajevo, Serbia, on June 28. They were unable to read German, however, and only Austrian newspapers were available. Little did they suspect the dire consequences of the archduke's death. The innkeepers, anxious to keep their guests as long as possible, played down any possibilities,

[25] Adelaide Nutting (Cortina, Italy) to Armine N. Gosling (St. John's), July 20, [1914], *ibid.*
[26] *Ibid.*

and no one that Adelaide consulted saw any reason why the three women should not continue their trip. On July 27 they left Cortina for Innsbruck, traveling partly by motor, partly by rail, over the beautiful Brenner Pass, arriving in Innsbruck shortly before sunset.

Noting that their train was two hours late, that several trains filled with soldiers seemed to have the right-of-way, that all bridges and tunnels were guarded, and that soldiers were everywhere in evidence, Adelaide became apprehensive. At Innsbruck the great square was filled with people shouting and singing as they bade a train full of soldiers goodbye. Notices had been posted in public places, and, despite her limited knowledge of German, Adelaide caught enough words to understand that they related to mobilization and had been issued by the emperor. The hotel keeper said only that a few regiments were being sent to guard certain bridges. Either ignorant of the situation or indifferent, he saw no reason why they should not continue, and he even allowed them to consign their baggage to Vienna.

On Thursday, July 30, the three women left Innsbruck by train for Salzburg, arriving in mid-afternoon to stay two or three days before going on to Vienna. Adelaide was uneasy, yet she had no definite reason beyond the scrappy news one read in occasional British newspapers or gathered from conversations with other travelers. No one thought there was any immediate danger, and Miss Goodrich and Miss Nevins wanted to visit Vienna and were willing to take the risk.

On Friday Adelaide began in earnest to dissuade them from going and finally said that if they persisted she would withdraw from the party. She was convinced from every fragment of information they received that a great upheaval was beginning. That afternoon, when they consulted a banker, he told them that if they waited another day they would not be able to go to Vienna or to get out of Austria. No one explained that on July 29 Austria had declared war on Serbia or that on that day Russia was mobilizing for war. The women then decided to take the next train for Munich. There they learned that the Hamburg-American Line had withdrawn all its steamers and that not only had their passage been lost but there was no certainty their money would be refunded. In Munich they were fortunate to secure first-class coach tickets on a through train to Flushing, where they could take a channel boat to England. They sat up all night with no food except some sandwiches and cherries purchased from a vendor at a station platform. Men and women were crowded into the compartment, and many had to stand all night in the train's corridors. The train was scheduled to arrive in Cologne early in the morning and at Flushing five hours later in time to catch the channel boat at

10:00 A.M., but the train arrived in Cologne several hours late and it took fourteen more hours to reach Flushing. At the German frontier, the through train became an accommodation train, and Adelaide, Annie, and Georgia found themselves dumped off unceremoniously at all sorts of strange, out-of-the-way places. They changed cars four times going through Holland, and at no place could they get a meal, only some sweet biscuits and a bottle of mineral water. At the last change they were able to buy some ham and eggs and hot tea.

At ten that night the weary travelers arrived at Flushing and boarded the channel boat, which was due to sail at midnight. It waited for one or two late trains loaded with refugees, however, and did not sail until 7:00 A.M. on Sunday, August 2. "There were hundreds on board, coming on all night, tired, hungry and anxious. The food gave out but with London in sight, no thought of that." They reached London at about three o'clock Monday afternoon and went immediately to the Kingsley, the small hotel where Adelaide had stayed before. She rushed out to buy a paper and cabled her sister to wire Charlie that she was safe.[27]

Everyone was in a dither in London. On August 1 Germany had declared war against Russia, an ally of Serbia. France was also an ally and would undoubtedly declare war. Britain was sworn to protect the neutrality of Belgium. While Adelaide, Annie, and Georgia were traveling from Cologne to Flushing, German troops were being rushed to the French and Belgian borders. Britain would have to act quickly, while the German fleet was still in the Baltic. The moment Belgium was forcefully invaded, Britain would declare war.

Adelaide had a large amount of Austrian money, which was worthless, and some American Express notes, which she feared might turn out to be worthless too. Annie Goodrich had a substantial letter of credit at Brown and Shipleys, but by special proclamation the British banks were to be closed until Friday. The women had only a few shillings until Adelaide found a former student working in a London hospital and borrowed five pounds. She also wrote to Dr. Osler at Oxford, and their immediate needs were met. When Adelaide went to the Hamburg-American office a crowd was outside and the blinds were down. The line of people at the American Express office extended nearly three blocks. The hotels overflowed with Americans carrying traveler's notes and letters of credit but no cash. Hundreds

---

[27] Adelaide Nutting (London) to Armine N. Gosling (St. John's), August 3–4, [1914], *ibid.*; to be sent on to Lizzie.

were trying to get home and were willing to go by steerage. Adelaide wrote her sister:

> I haven't been here long enough to get the general feeling but there seems to be a feeling that England can hardly help being drawn into it. The Germans appear to be war-mad, and to be anxious to fight the world. If they have Russia, France and Great Britain at one time, perhaps it may occupy them. . . . Think of us in London with no clothes but what we have carried for a week in a dress suitcase. Everything in our trunks and no hope of getting them for weeks . . . both trunks and mail bags are stacked up in railway sheds along the German frontier, trains all needed for mobilizing troops.[28]

Adelaide did not know that Germany had already violated Belgium's neutrality and had crossed the frontier to invade France from a vulnerable spot. In a few hours Britain would declare war on Germany, and three days later British Expeditionary Forces would land in France.

On Tuesday morning Adelaide, Georgia, and Annie stood for three hours in the rain with hundreds of other stranded Americans waiting to get inside the American Express office, where traveler's checks were being honored dollar for dollar. All week long thousands of other tourists would pour into London, wondering how and when they would get home.

At Teachers College many inquiries were being made about the safety of Miss Nutting and Miss Goodrich. As late as August 10 no word had been received. On the assumption that they might still be in Austria, Isabel Stewart wrote to their Salzburg address, confident that if Adelaide kept well and had enough money she could look after herself. From Newfoundland, Gilbert Gosling wired Dean Russell that he would send funds to Adelaide when and where they were needed. Miss Stewart then proceeded to outline arrangements for fall classes, in case Adelaide was long delayed.[29]

After what seemed like endless days of telephoning, telegraphing, and cabling, Gilbert Gosling secured passage for Adelaide on the S.S. *Parthenia*, a Donaldson vessel with a cargo of coal bound from Glasgow to Botwood on the Bay of Exploits, Newfoundland, about 160 miles northwest of St. John's. From there she could travel to her sister's home by train.

At the station in London, Georgia and Annie bade Adelaide a fond and brave goodbye as she left for Scotland. Although rough and

---

[28] *Ibid.*
[29] Isabel Stewart (New York) to Adelaide Nutting, [Salzburg, Austria], August 10, 1914, MAN–IMS Correspondence.

anxious, the crossing was uneventful, and she arrived safely at her sister's home on Wednesday, August 26.[30] Never had family seemed so dear, Minnie, Gilbert, Ambrose, Armine, Frances, and Arthur. Adelaide kissed each one and found herself starting all over again with Minnie. She was relieved to learn that, after tramping for a week from one steamship office to another, Annie Goodrich and Georgia Nevins had finally secured passage on the *King George*, of the Canadian Northern Lines, sailing from Bristol.[31]

When word reached Teachers College on August 15 that Adelaide was in London safe and sound, Isabel Stewart dispatched a letter to St. John's, telling her about the close of the summer session, with its fifty-one students in nursing education, and bringing her up to date on the staff. The most exciting news was that "Helen Scott Hay is organizing Red Cross nurses in New York, and it is quite probable they will go to the front."[32]

After a few days' rest, Adelaide continued her journey to New York aboard the R.M.S. *Stephano*, of the Red Cross Lines, which plied between St. John's and Halifax, Halifax and New York.[33] As the passengers talked aboard the *Stephano*, the Battle of the Marne was being fought in France, where only the combined forces of the British and the French were able to hold back the kaiser's legions. It was not until the pilot came aboard the ship as it entered the Narrows that they learned of the Allies' first victory and that, at least for the time being, Paris had been spared. Once again Adelaide stood on deck watching for the Statue of Liberty and feeling how good it was to be home again.

Classes began at Teachers College in an awesome way the fall of 1914. Since September 7 a Red Cross ship, staffed by nurses and doctors ready to go to Europe, had been waiting in the Hudson River. It did not sail for nearly a week. Meanwhile, everyone talked about the war in Europe. At the first noon-day convocation in Millbank Chapel, Dean Russell addressed himself particularly to the foreign students, reminding them that they were the guests of a neutral country. Residence in the United States was a privilege that carried with it responsibilities.[34]

[30] Clipping from the *Evening Herald* (St. John's), August 29, 1914, scrapbook, MAN Papers.

[31] *Ibid.*

[32] Isabel M. Stewart (New York) to Adelaide Nutting (St. John's), August 15, 1914, *ibid.*

[33] Adelaide Nutting (aboard the R.M.S. *Stephano*, en route to New York) to Armine N. Gosling (St. John's), September 7, 1914, *ibid.*

[34] Ethel Johns, "Opening a Door," *The Johns Hopkins Nurses Alumnae Magazine*, April, 1958, p. 26.

Seventy-one students had enrolled in nursing education, almost 50 percent more than the year before. Adelaide cast a discerning eye over the list of students; among them were a number of Canadian nurses. Soon, she feared, there would be wartime jobs to do, but for the present the students must dedicate themselves to improving their knowledge, grasping the significance of their work, and advancing their profession. Mounting the platform for the first meeting with her students, she calmly looked them over, her cool, level gaze moving from one to another, as though she wondered what they were seeking and whether they would know what to do with it if found. She spoke of the standards that had been set in nursing education. To many they seemed unattainable. "Stringent requirements," she said, "must be met before recognition would be granted to schools of nursing in any university." Collegiate schools were now the great objectives of nursing leaders, but, before attaining this status, the nursing faculty would have to show academic qualifications comparable to those of other departments. There might be compromise at first, but not for long.[35]

Adelaide had given much thought to collegiate schools. Even before she left Johns Hopkins she had discussed the matter with Dr. Hurd, and they had been in agreement on the inequities of a system which placed on students not only the burden of financing their schools but that of contributing to the upkeep of the hospital through long hours of service, and which failed to give the school a definite allocation of funds to carry out its program of education. The September, 1906 issue of the *American Journal of Nursing* carried a significant address by Dr. Hurd on the question "Shall Training Schools be Endowed?"[36] In this paper he set forth the evils of the existing system and the advantages of endowment to both hospital and school.

Adelaide kept in close touch with Louise Powell, a former student at Teachers College who in 1910 had taken over the direction of the University of Minnesota Training School, where she became convinced that, if nursing schools were to develop on a par with the professional schools of medicine, law, and theology, and do so with true academic freedom, financial independence was necessary.

The Johns Hopkins Training School, where Adelaide had studied and served as superintendent, was dear to her. She knew its strengths and weaknesses, its constant struggle against a limited staff and overworked student nurses. She longed to see it attain the stature of Isabel Hampton's dreams. Only with an endowment could the school

[35] *Ibid.*
[36] Henry M. Hurd, "Shall Training Schools be Endowed?" *American Journal of Nursing*, September, 1906, pp. 843–54.

achieve freedom and the high goals of a collegiate program. She believed the time had come for the school to seek that endowment.

Speaking at the twenty-fifth anniversary celebration of the Johns Hopkins Hospital and Training School, Adelaide said that, despite the progress made in nursing education, some of the most fundamental problems remained unsolved, most significant of which was the financial support of training schools.

> There is not a single endowed training school in the whole wide world. All training schools are self-supporting institutions. This should not be. A sounder economic basis eventually all schools should have. Every training school should have its own appropriation, prepare its own budget and be accorded an established and dignified position. . . . The hospital should not be constantly under the painful necessity of weighing every request from the training school against obviously needed things, improvements or appliances, which are the very life of the hospital. . . . Could the Twenty-fifth Anniversary of the Johns Hopkins Hospital Training School be more appropriately or justly celebrated than by beginning to provide her with a suitable endowment.[37]

Adelaide's challenge was answered. At its November meeting the Hopkins Alumnae Association responded by going on record as desiring to mark the occasion of the twenty-fifth anniversary by collecting a fund for the hospital's training school. At the annual alumnae meeting on May 27, 1915, the president, Mrs. Isabelle Stevens Hunner, class of 1900, announced that Miss Nutting had agreed to serve as chairman of the Endowment Committee on the condition that she be allowed to choose the other members of the committee. While recruiting her committee she made a study of the techniques and procedures of fund raising. Harvard was then conducting a campaign for $15,250,000, and not a facet of its drive failed to come under Adelaide's scrutiny.[38]

On December 3, 1915, the Alumnae Committee of The Johns Hopkins Training School Endowment Fund held its first formal meeting in Baltimore, each member paying her own expenses. The committee set $1,000,000 as its goal and invited Judge Henry D. Harlan, president of the Board of Trustees, Dr. William H. Welch, and Dr. Winfred H. Smith, Dr. Henry Hurd's successor, to constitute an advisory

[37] *Baltimore Sun*, October 6, 1914, p. 8, col. 1; M. Adelaide Nutting, "The Work of The Johns Hopkins School for Nurses," *The Johns Hopkins Nurses Alumnae Magazine*, January, 1915, pp. 6–18.

[38] M. A. Nutting, "Notes on Endowments: The Johns Hopkins Alumnae Fund," [1915–16], MAN Papers.

committee.[39] A circular letter was soon sent to all 716 graduates. The first appeal brought in $11,383.59 in pledges and cash. Helen Jenkins, nursing education's good friend, sent a check for $500. Meanwhile, the committee made a survey of other endowments and foundations to whom an appeal might be directed. For the next ten years Adelaide would give her energies unstintingly to the Hopkins Endowment Fund.[40]

After the meeting of the Endowment Committee, Adelaide stayed over to address the Teresians, the history of nursing club she had started ten years before. It was always a delight to address this group, to tell of the early history of the training school, to pay tribute to Isabel Hampton, Dr. Hurd, Dr. Osler, and Lavinia Dock, and to speak of the graduates scattered throughout the world who had distinguished themselves in the profession and brought honor to Hopkins. Adelaide believed that Hopkins nurses had a special mission, and she tried to imbue the students with a sense of loyalty to the school as well as to the profession.

> I wish I could find words to show nursing to you as I see it. It is one of the most tender and beautiful of arts. . . . If our work means anything, it means the reverse of anything cold, hard, callous, starched and official. Nursing is something warmer, kindly, sympathetic, generous, something to lean on, abounding in helpfulness, genuine. . . . Firmness is not to be mistaken for harshness and severity.[41]

Adelaide was especially impressed with the president of the Teresians, Lillian Hudson, a beautiful Canadian girl, charming and well poised, deft of hand and quick of mind. She was interested in public health and knew of the work being done by the Henry Street nurses. Lillian Hudson was equally attracted to the inspiring professor from Teachers College. This was the beginning of another of Adelaide's teacher-student friendships that would bring mutual strength and joy throughout the years.

The campaign for a million-dollar endowment was an ambitious undertaking, yet private philanthropy had given millions to institutions of higher education such as Harvard, Princeton, Cornell, Smith,

[39] Among others listed were Dr. Richard Olding Beard, University of Minnesota Medical School; Drs. James Murphy and George Dock, Washington University; and Dr. C.-E. A. Winslow, Columbia University. See Sara E. Parsons, "Encouraging Signs in Nursing Education," *American Journal of Nursing*, January, 1915, p. 274.

[40] "Report on the Endowment Fund of The Johns Hopkins Nurses Alumnae Association," n.d., MAN Papers.

[41] Penciled notes, December 3, 1915, "Book of the Teresians," *ibid.*

She pointed out opportunities in public health and commended the from Baltimore, Adelaide settled down to write a paper or pamphlet which would open the drive for funds. She entitled her article "A Sounder Economic Basis for Training Schools for Nurses," and wisely pleaded the cause of all nursing schools, not merely Johns Hopkins. She built her case logically and forcefully. In 1915 there were between 30,000 and 40,000 students in 1,100 training schools. She struck out against the exploitation of student nurses in hospital schools, at the long hours of repetitive tasks that had no educational value. Why should not schools rendering an important public service secure substantial aid from public funds? The article, first published in the *American Journal of Nursing* in January, 1916, was later reprinted by the National League of Nursing Education and sold in pamphlet form.[42]

Adelaide did not attend the International Council of Nurses' congress in San Francisco in 1915, nor did Lavinia Dock, the honorable secretary, who had arranged the grand tour west for American nurses and the visiting foreign delegates. The war had restricted foreign travel, and Lavinia could not bring herself to face the decimated ranks of the council. She decided to throw her strength and energy into the suffrage movement.[43] Adelaide concerned herself with the Hopkins Endowment Fund and advancing the idea of the university school.

On January 5, 1916, Adelaide read a significant paper on "The Education of Nurses" before a section of the Pan American Scientific Congress. In it she said that the ideal school of nursing was the university school. In May she gave the commencement address at the Lakeside Hospital in Cleveland. Speaking on "The Obligations of Opportunity," she pointed out that persons of high birth and social position, great riches, and great knowledge have heavy obligations to society. Wealth, she said, imposes the obligations of philanthropy, but the "supreme opportunity in this world is intellectual. The world expects much of certain professions."

> If you want to get out of prison, what you need is the key to the lock. . . . No higher obligation rests upon nurses today than to give serious and intelligent study to problems of various kinds, educational, economic and professional which have arisen in the field of nursing.

[42] M. Adelaide Nutting, "A Sounder Economic Basis for Training Schools for Nurses," *American Journal of Nursing*, January, 1916.

[43] Annie W. Goodrich (New York) to Margaret Breay (London), April 17, 1915, quoted in Margaret Breay and Ethel Gordon Fenwick, *History of the International Council of Nurses* (Geneva: International Council of Nurses, 1931), p. 114; Lavinia Dock, "Foreign Notes," *American Journal of Nursing*, July, 1915, p. 847.

She pointed out opportunities in public health and commended the efforts of Massachusetts General Hospital to secure endowments.[44]

Instead of holding annual reunions at commencement time, which was largely given over to receptions and dinners, Teachers College for many years sponsored an annual alumni educational conference in February. In addition to general convocations, some departments held sessions with informative addresses by alumni and staff, bringing the graduates up to date on developments within the department and the field.

From her experience at Johns Hopkins and with the Associated Alumnae, Adelaide knew the value of an alert, active alumnae association. In 1911, with her blessing and the assistance of Isabel Stewart, Miss Tracy, an early nursing student at Teachers College, had invited a number of graduates of the old home economics course who were living in the New York area to meet on the grounds of the Adams Nervine Hospital, Jamaica, Long Island, on the afternoon of June 6, 1911, to form the nucleus of an alumnae association of the new Department of Nursing and Health. Twenty nurses had attended and had decided that any graduate receiving either the certificate or the diploma was eligible for membership. Mary C. Wheeler, soon to become a prominent figure in American nursing, had been elected president.

Consequently, at the Teachers College alumni conference held in February, 1915, the Nursing and Health Department was well represented. Among the topics the graduates discussed were "The Teaching Problems of the Public Health Nurse," "Shorter Hours," "Existing Affiliations between Nursing Schools and Universities," and "The Training of Social Workers." Adelaide closed the session by summarizing the work that had been done in nursing education at Teachers College.

Such departmental conferences did yeoman's service for the nursing profession by anticipating issues, providing calm and dispassionate discussions, and putting facts before a large number of nurses. Later, when a decision had to be reached, informed graduates of Teachers College were prepared to advance proposals. Publicity in professional journals and newspapers heralded far and wide the leadership coming from Teachers College.

Adelaide strengthened her staff as this was needed. Mrs. Jenkins' offer of $2,000 to pay the salary of an assistant professor had enabled the department to employ Miss Goodrich. By 1915 the staff consisted

[44] M. Adelaide Nutting, "The Obligations of Opportunity" (Address given at the sixteenth commencement, Lakeside Hospital, Cleveland, Ohio, 1916), p. 12.

of Adelaide, Annie Goodrich, Isabel Stewart, and Anne Harvey Strong, who divided her time between the Henry Street Nursing Service and Teachers College. There were special lecturers, and the students also took courses from instructors in other departments.

Illustrative of the lectures was a series of five given by Emily Dinwiddie, sanitary inspector for Trinity Corporation Tenements: "Sanitary Inspection and Housing Administration"; "Inspection by Nurses, Visiting Housekeepers and Others Working with Families in Neglected Homes"; "How to Inspect and What to See in a House"; "Sanitary Problems of Rural Districts and Small Towns." The latter called attention to disposal of garbage and refuse, water, milk supply, household pests, and relations with health boards.[45] Although the lecture budget was small, devoted and interested persons such as Lavinia Dock, Carolyn Van Blarcom, whose new field was the prevention of blindness, Clara Noyes, Florence Johnson, and Lillian Wald lectured for as little as ten dollars. Adelaide insisted that a lecturer be paid something, even if she had to pay the fee from her own purse.

The New York League of Nursing honored Adelaide for her services to nursing education with a dinner on November 11, 1915, at the Cosmopolitan Club. Lillian Wald was toastmistress, and speeches were made by Dr. Rufus Cole, director of Rockefeller Hospital; Dr. C.-E. A. Winslow of the Yale School of Public Health; Dr. Maurice Bigelow, Teachers College; Dr. Wright, deputy commissioner of New York; Dr. Haven Emerson, commissioner of health; Mrs. Cadwalader Jones of the Metropolitan Hospital Board; and Beatrice Kent, assistant editor of the *British Journal of Nursing*. Dr. S. S. Goldwater spoke of Adelaide's influence on nursing and endorsed her position on endowments. Mrs. Jenkins told of her work with Miss Nutting and Mrs. Robb, and Annie Goodrich spoke as a colleague. At last it was Adelaide's turn to respond. The previous speakers had talked of nursing's debt to her; she spoke of her debt to the profession. First of all, it had brought her to the United States.[46]

> My great sympathy with American ideals, my profound belief in her principles of government have made it a delight to live among you. I hasten to add that my love for my own country and race remains untouched—a vital part of my being, rooted more and more deeply as the years pass. The debt I owe to my profession can not be measured but these are some of the things it has done for me. It first opened my eyes a little to the real things of life. It built up within me certain ideals of

[45] Correspondence between Adelaide Nutting (New York) and Emily Dinwiddie, [New York], 1912, 1913, 1914 (otherwise undated), MAN Papers.
[46] *The Johns Hopkins Nurses Alumnae Magazine*, February, 1916, pp. 26–30.

service. It set free such energies as I possessed and it revealed to me, in an entirely new way, the purpose of self-discipline and the need for it in life. It gave me the best and most enduring friendships I have ever had.

She spoke of Isabel Hampton Robb, Lavinia Dock, Dr. Osler, and Lillian Wald. "A blessed thing in my life," she said, "is to have known the House on Henry Street." Also there were Dean Russell and Mrs. Jenkins, whose gift had enabled all divisions in the department to develop simultaneously. Since 1899, students from 150 training schools, 29 states, and 6 foreign countries had come to Teachers College to study nursing education.[47]

Honors were sweet, but to Adelaide they brought new demands. On one of the small, penciled slips found among her papers she confessed she had always driven herself. Too many people had attributed to her qualities she did not feel she possessed, and she had pushed herself lest she disappoint those who trusted her.[48]

In June, 1916, Adelaide's brother-in-law, Gilbert Gosling, was elected mayor of St. John's, Newfoundland. He had always been civic-minded and had often discussed matters relating to public health on her visits to the Gosling home. As mayor, one of his innovations was Baby Week. He asked Adelaide to recommend a nurse who could give lectures, instruction, and demonstrations in the care of infants and young children. She sent Lillian Hudson, who had come to Teachers College after completing her course at Johns Hopkins and was just beginning a long and distinguished career in public health. Miss Hudson did her work well, and, following her departure, a full-time, experienced welfare nurse was employed to do visiting nursing among the needy and to inaugurate a health program in the schools.[49]

Each month the war in Europe became more threatening. The sinking of the Lusitania in May, 1915, had brought the United States dangerously close to war with Germany. Since the outset of the war the unique role of the American Red Cross in sending volunteer units abroad had alerted American nurses. In September, 1916, Clara Noyes resigned as superintendent of the Bellevue Training School to become director of the Bureau of Nursing, American Red Cross, under the chairmanship of Jane Delano. The National Defense Act of 1916 brought fear to many Americans. Lavinia Dock, Lillian Wald, and their friend Jane Addams joined the ranks of those who opposed the war and advocated peace at any price.

[47] *Ibid.*
[48] Adelaide Nutting, "Miscellaneous Notes," MAN Papers.
[49] Armine N. Gosling, *William Gilbert Gosling: A Tribute* (New York: Guild Press, 1935), pp. 84–91.

Adelaide maintained a discreet silence, but that did not mean she was not concerned. One of Jim's boys, Harold, was a bombardier in the Canadian Expeditionary Force. Keith would soon be going, and so would Armine's son, Ambrose. Adelaide's other nephews, Bruce and Arthur, were too young to serve. Her nieces, Armine and Frances, who had spent the fall semester studying in New York, returned to their home in Newfoundland; in January, Armine, who had lived at Adelaide's apartment, sailed for France with an ambulance outfitted by her father.[50]

Events moved swiftly in 1917. On January 22 President Wilson delivered his "Peace without Victory" speech before the Senate. Despite Germany's pledges, submarine activities were renewed, and on February 3 the United States broke off diplomatic relations. On February 26 the American policy of armed neutrality was announced. A feverish month followed, and on April 6 the United States declared war on Germany.

[50] Armine Gosling Campball (Mangrove Bay, Bermuda) to Helen E. Marshall (New York), October 15, 1965; and Ambrose G. Gosling (Victoria, British Columbia) to Helen E. Marshall (New York), November 2, 1965; Marshall Papers.

XVIII

Apprenticeship to Duty, 1917–1919

When the headlines of the New York papers screamed the imminence of war, Adelaide telephoned Isabel Stewart, asking her to come at once to her apartment. There were important things to be discussed. Was the nursing profession ready for war?[1]

Before the National Defense Act of 1916, which provided for expansion and reorganization of the army and the creation of a council of national defense to coordinate the military and industrial resources of the nation, had been passed, the Medical Department of the Army, in conjunction with the Red Cross, had worked out a plan for the creation of fifty base hospitals with staff to be recruited from civilian hospitals. The local chapter of the Red Cross would provide the equipment for each, at a cost of from $25,000 to $75,000, and the staff of 25 doctors and 50 nurses, a number which later doubled; 25 nurses aides; 15 reserve nurses and 25 reserve nurses aides; and other personnel needed to care for a 500 (later raised to 1,000) -bed hospital. All nurses were to be recruited through the Red Cross Nursing Service.[2] The organization of 25 of these base hospital units was already well under way. Adelaide was quite familiar with Base Hospital No. 18, the Johns Hopkins unit. Dr. Winford Smith, superintendent of The Johns Hopkins Hospital, was the director, and her own physician, Dr. John M. T. Finney, was chief surgeon.[3]

By the time Isabel Stewart arrived at the apartment, Adelaide had a course of action in mind. She asked Isabel to telephone Lillian Wald and Annie Goodrich (then president of the American Nurses Association), asking them to come as soon as they could to the library at Teachers College. Ella P. Crandall, director of the National Organiza-

[1] Isabel M. Stewart, *Oral History*, 2 vols. (New York: Columbia University, Butler Library, 1958), 1: 183.
[2] Portia B. Kernodle, *The Red Cross in Action, 1882–1948* (New York: Harper & Bros., 1949), pp. 108–9.
[3] *The Johns Hopkins Nurses Alumnae Magazine*, May, 1916.

tion of Public Health Nursing, was also invited to join them. Adelaide began: "Now we know just what will happen if war really comes. In the first place there will be a need for larger numbers of nurses to go abroad, and then we will have a great lack at home. We are already short of nurses, and particularly in our schools. We'll have to be careful because a good many college women have already signed with the Red Cross thinking they would get jobs abroad."[4] She proposed that the nursing group see what could be done to get college women to take training for future needs, and that nursing schools be asked to reduce the training period from three years to two years and four months for college women. Miss Nutting and Miss Goodrich were adamant that standards be maintained, and both were confident that reducing the training period for women who had taken science courses would not lower the quality of nursing graduates.

That same afternoon telegrams were sent to a number of schools, asking their reaction to these proposals. In addition, a public letter signed by Lillian Wald was addressed to college-trained women, urging them to enroll in nurses training and stressing the need for visiting nurses in the conservation of child life, in hygiene, and in sanitation. Miss Wald stated emphatically that no contribution to the problem could be made by the short, popular courses in nursing so widely publicized. Training could be accelerated, however, for women whose college courses had given them a good scientific background. She appealed to college presidents and others to bring the matter to the attention of graduating seniors before they dispersed to their homes.[5]

The next step was the organization of an emergency council composed of leaders in nursing, public health, and medicine who were concerned about the quality of nursing. A tentative list of persons who might be expected to serve on such a committee was drawn up, and others were added to it after telephone conferences. While the committee was being assembled, Miss Nutting, Miss Stewart, and Miss Crandall gathered statistics on nurses in the United States. In 1917 there were 88,000 registered trained nurses and approximately 17,000 who were not registered. About 14,000 nurses would be graduating in 1918.[6]

    [4] Stewart, *Oral History*, 1: 183.
    [5] Circular letter, signed by Lillian Wald, [early spring, 1917], Department of Nursing Education Archives, Teachers College.
    [6] M. Adelaide Nutting, "How the Nursing Profession is Trying to Meet the Problems Arising Out of the War," MAN Papers.

On April 8 Clara Noyes, director of the new Red Cross Bureau of Nursing, wrote to Adelaide:

> Surely we need your prayers. There are moments when I wonder whether we can stem the tide and control the hysterical desire on the part of thousands, literally thousands to get into nursing or their hands upon it.
>
> Tell Anne of Albany (Annie Goodrich) that if I were not convinced before, I should be now that the most vital thing in the life of our profession is the protection of the use of the word *nurse*. Everyone seems to have gone mad. I talk until I am hoarse, dictating letters to doctors and women who want to be Red Cross nurses in a few minutes, the meaning of the word *nurse* and what a Red Cross nurse is. I am for Red Cross Headquarters conducting the biggest educational campaign that has ever been taken in this direction. . . . From nine stenographers we now have between 25 and 30. . . .
>
> Do support us, as I know you are, in opposing six month courses as suggested by St. Luke's.[7]

Adelaide and her colleagues understood Miss Noyes's concern. They were well aware of the unsuccessful protest of the professional nurses in England against the patriotic socialites who clamored to get into military nursing, seeking what Lavinia Dock called "tinsel glory" at the expense of men who needed expert nursing, not trial-and-error care. Criticisms by English nurses appeared in the *American Journal of Nursing* because they were too scathing for the British Journals to print. Isabel Stewart had visited hospitals in England in the summer of 1915 and had seen for herself that short-term nurses and aides must not be allowed to substitute for qualified registered nurses.

On April 17 Miss Noyes wrote Adelaide that for more than eight years Jane Delano had stood firmly for the maintenance of proper nursing standards against tremendous social and financial pressures. Consequently, the Red Cross had not offered a short course in war nursing, and the arrangement for admitting a group of women to assist in base hospitals as nurses aides was made in fear and trembling.[8]

Adelaide replied that the poorly written prospectus for St. Luke's six-month course was designed for volunteers who would work only at St. Luke's, in the event the regular staff of nurses was depleted by the war.[9]

---

[7] Clara Noyes (Washington, D.C.) to Adelaide Nutting (New York), April 8, 1917, Department of Nursing Education Archives, Teachers College.

[8] Clara D. Noyes (Washington, D.C.) to Adelaide Nutting (New York), April 17, 1917, *ibid.*

[9] Adelaide Nutting (New York) to Clara Noyes (Washington, D.C.), April 19, 1917, *ibid.*

It was several weeks before personnel for the National Emergency Council could be fully recruited, but on June 4, 1917, an organization meeting was held at the offices of the NOPHN in New York City. Only Adelaide Nutting, Lillian Wald, Annie Goodrich, Ella Crandall, Mary Beard, and Lillian Clayton were present. Miss Nutting was elected permanent chairman, and Miss Crandall was elected secretary. To start the committee's work, Miss Goodrich and Miss Wald each contributed $100. On June 6 the members of the committee were announced: M. A. Nutting, professor of nursing and health, Teachers College, Columbia University; Ella Phillips Crandall, executive secretary of the National Organization of Public Health Nursing, secretary; Mary Beard, president of NOPHN; Dr. Herman Biggs, commissioner of public health, New York State; S. Lillian Clayton, president of the National League of Nursing Education; Jane A. Delano, chairman of the National Committee on Nursing Education; Dr. S. S. Goldwater, Mt. Sinai Hospital; Annie W. Goodrich, president of the American Nurses Association; Dr. Winford Smith, superintendent of The Johns Hopkins Hospital; Dr. C.-E. A. Winslow, professor of public health, Yale University; and Lillian Wald, superintendent of the Henry Street Settlement. Later added were: Mary S. Gardner, director of the Bureau of Public Health Nursing, American Red Cross; Mrs. John Hughie, superintendent of the Navy Nurse Corps; and Dora E. Thompson, superintendent of the Army Nurse Corps. Subsequently, these eleven nurses also served on the Committee on Red Cross Nursing.[10]

At an informal conference on June 13, the New York members of the committee decided to send letters to the presidents of women's and coeducational colleges, asking them for a roster of their 1917 graduating classes. Miss Nutting and Miss Goodrich were asked to draft the letters. With its personnel carefully chosen and a program of action outlined, the committee was ready to offer its services to Dr. Franklin H. Martin, who had been authorized by the Council of National Defense to organize the General Medical Board. Two other nursing committees were already functioning under the Council of National Defense: the Subcommittee on Public Health Nursing, of which Mary Beard was chairman; and the Committee on Home Nursing, headed by Lillian Wald. The Public Health Nursing Subcommittee was especially concerned with venereal diseases, the children's year campaign, and protective health measures in industry.[11]

At the meeting of the General Medical Board on June 24, Dr. Welch

[10] "The National Emergency Committee on Nursing" (by Adelaide Nutting or Isabel Stewart), *ibid.*
[11] *Ibid.*

presented the proposal of the Public Health Nursing Subcommittee of the Committee on Hygiene and Sanitation that in times of crisis the National Emergency Committee on Nursing make available to the United States certain facts essential to the efficient use of nurses and to devising the wisest methods possible in meeting the problems of the sick in civilian hospitals and homes, as well as the need to increase the number of student nurses. When the matter was taken up the next day at the board's executive meeting, these services were accepted.[12]

Ella Crandall was loaned by the NOPHN to become secretary for the government-sponsored committee. The Council for Defense provided office space in Washington, office equipment, secretarial help, and franking privileges. Friends of nursing contributed $10,750 to speed the publication of costly pamphlets and to launch a publicity campaign.[13]

When the Medical Board met on Sunday, July 29, Miss Crandall reported that 7,000 letters had been sent to the 1917 graduates of women's and coeducational colleges and that 700 letters had been sent to hospitals for data on their training schools and nursing services. Letters were soon to be sent to the superintendents of accredited training schools, recommending that all nurses graduating in 1917 join the Red Cross. The committee proposed that the American Nurses Association conduct a complete survey of the nursing situation.[14]

Meanwhile, Adelaide Nutting was serving on the Mayor's Committee on the Study of the Nursing Situation in New York. Helen Boyd, in a survey of the nurses in the city, arrived at a total of 10,308, of whom 1,701 were enrolled in the Red Cross.[15]

On July 2, as chairman of the National Emergency Committee on Nursing, Adelaide authorized Annie Goodrich to direct a complete census of nurses in the United States through the ANA and to place responsibility for conducting the survey on the state nursing organizations.[16]

Ever on the horizon hovered the specter of nurses aides. Would the country throw its weight behind preparing nurses who were qualified

[12] "Report from the Meeting of the General Medical Board, Council of Defense, Mussey Building, Washington, D.C., June 24–25, 1917," vol. 1, pp. 137–39, National Archives.
[13] "The National Emergency Committee on Nursing."
[14] Ibid.
[15] "Report of the Mayor's Committee on the Study of the Nursing Situation in New York as of July and August 1917," ibid.
[16] M. A. Nutting (New York) to Annie W. Goodrich (New York), July 2, 1917, National Archives and Department of Nursing Education Archives, Teachers College.

to meet military and civilian needs, or would it rush into a scheme quickly to train aides ill-prepared for actual nursing? From the outset, some hospital superintendents—notably, Dr. S. S. Goldwater of Mt. Sinai Hospital—feared the effect the war would have on hospital staffs if the Red Cross took only graduate nurses for military service.

Following the passage of the National Defense Act on June 3, 1916, the Red Cross had inaugurated brief courses to train nurses aides for the protection of the civilian population in homes and hospitals and thereby to insure continuous and adequate provision for the needs of the army. Miss Nutting and other nursing leaders were well aware that there were many repetitive duties and non-nursing duties about the hospital of which graduate nurses should be relieved, but they were apprehensive that as soon as aides were brought into the hospital they would be asked to perform duties ordinarily performed by highly skilled nurses rather than to relieve the nurses of non-nursing duties; they also believed that the nurses themselves would not be prepared to accept or supervise aides.

The Committee on Nursing believed that the problem of keeping up the kind of supply needed could best be met by greatly increasing the number of students in the training schools. In cases of necessity, senior student nurses of the third-year classes could be transferred to military service. Isabel Stewart was set to work writing pamphlets and leaflets to be distributed to high-school and college graduates, principals and superintendents. The first of these was a forty-seven-page pamphlet, *Opportunities in the Field of Nursing,* 13,000 of which were distributed; the second was a four-page leaflet entitled *Nursing,* 70,000 copies of which were made; the third was *Nursing—A National Service,* a fifteen-page pamphlet with a printing of 30,000 copies. During the next eighteen months 210,000 pamphlets and leaflets were distributed.

The work of the Committee on Nursing was financed largely by gifts from four of the state branches of the League of Nursing Education and by substantial donations from Mrs. Felix Warburg ($5,000), Mrs. Helen Hartley Jenkins ($2,000), Mrs. J. Everitt Macy, and Mrs. R. L. Ireland.[17]

The response from hospitals to the idea of reducing the period of residence for college women with a good science background was favorable enough to warrant a press release, and Adelaide told a *New York Evening Sun* reporter of the special inducements offered to college women to take up nursing.

[17] "Report of the Committee on Nursing, General Medical Board, Washington, D.C., April 1, 1919," pp. 11, 21, National Archives.

Do not get the idea that by shortening the course to two years on the hospital side by giving credit for a year of work accomplished on the college side that the hospital work will be any less thorough. It will be as hard, intensive and thorough as that any nurse ever received. . . . The first eight months of a nurse's training are largely given over to ground work in science and academic work. The girl with college training who has had chemistry, biology, psychology, botany has already that first eight months done.

Commenting on the Red Cross, Adelaide said that its foresight had made the United States, with its 9,000 nurses enrolled for active duty, better equipped to meet an emergency than any nation had ever been. She emphasized that the Red Cross's purpose in offering short courses was not to prepare women for a profession but to help them in their own homes to conserve the health of their families and to give intelligent care in cases of minor and chronic illnesses. The courses might help in relief work, but it had never been intended that those who took them should take the place of the trained nurse in cases of serious illness. Red Cross nurses aides had been given courses so that in emergencies they might assist nurses in simple routine duties in hospitals and convalescent homes, but hospitals were not yet calling for this kind of help.[18]

At Teachers College the courses in nursing education were geared to wartime needs. They included first aid, care of children, surgical dressings, occupations for invalids, and emergency short courses such as those for volunteer health visitors and visiting nurses aides, April 16–May 27, and cookery, May 21–June 8, 1917, which would help agencies at the Henry Street Settlement and the Association for Improving the Conditions of the Poor. Volunteers were trained to take records and were taught the elementary principles of cookery, nutrition, hygiene, and massage.[19]

Hospitals began seriously to consider the problem of training additional nurses. Dr. William Welch, realizing that an increase of from twenty to fifty students would place too great a burden on the existing facilities at Johns Hopkins, wrote to Adelaide for suggestions. She replied that nearby homes and buildings might be rented and outfitted as dormitories. She recommended that from twenty-five to forty or fifty of the present training schools undertake the accelerated program, and estimated that the maintenance of one student nurse would

18 "Plea for More Expert Nurses," *New York Evening Sun*, June 30, 1917.
19 "Emergency Courses, World War I," Department of Nursing Education Archives, Teachers College.

cost between $400 and $450. She thought a grant of from $15,000 to $20,000 a year from one of the educational foundations might provide for 800–1,000 extra nurses.[20] She had already solicited the Rockefeller Foundation for funds to assist in educating college women to take their place in nursing and was waiting for a reply.[21]

On August 12, 1917, Adelaide attended her first meeting as chairman of the Committee on Nursing, General Medical Board, Council for Defense. She estimated that only 80,000 nurses of the 200,000 women engaged in nursing were actually registered, and that there were at least 17,000 qualified graduates who were not registered. She reported that 13,000 letters had been sent urging 1917 training school graduates to join the Red Cross Nursing Service.[22]

At the meeting of the General Medical Board on September 9, the Committee on Nursing had more significant data to report. Of the 500 replies received from letters sent to 1,000 training schools, 51 percent reported no shortage of nurses in their communities; 44 percent reported only a slight shortage. Most of the schools favored public health training in the senior year. Local publicity was being used to attract young women to nursing. A survey of registries was being made, and 2,300 agencies were ready to assist in the application of the selective draft. As a last resort, Adelaide said, graduation could be advanced from four to six months ahead of schedule. It appeared that Red Cross nurses aides would provide enough extra women to care for the nation's home needs if the supply of nurses failed. A cordial response had been received to the 700 letters sent out over the signatures of Dr. Franklin Martin and Dr. W. G. Simpson, assistant surgeon general, urging hospitals to increase the number of trainees. Of the 335 replies tabulated, 30 hospitals had increased their classes and 53 had increased housing, 28 replied that housing was an obstacle, 8 would accept non-residents, and 5 would reduce the hours of work. The increase in nursing trainees in the fall of 1917 was estimated at 1,500.

Fourteen hundred letters to principals of training schools brought in 24,000 names and addresses. A direct appeal was sent to 10,000 of the women graduating from college in 1917, and 14,000 letters went out to high-school graduates. The appeal of the Committee on Nurs-

[20] William H. Welch (Baltimore) to Adelaide Nutting (New York), July 18, 1917; and Adelaide Nutting (New York) to Dr. William Welch (Baltimore), July 31, 1917, MAN Papers.

[21] Adelaide Nutting (New York) to George Vincent (New York), July 10, 1917, ibid.

[22] "Minutes of the General Medical Board, Council of National Defense, Meeting at Rockefeller Institute, New York, August 12, 1917," National Archives.

ing was reinforced by articles in national magazines and newspapers. Next the committee would consider the necessary preparations for nurses in convalescent hospitals.[23]

In the fall of 1917 Adelaide was also deeply involved in starting an experimental five-year course at Teachers College in cooperation with Presbyterian Hospital, a project which she and Miss Maxwell had discussed as early as 1911. Adelaide and her staff had long desired the opportunity to develop a bona fide university school of nursing and hoped to attract into nursing many of the well-qualified young women who were enrolling in colleges and universities. Because of the educational opportunities afforded them, students completing the course would qualify for a bachelor of science degree and a diploma in nursing.[24] At the same time, an eight-month course combining practical and theoretical courses in public health nursing was arranged with the Henry Street Nursing Association. Work in occupational therapy, begun in 1912 with a single course, took on new significance with the war and later developed into a major.

The war brought numerous changes in the staff. Annie Goodrich, who had been dividing her time between Teachers College and directing the Henry Street Visiting Nurse Association, was released for service in army hospitals. Anne Strong was called to Simmons College to direct the Public Health Nursing Department, and Florence Johnson, who succeeded her, soon left to direct the Atlantic Division of the Red Cross Nursing Service. In 1918 Lillian Hudson joined the staff. In addition to their regular courses, the staff was called on from time to time to teach emergency courses for occupational therapy aides, naval corpsmen, and home nursing groups.

Despite additional wartime demands and her work as chairman of the education committees of the International Council of Nurses and the NLNE, Adelaide managed to take on new responsibilities. In June, 1917, she signed a contract with Commissioner P. P. Claxton, Bureau of Education, Department of Interior, to revise the *Educational Status of Nursing*,[25] and the following December, after thinking the matter over for a week, she decided to accept a position on the Nursing Com-

[23] Ella Crandall, reporting for the Committee on Nursing, "Minutes of the General Medical Board, Council of National Defense, September 9, 1917," *ibid.*

[24] Isabel M. Stewart, "An Outline of the History of the Department of Nursing Education," *Twenty-five Years of Nursing Education in Teachers College, 1899–1925* (*Teachers College Bulletin*, 17th ser., February, 1926), pp. 11, 13; *idem*, "Five Year Course," *ibid.*, pp. 30–37.

[25] "Contract between Adelaide Nutting, Teachers College, New York, and P. P. Claxton, Commissioner, Bureau of Education, Washington, D.C., June 23, 1917," MAN Papers.

mittee of the Henry Street Settlement, to which she had been unanimously elected.[26] This would mean one more monthly meeting in addition to those of the General Medical Board's Committee on Nursing
and the Red Cross Committee on Nursing, operating in conjunction
with the Department of Labor and the General Medical Board, but,
realizing how much the public health work at Teachers College was
indebted to the Henry Street Settlement, she wrote Miss Wald: "I am
happy indeed to become one of your members and in being given the
privilege of sharing in so far as I am able the devoted labors of yourself and your associates."[27]

No other accomplishment of Adelaide Nutting's career was so
remarkably geared to the hour and to the need of America as the
completion and publication in 1917 of the NLNE's *Standard Curriculum for Schools of Nursing*.[28] It provided the guidelines and standards
to be upheld in the critical months ahead. Since 1914 its preparation
had occupied much of Adelaide's time, as well as that of Isabel
Stewart.

In 1914 the Education Committee of the NLNE had begun to prepare a series of guidelines designed to help nursing schools move
toward a professional status comparable to that enjoyed by school
teachers and social workers. The first studies dealt with shorter hours
and the elimination of non-educational activities in training schools.
Despite Adelaide's ideal of autonomous nursing schools, the new curriculum guide was designed primarily for use in hospital training
schools. It defined the size and type of hospital which provided the
appropriate training field.[29] The procedure followed in preparing the
Standard Curriculum was typical of the careful, diplomatic, and logical way in which Miss Nutting and Miss Stewart worked. When the
American Journal of Nursing opened its Department of Nursing Education in 1915 under the direction of Isabel Stewart, its columns were
used to promote standards. Among the topics discussed were "What
Is Expected of Nursing?" "Is the Nurse a Scientifically Trained Assistant or Servant to the Physician?" and "What Constitutes Good Nurs-

[26] Lillian Wald (New York) to Adelaide Nutting (New York), November 28,
1917; and Adelaide Nutting (New York) to Lillian Wald (New York), December
6, 1917; *ibid*.

[27] *Ibid*.

[28] Committee on Education, National League of Nursing Education, *Standard
Curriculum for Schools of Nursing* (New York: National League of Nursing Education, 1917).

[29] Isabel M. Stewart and Anne L. Austin, *A History of Nursing from Ancient
to Modern Times: A World View* (New York: G. P. Putnam's Sons, 1926), p. 210;
Mary M. Roberts, *American Nursing: History and Interpretation* (New York:
Macmillan, 1954), pp. 100–102.

ing Service?" All the outlines in the *Standard Curriculum* were first published in the *Journal* and were thereby subjected to the scrutiny and criticism of the nursing profession. Most of the "standards" had been tested previously by a few schools equipped with good teaching and clinical facilities and capable faculties.[30]

The curriculum guide, so urgently needed by nursing schools, was welcomed by most state boards of nurse examiners and the better schools. It proved an admirable blueprint for the thirty-one units of the Army School of Nursing organized the following year. The *Standard Curriculum*, revised and reprinted in 1927 and in 1934, established the NLNE as an inexhaustible source on nursing education.[31]

The war was brought close to Adelaide again when her nephew Harold Nutting, son of Jim and Claire, enlisted in the Canadian Expeditionary Force, and again when his brother Keith enlisted. Dr. Osler asked Adelaide to let him know at once if either of her nephews were wounded in the war. "I am at hospitals all over the country." When Claire sent word that Harold, a bombardier, had been wounded on November 6, 1917,[32] Adelaide wrote to Dr. Osler at once. Before a month had passed Claire wrote that Keith was in the hospital at Taplow, Bucks, ill with severe bronchial trouble.[33] Not long afterward a letter came from Grace Osler saying that Keith had spent several days in the Osler's home recuperating.[34]

By November, 1917, 15,000 nurses had placed their services at the disposal of the Red Cross (more than 7,000 since the declaration of war),[35] and thousands of women were besieging the Red Cross, asking to do volunteer work. The nation's army of 200,000 men was rapidly expanded. Thirty-two camps and cantonments, with facilities for 1,800,000 trainees, were set up, and in less than a year half a million American soldiers were in France.

[30] Isabel M. Stewart, "Department of Nursing Education," *American Journal of Nursing*, October, 1915, pp. 319–37.

[31] Roberts, *American Nursing*, p. 100.

[32] William Osler (Oxford) to Adelaide Nutting (New York), [1915–17]; Claire Nutting (Ottawa) to Adelaide Nutting (New York), March 7, 1917; and Claire Nutting (Ottawa) to Adelaide Nutting (New York), November 6, 1917; MAN Papers.

[33] Claire Nutting (Ottawa) to Adelaide Nutting (New York), December 3, 1917, *ibid.*

[34] Grace Osler (Oxford) to M. A. Nutting (New York), [1917], *ibid.*

[35] The Red Cross Nursing Service was restricted to women between the ages of twenty-three and forty who were graduates of fifty-bed hospitals serving both men and women. See "Information for Applicants," *American Red Cross Bulletin no. 703*, November, 1917, superceding *American Red Cross Bulletin no. 150*, American Red Cross Nursing Service, Washington, D.C.

The army insisted that there should always be available more than a sufficient number of nurses. Surgeon General William C. Gorgas did not object to aides, but the chief surgeon of the American Expeditionary Forces in France did not favor using them overseas. The matter of aides came up often in the meetings of the General Medical Board. Adelaide insisted that trained nurses could be provided as rapidly as the army needed them. Annie Goodrich's survey, released in March, 1918, revealed no shortage of nurses as late as January, 1918; in fact, it reported idle nurses. The Medical Board's Committee on Nursing estimated that 98,162 graduate nurses would be available by the end of 1918, almost double the number the Medical Department had requested[36] (15,000–20,000 nurses per 1,000,000 men[37]).

Two other projects occupied the attention of the Nursing Committee. One of these was Vassar Camp, to be developed by Miss Nutting, and the other was the Army School of Nursing outlined by Miss Goodrich but not authorized by the War Department until May 25, 1918. Not everyone on the committee approved of the Army School of Nursing. Dr. Goldwater called it a national blunder whose only redeeming feature was the appointment of Annie Goodrich as director, but Dr. Martin and the nurses of the committee unequivocally endorsed the plan.[38]

In December, when Dr. Henry Noble McCracken, president of Vassar College, offered facilities to the Red Cross for patriotic use, Adelaide quickly saw the possibilities.[39] Mrs. John Wood Blodgett, an alumna and trustee who conceived the idea of using the campus to train aides, thought the college could accommodate 1,000 young women, but Dr. McCracken estimated only 500. When he met with Adelaide, she convinced him that the Vassar facilities might be more profitably used to give college graduates a three-months' intensive course before sending them on to complete nurses training in the outstanding schools of nursing.[40] From the survey the National Emergency Committee had made at the outset of the war, she knew which

[36] Kernodle, The Red Cross in Action, p. 126.

[37] Announcement, "The Training Camp for Nurses at Vassar College," [1918], MAN Papers.

[38] "Minutes of the Nursing Committee, General Medical Board, Council of Defense, May 20, 1918," Department of Nursing Education Archives, Teachers College.

[39] M. Adelaide Nutting, "Notes on Interview with Dr. Henry N. McCracken, President of Vassar College, at Manhattan Hotel, December 10, 1917," MAN Papers.

[40] M. Adelaide Nutting (New York) to Mrs. John W. Blodgett (Grand Rapids, Mich.), December 19, 1917, ibid.

schools would be willing to allow credit to the entering student with a strong background in science.

Jane Delano approved the general idea.[41] The Red Cross contributed $75,000 to the project and asked Adelaide to develop the plan. Miss Nutting selected her committees from the three nursing organizations, Vassar's trustees, faculty, and alumnae, the Red Cross, and the General Medical Board. Isabel Stewart, representing the NLNE, was appointed chairman of the Committee on Curriculum. The teaching staff was largely selected by Adelaide, and the assistants were chosen by Dr. Herbert Elmer Mills, professor of economics at Vassar, who was to serve as dean of Vassar Camp.

While Adelaide recruited her faculty and worked out other details, a vigorous publicity campaign was undertaken. Vassar Camp, open to 1909–18 graduates of approved colleges between the ages of twenty-one and thirty-one, would begin June 24 and close September 13. There would be two terms, with classes six days a week and a half-holiday on Saturday. Expenses would be $25 for tuition and $70 for room and board. Students could choose schools of nursing they wished to attend from a list of cooperating hospitals at which their training would be completed in two years and three months.[42]

A letter of information explaining the over-all scheme of Vassar Camp was sent to the presidents and deans of colleges, asking their cooperation. It was signed by Lillian Wald, Julia Lathrop, Adelaide Nutting, and Annie W. Goodrich. Newspapers carried stories about the proposed camp; the *Literary Digest*, *The Survey*, *Independent*, and other magazines also publicized it.[43] In an article in *Independent* Dr. McCracken declared, "Nursing is the front line trench for women."[44]

Adelaide designed Vassar Camp after Plattsburg Military Camp, where college men were given intensive officer training. The Vassar brochure proclaimed:

This country is facing a serious shortage of nurses, a shortage that will be more acute before the war is over. With every million of our soldiers, fifteen to twenty thousand nurses must go. The need of nurses for reconstruction work cannot be exaggerated. This need will continue for the care of convalescents and the permanently crippled and against the many forms of disease which war brings in its train.

[41] M. Adelaide Nutting (New York) to Lillian S. Clayton (Philadelphia), December 22, 1917, *ibid.*
[42] "The Training Camp for Nurses at Vassar College."
[43] *Literary Digest*, April, 1918, p. 33; *Survey*, April 27, 1918, pp. 94–95.
[44] *Independent*, May 11, 1918, pp. 242–58.

There are almost unlimited opportunities for patriotic, ambitious and capable nurses. About thirty district branches of nursing, many of them in the big new field of public health nursing, are calling them. College women are wanted because their previous education facilitates intensive training and more rapid advancement to posts of urgent need.[45]

While the Vassar plan took shape, the matter of the Army School of Nursing was still hanging in the balance. Annie Goodrich waited impatiently for Surgeon General Gorgas and Secretary of War Newton D. Baker to make up their minds. Dr. Goldwater continued to bring up the matter of aides.[46]

As outlined by Miss Goodrich, the Army School of Nursing would be directed from the surgeon general's office, while its training units would be located in various camp hospitals. Student nurses would provide much of the care for patients in these hospitals and thus would release army nurses for other posts. Annie Goodrich believed that care by student nurses directed by trained supervisors would be far superior to care given by aides; furthermore, graduates of the army school would be permanent, well-prepared additions to the nursing profession.

When the three national nursing organizations (ANA, NLNE, NOPHN) convened for a joint annual meeting in Cleveland, May 7–11, 1918, the issue was discussed. Colonel Winford H. Smith read a paper on the "Army School of Nursing," and Dr. S. S. Goldwater, speaking on "The Nursing Crisis," appealed for laymen to supplement the trained nurse staff. Jane Delano spoke on the "Red Cross Aide versus the Short Term Course." She was followed by Annie Goodrich, who spoke on the army school plan. Miss Goodrich was thoroughly opposed to aides and was convinced that the War Department had not endorsed the army plan because of the pressure for aides. Miss Nutting and Mrs. Chester Bolton, a prominent citizen of Cleveland and a neighbor of Secretary of War Baker, supported Miss Goodrich's plan. When a concensus of the three organizations was called for, the vote was overwhelmingly in favor of the army school.[47]

Meanwhile, in Washington, the War Department rejected the pro-

[45] "The Training Camp for Nurses at Vassar College"; Gladys Bonner Clappison, *Vassar's Rainbow Division, 1918* (Lake Mills, Iowa: Graphic Publishing Co., 1964), p. 15.

[46] Annie Goodrich (Washington, D.C.) to Adelaide Nutting (New York), April 24, 1918; and S. S. Goldwater (New York) to Ella P. Crandall (Washington, D.C.), April 16, 1918; MAN Papers.

[47] *Twenty-fourth Annual Report of the National League of Nursing Education*, May, 1918; Kernodle, *The Red Cross in Action*, pp. 135–39; Roberts, *American Nursing*, p. 137.

posed army school. Miss Nutting and Miss Goodrich quickly rallied a
special committee, which included Mrs. Bolton and Surgeon General
of the Army Gorgas. Secretary of War Baker granted the delegation
a special hearing on May 25 and approved the army school program
after he was assured the Student Nurse Reserve would also provide
students for civilian schools of nursing.[48]

Jane Delano accepted the verdict of the nursing organizations and
promptly doubled her efforts to meet the military's demands by holding an enrollment campaign from June 3 to July 17. Her magnanimity
can be seen in a telegram to Adelaide Nutting: "Greatly desire appeal
for enrollment of graduates and applications for Army School of
Nursing to use in connection with our enrollment campaign beginning
June 3. Will you kindly wire message about 300 words collect, as
Chairman Committee Council National Defense."[49] Adelaide com-
plied.

> The appeal of the Red Cross to our nurses to enroll for service is a
> call to arms. It comes straight to every one of us as a summons to duty.
> Our country in her hour of great need is turning to her trained nurses
> in full confidence that we will hasten to answer her call, and that we will
> bring our entire strength to whatever service is required of us, thinking
> no effort, no sacrifice too great to make. The men of our army are
> offering all that they have—their lives. When they are wounded, sick
> and suffering, we must be there to sustain them with our best skill and
> strength. Their families at home and the workers in a thousand fields
> who supply the sinews of war and our daily needs must be cared for
> in illness, safe-guarded in health and kept at their greatest productive
> power. Hospitals and training schools must increasingly labor at their
> life-saving tasks; and in training new nursing forces that our ranks may
> always be kept full. Let us dedicate ourselves anew to whatever service
> our country most needs of us. When every available nurse is at her
> post of honor and of duty, we shall have met our call to arms. So far
> the test has been met. Nurses have been ready. They have answered
> their summons in thousands and have met dangers and hardships as
> bravely and quietly as any soldier. They are piling up tradition of real
> moral splendor. We know they will not fail. To the young women who
> wish to enter this great branch of national service, a new opportunity
> comes in the Army School of Nursing, which the government has just
> established. Here in training, wearing the hospital uniform, they are in
> the active service of their country and no more direct, useful and fruitful
> way of serving could be given them. Every student nurse becomes a part
> of the nation's army of home defense.[50]

[48] Roberts, *American Nursing*, p. 139.

[49] Telegram, Jane A. Delano (Washington, D.C.) to M. Adelaide Nutting (New
York), May 28, 1918, Department of Nursing Education Archives, Teachers
College.

[50] Telegram, A. Nutting (New York) to Jane A. Delano (Washington, D.C.),
May 31, 1918, *ibid.*

On June 24, 1918, Vassar Camp opened with a public convocation in the chapel.[51] President McCracken presided at the flag-draped lectern. Solemnly he faced the 437 eager young women in the freshly starched, varicolored probationer uniforms of the thirty hospitals that had accepted them for training. Some wore pink, some gray; others wore blue and white checks, blue and white stripes, buff and tan, or light blue and dark blue. Some uniforms had white collars; all were three inches from the floor. All the trainees wore black oxfords and black cotton stockings; white aprons and kerchiefs would be added later, as would the white caps. Each girl carried a writing tablet and a fountain pen. Sitting in separate sections were the faculty, and the graduate nurses in their stiff, white uniforms.

"This," said Dr. McCracken, "is the first camp of its kind in America. It is a milestone in nursing history." There were other speakers from the Red Cross, the Council of Defense, then Mrs. Blodgett, Miss Goodrich, and Dean Mills. Adelaide had sent her own greeting to be read:

> The opening of the school of Vassar has come to seem to me one of the greatest events of the history of nursing. And I wish I could be present to see with my own eyes the wonderful sight. How deeply indebted the whole profession of nursing must always be to you for your labors in support of the standards we have struggled so long to uphold.[52]

Fervently the group sang the last stanza of "America." Then, with his gavel, President McCracken signaled the opening of the camp's first session.

Adelaide did not visit the camp until later, but from the Hillcrest Inn, Ogunquit, Maine, where she vacationed with Georgia Nevins, she kept in close touch with it through Isabel Stewart, who was doing double duty directing the summer session in nursing education at Teachers College and teaching a term at Vassar. The Vassar camp faculty was outstanding and included such distinguished teachers and scientists as Dr. Florence Rena Sabin, The Johns Hopkins University School of Medicine; Charles-Edward Amory Winslow, professor of public health, Yale School of Medicine; Dr. Otto Knut Olaf Folin, professor of biological chemistry, Harvard Medical School; Helen M.

---

[51] Other institutions offering similar courses were Western Reserve University, Cleveland, Ohio; University of Cincinnati, Ohio; University of Iowa, Iowa City. See M. A. Nutting (New York) to Mary E. Botler (Philadelphia), June 3, 1918, *ibid.*

[52] Clappison, *Vassar's Rainbow Division*, pp. 32–34.

Pope, assistant professor of nutrition, Margaret Morrison Carnegie School, Carnegie Institute of Technology; Nina D. Gage, superintendent of nurses, Hunan-Yale Hospital, Changsa, China; Anna D. Wolf, Johns Hopkins; Nellie X. Hawkinson, a graduate student at Teachers College and former superintendent of the Union Avenue Hospital of Framingham, Massachusetts; Bertha Harmer, St. Luke's Hospital Training School for Nurses; Mary M. Marvin, graduate student at Teachers College; and Grace Watson, an instructor at Bellevue Hospital, New York. Isabel Stewart and Anne Harvey Strong, assistant professor of public nursing, Simmons College, Boston, taught the history of nursing. A number of Vassar faculty members served as assistants.

Vassar's gymnasium was converted into a hospital with rows of beds and bedside tables, while the museum was transformed into a kitchen and laboratory. Four residence halls were assigned to students, and one was reserved for the faculty. The camp was divided into companies, the companies into squads, and a sergeant commanded four squads. Although the discipline was military, with emphasis on promptness, regularity, and obedience, self-government was an important feature of the camp.

The campers soon joined forces with the 200 Farmerettes, the Vassar girls who had stayed on to till the 675-acre farm, tend the grounds, and milk the dairy cows, and together they edited a weekly newspaper called *The Thermometer*. It featured sketches of the neophytes of ward and farm, their amusing ignorance, abiding humor, and sound convictions. Both groups were trying to meet their country's need. Copies were mailed regularly to Miss Nutting and to President Wilson.[53] Adelaide read her copy avidly, looking for indications that the camp was fulfilling its mission of dedicating college women not only to the service of their country but also to the profession of nursing.

The summer passed quickly for the young women in Poughkeepsie. At Ogunquit, by the sea, Adelaide spent the mornings in her room or in a sheltered corner of the veranda writing letters, reading her mail, and attending to committee work. Following an afternoon nap, she and Georgia would alternate reading with needlework and then take a short walk along the beach or an occasional drive with friends. In the evenings Adelaide read, wrote, or, if no one else was available, made a fourth with Georgia and another couple for a quiet hour of auction

[53] *The Thermometer*, published by Vassar Campers and Farmerettes, 1918–21, Department of Nursing Education Archives, Teachers College.

bridge. She kept in close touch with Ella Crandall in Washington concerning matters relating to the Committee on Nursing of the General Medical Board, Council of Defense.

As American troops began to move toward France at the rate of 300,000 a month, Dr. Will Mayo of the General Medical Board and president of the College of Surgeons and Dr. Goldwater of the Nursing Committee became alarmed about the supply of nurses. Secretary Baker stood firm: "Under no circumstances is the Army to call out of civil hospitals second and third year pupils. That would be a body blow to civil hospitals and is unnecessary."[54]

Dr. Franklin Martin, chairman of the Medical Board, was loath to do anything that would interfere with building up the Student Nurse Reserve, and the Red Cross appealed to the public to forego the use of the trained nurse. Martin was very anxious that 25,000 reserves be enlisted who could be called up for civilian use.

When it became apparent that there would again be great pressure for aides, Adelaide cut her vacation short on August 13 and returned to New York to assemble facts and figures for the meeting of the Committee on Nursing with the General Medical Board in Washington on August 17.[55]

Dr. Martin called the meeting for 8:30 A.M. The agenda, the formulation of a program of nurse procurement upon which the Army and Navy departments, Public Health Service, and civilians could agree, was itself the portent of a stormy session. Colonel J. M. T. Finney, formerly of The Johns Hopkins Hospital and now chief surgeon of the American Expeditionary Forces, had just returned from the battlefields of France and wanted to know what surgeons abroad could expect. Deeply concerned for civilian and military hospitals, Dr. Will Mayo was convinced that aides were the solution.

Would this meeting turn into a clash between men and women, doctors and nurses, "Trained Nurses versus Aides"? Nursing had always had a good friend in Dr. Welch. As early as May he had recommended military rank for army nurses.[56] Adelaide adjusted her pince-nez glasses and surveyed the group. The nursing profession was well represented: S. Lillian Clayton, president of NLNE; Mary Beard, president of NOPHN; Ella P. Crandall, secretary, and Paul

[54] Newton D. Baker (Washington, D.C.) to Dr. S. S. Goldwater (New York), n.d., Office of American Red Cross, Washington, D.C.

[55] (Copy) S. S. Goldwater (New York) to Jane A. Delano (Washington, D.C.), June 12, 1918; and (copy) S. S. Goldwater (New York) to Ella P. Crandall, (Washington, D.C.), June 17, 1918; MAN Papers.

[56] "Minutes of the General Medical Board, Council of National Defense, May 5, 1918," National Archives.

Brathwaite, assistant secretary, of the Committee on Nursing, General Medical Board, Council of Defense; in the uniform of their respective services, Mrs. Lena S. Higby, Navy Nursing Corps; Annie W. Goodrich, Army School of Nursing; Dora Thompson, Army Nurse Corps; and from the Red Cross, Jane Delano of the Nursing Department, and Clara D. Noyes of the Bureau of Field Nurses. Civilian interests were represented by Hannah Patterson, secretary of the Women's Committee. Speaking for the medical services and wearing army insignia were Colonel Finney, Dr. Welch, Colonel Will Mayo, General Robert Noble, and Colonel Robert Dickinson, all from the surgeon general's office, and Colonel Martin, chairman of the Medical Board, Council of Defense. Annie Goodrich looked pale and worn, but Adelaide knew she could depend on her to give her last ounce of energy in behalf of a cause in which she believed.[57]

After Dr. Finney had given firsthand information on the nursing situation in France and had estimated that an army of 3,000,000 would need 50,000 nurses, Ella P. Crandall reported that during the first year of the committee's existence 7,000 more students had enrolled in training schools than at any previous time. She reiterated that it was the obligation of the committee to see that civilian as well as military needs were met.

Then it was Miss Nutting's turn to speak. She was dressed in a dark, ankle-length, gored skirt, a white shirtwaist with high collar, a long, dark, and narrow ascot tie tucked in at her waist, a long, gold watch chain around her neck, with its watch anchored in her belt, and, on her head, a pointed Breton sailor of dark straw trimmed with an upright band of glistening cock feathers and a single rose in front. Leaning forward, with her hands on the table, she clearly and concisely reviewed the work of the committee, the appeals it had made to high schools, private schools, colleges, hospitals, and training schools, the press releases, and other publicity.[58] A million men in France, she said, did not mean a million men on the firing line, and she had confidence in the response of American women to their country's need. Nurses would be available when the government had housing and hospitals ready to receive them. She then turned to Hannah Patterson of the Women's Committee, who reported on the campaign to raise a reserve force of 25,000 U.S. student nurses for civilian hospitals, training schools, and the Army School. Many states

[57] Franklin Henry Martin, *Digest of Proceedings of the Medical Board, Council of National Defense, during World War I* (Washington, D.C.: Government Printing Office, 1934), pp. 378–80.
[58] *Ibid.*, p. 478.

had exceeded their quota. Mrs. Higbee said the navy was adequately cared for as far as nurses were concerned. Jane Delano reported that the Red Cross enrollment campaign had already brought in 50 percent of the 25,000 nurses the army sought. Registration had been waived, and any nurse who qualified for the Army Nurse Corps could be enrolled. There were 5,600 nurses overseas and 2,000 more ready to go, many of them in New York awaiting transportation.

Dr. Finney suggested that student nurses be assigned to hospitals in the rear of the fighting lines and that base hospitals be used as teaching hospitals; he said that General Pershing and General Ireland approved of sending second- and third-year students from the United States to complete their training in base hospitals and that head nurses in Europe favored the plan. The nurses present raised their eyebrows and looked from one to another. General Noble quickly interposed that Secretary Baker's letter to Dr. Goldwater contradicted such a plan.

In answer to Dr. Welch's question whether an effort was being made to adjust the supply of nurses to the need, Miss Crandall and Miss Delano described the methods being used to conserve nursing resources. Colonel Dickinson called for statistics. Miss Goodrich replied that 15,000 letters of inquiry had been received since the announcement of the army school in May. Seeing an opportunity to drive home her point, Miss Nutting proposed that a chart be prepared showing the figures then available.

Colonel Mayo asked why student nurses should not be drafted for overseas duty just as men were. Turning to the astonished women, he lashed out that their slogan seemed to be, "The trained nurse first, God and country afterward." Dr. Finney was adamant that only the "right kind of women be sent overseas." When confronted with the fact that, if nurses were sent over at the same rate as men, 1,000 women would have to be sent each week, Colonel Mayo was forced to admit that the army did not have adequate quarters for that number. Finally, Dr. Martin adjourned the meeting until Wednesday, August 21, when the women would bring in figures that the men would go over, bring back to the committee, and then send to the secretary of war and the secretary of the navy.[59]

It was a tense and exhausting meeting. Colonel Dickinson had challenged every figure presented. There had been near clashes of temper, and the nurses had been rankled by Dr. Mayo's insinuations

[59] "Minutes of the Meeting of the General Medical Board and the Committee on Nursing, August 17, 1918," Department of Nursing Education Archives, Teachers College.

that the nurses were more selfish than patriotic. Although their voices sometimes betrayed their excitement, Miss Nutting and Miss Goodrich tried to speak with calmness and self-assurance. They were grateful for the support of Dr. Welch, who knew when to inject a diplomatic word in order to avert an explosion.

When the committee reassembled on August 21, 1918, the nurses had prepared their charts. Since Dr. Martin was vacationing in the Midwest, Miss Nutting presided. Colonel Dickinson presented a statement on the status of the Army Nurse Corps, civilian and army hospital needs, and the availability of supply. Miss Delano suggested that 50,000 nurses be sent overseas for duty and that 20,000 remain in the United States. Dr. Mayo insisted on 25,000 civilian nurses. Miss Goodrich protested, and the number was cut to 20,000. Miss Nutting reminded the committee that Secretary Baker did not want third-year students taken out of school. Colonel Dickinson said it would cost $50,000,000 to construct barracks for training schools, and that additions to hospitals in the United States would cost $1,220 a bed, while Dr. Mayo insisted they could be built for $500 per bed.

On September 4 a *New York Times* reporter interviewed Miss Nutting relative to the nursing situation. She carefully explained that the most recent survey showed about 100,000 graduate nurses, registered and unregistered, in the United States. From this number perhaps 25 percent should be deducted because of age or disability. In 1918, 1,579 training schools had graduated 14,000 nurses. In response to Surgeon General Gorgas' call for 25,000 graduate nurses by January, 1919, 26,000 nurses had been enrolled by the Red Cross and 15,000 were in military service. These figures were interpreted too enthusiastically by the reporter, however, and, to Miss Nutting's chagrin and that of the Medical Board, the *Times* declared the next day that the nursing problem had been solved.[60] The facts were further distorted when the *Illinois Medical Journal* reported that Miss Nutting had announced on September 4 that there would be enough nurses to care for an army of 5,000,000 men.[61]

Seeing the article in the *Times*, Dr. Martin sent a note to Miss Nutting, challenging her statistics, and Brigadier General Charles Richards released a press statement on September 14, denying that the supply of nurses was adequate, and saying that 25,000 nurses must be available by the end of the year. Two days later the *Pittsburgh Gazette* stated editorially that "the statement of the woman connected with the enrollment of nurses," to the effect that enough nurses had been enrolled, was damaging to the cause, that Miss Nutting's statement was not correct, and that Brigadier General Charles Richard said 50,000 nurses must be raised by July 1, 1919.[62]

In the midst of the controversy, Adelaide went to Poughkeepsie for the final convocation of the Vassar campers the week before they were to leave for their respective hospitals. In France, American soldiers were in the thick of the fighting, on the Aisne-Marne, Somme, Oise-Aisne, and Ypres-Lys offensives; at home, families scanned the daily casualty lists for the names of relatives and friends. Miss Nutting had been asked to give the principal address to the departing campers. With her on the platform of the chapel sat Ella Crandall, representing the Council of Defense, Mrs. John Wood Blodgett, who had originated the idea of patriotic service at Vassar, and Dean Herbert Mills, who had carried out the plan.

Adelaide called her address "Apprenticeship to Duty."

The country knows what it wants of its men in wartime. For women, war complicates the situation. No country has really known what is really needed of its women in wartime. . . .

The Medical Department of the army is making a superb effort to clarify the whole nursing situation, and for the first time, to place and keep the care of its sick men in the hands of trained and skilled women, and partly because we are better understanding the real meaning and value of such training. It is our own president who has said, "This is no war for amateurs." . . . It is due to skilled nursing as well as to remarkable surgery that . . . 80 per cent of wounded men are said to have been returned to the front to fight again. . . . That we may be able to continue this kind of care for our men . . . was a part of the large purpose of the Vassar training camp. . . .

I wish I could find words to picture nursing to you as I see it. It is to me, one of the most beautiful and tender of all of the arts of life. . . . One cannot hand out the art of nursing to anybody. The tools of nursing are many of them simple enough, but the range of sources from which they are drawn must be very wide, and their uses perfected by long and arduous effort. Senses and perception must be trained to their finest adjustments. Behind that quick sure touch, that fine and delicate manipulation, must be months of toil and practice, experiment and failure, as well as progress. Behind that sure judgment lie long stretches of experience and careful study of persons and situations, of comparisons and results.[63]

[62] Clipping from the *Pittsburgh Gazette*, September 16, 1918, Clipping file, General Medical Board, National Archives.

[63] M. Adelaide Nutting, "Apprenticeship to Duty" (Address to students of the Vassar Training Camp for Nurses, September 9, 1918), pp. 1, 2, and 7, issued by the Committee on Nursing, General Medical Board and printed in the *American Journal of Nursing*, December, 1918.

She traced the history of nursing from 1889, describing its professional organizations, journals, textbooks, and advances in registration, nursing education, and public health. "The profession of nursing," she said, "stands . . . solidly on its record of achievement and devotion to the public good."[64] She paid high tribute to American nurses in military service, still "without the rank of which Canada and Australia have been unwilling to deprive their nurses," and to Edith Cavell, the British nurse who before her execution proclaimed, "Patriotism is not enough, we must hold no bitterness in our heart toward anyone."[65]

Adelaide then welcomed and commended the Vassar Camp trainees: to the company of valiant women "living and dying with high hearts and full measure of devotion."

> Knowing the roads in the journey ahead of you I am not without moments of anxiety and apprehension. I would that, like the convoy that encircle our transports and guard them on their perilous journey, we could somehow protect you, not against the hardships—never, but perhaps against yourselves. There will be days when everything will seem sordid, when you will be tired and disheartened and ready to give it all up. It will not seem to you worth the effort. But we are relying on you to still see, even though dimly, the "vision splendid," to listen to no voices of defeat and to realize that
>
> > Tasks in hours of insight willed
> > Can be through hours of gloom fulfilled.
>
> Let the thought of the sore needs of the people which await your ministry fortify you, and let me say, for the nurses of this country, they stretch out welcoming hands to you as you enter the apprenticeship to duty to which you have dedicated yourselves.[66]

The trainees finished their last week's work and, with a parting injunction from Annie Goodrich on August 14, left for the thirty affiliated hospitals where they were to complete their training.[67]

Adelaide returned to New York to prepare for the fall term at Teachers College and to seek new ways of augmenting the supply of nurses for military and civilian hospitals. One hundred seventy stu-

[64] *Ibid.*, p. 10.
[65] *Ibid.*, p. 11.
[66] *Ibid.*
[67] Of the 418 women who completed the Vassar course, 399 entered the thirty affiliated schools of nursing; some took up other forms of war work, and only 3 or 4 renounced their pledge to become nurses and returned to their families; 57 went to Bellevue; 21 to City Hospital, New York; 17 to Boston City; and 13 to the University of Michigan Hospital. See Dean Herbert Mills's speech in *The Thermometer*, March, 1921, quoted in Clappison, *Vassar's Rainbow Division*, p. 132.

dents enrolled in the Department of Nursing and Health; it was the largest number to date and an increase of 43 percent over the previous year.[68]

The controversy over nursing statistics and civilian and military needs continued. On September 21 the press announced nationwide that, at the request of Secretary of War Baker and Surgeon General Gorgas, the American Red Cross would make a comprehensive survey of nursing resources, cataloging graduate nurses, both registered and unregistered, pupil nurses, nurses' aides, semitrained aides, attendants, midwives, and practical nurses. With the cooperation of Jane Delano, Frederick C. Monroe of Boston would conduct the survey through local chapters of the Red Cross.[69] The *New York Times* struck a note of optimism when it quoted Miss Nutting's statement that 4,000 applications had been received for the Army School of Nursing and that student nurses were thronging training camps and hospitals.[70]

The matter of aides remained a touchy subject. Rather than incur the ire of nursing leaders, the American Hospital Association discreetly went on record in favor of the training of hospital helpers, calling them assistants rather than aides. Dr. Goldwater, who had recently resigned from the General Medical Board's Committee on Nursing, sent the committee a letter and a copy of the resolution that civilian hospitals having the necessary facilities set up a training program for hospital assistants according to the plans and qualifications which might be developed by the Army School of Nursing.[71]

Meanwhile, the Allies had launched the great fall offensive in France. After the victory at St.-Mihiel, American troops were concentrated in a sector between the Meuse River and the Argonne Forest; their objective was to attack the Sedan-Mézières railroad, the main line of supply for the Germans on the western front. The American offensive, part of Foch's master plan to oust the Germans, involved 1,200,000 U.S. troops. As the Allies moved forward, Spanish influenza struck at home and on the lines. Between October 1 and October 4, 1918, more than 500 cases were reported to the Henry Street Visiting Nurse Association alone.[72] So acute was the situation in the eastern United States that on October 3 the transportation of nurses

[68] Stewart, *Twenty-five Years of Nursing Education in Teachers College*, p. 16.

[69] Clipping file, Council of National Defense, National Archives.

[70] Clipping from the *New York Times*, September 22, 1918, *ibid*.

[71] "Minutes of the Special Committee, Medical Board, October 3, 1918," Department of Nursing Education Archives, Teachers College.

[72] R. L. Duffus, *Lillian Wald: Neighbor and Crusader* (New York: Macmillan, 1938), p. 200.

and nurse's aides from the United States to American hospitals in France was halted.[73] Lillian Wald asked Miss Nutting to meet with nursing leaders and hospital administrators on October 11 for the purpose of organizing the Emergency Nurses Council for New York to recruit and allocate nursing services where they were most needed.[74]

The flu spread across the country like a prairie fire; theaters, churches, and schools were closed. Churches and gymnasiums became improvised hospitals, and volunteer nurses were recruited without reference to training. For doctors and nurses, sleep was rationed. Many people wore surgical masks on the streets, and in some communities the demand for caskets exceeded the supply. When the troopship *Olympic* docked at Southampton, England, it reported 2,300 aboard, hundreds ill, and 119 deaths. Among the American Expeditionary Forces, the ratio of deaths from influenza to those caused by battle wounds was ten to one.

This was "the baptism of fire" to which Vassar Camp trainees were subjected two weeks after they entered their respective hospitals. The flu epidemic settled the question of aides as far as Miss Delano was concerned. On October 17 she wired Florence Johnson in New York to start training at once. Some of the aides might be used in caring for victims of the flu epidemic. Two days later newspapers in New York and other cities announced the call for 15,000 nurse's aides for duty in France.

The New York County chapter of the Red Cross announced it would provide nurse's aide training consisting of fifteen lessons and 240 hours of hospital work. Persons between the ages of thirty-five and forty-five were sought. Two letters of recommendation were to accompany each application. Those accepted would be paid $30 a month, plus expenses, transportation, and equipment.[75] Canadian women were eligible, but no Austrian- or German-born women would be accepted. Undergraduate college students could enlist if they had had six months of nurses training. Instruction for aides was accelerated to the point that it could be completed in five days. Aides were to be sent to France in groups of twenty-five or fifty.

[73] Clipping from the *New York Sun*, October 4, 1918, Clipping file, General Medical Board, National Archives.

[74] Lillian Wald (New York) to Adelaide Nutting (New York), October 11 and December 12, 1918, MAN Papers.

[75] (Copy) telegram, Jane Delano (Washington, D.C.) to Florence Johnson (New York), October 19, 1918; and Letter 3194 A.R.C., Jane Delano to All Division Directors of Nursing, October 31, 1918; Department of Nursing Education Archives, Teachers College.

Adelaide had disapproved of the plan when it was suggested in February and had complained to Jane Delano.[76] Sick, wounded, and dying men should not be left to the care of inexperienced nurses. Again she quoted President Wilson: "War is not a job for amateurs."

In France the final phase of the Meuse-Argonne offensive began on November 1. Within a week the American army reached Sedan, cut off the railway, and made the German position there untenable. Bulgaria had surrendered. The German navy at Kiel had mutinied, and a revolution had taken place. Kaiser Wilhelm had abdicated and fled. A republic described as the German Peace Commission sent representatives to meet with General Foch in the Forest of Compiègne.

The flu epidemic in America had abated somewhat when news of the armistice came, but there was barely time for a shout of joy or a prayer of thanksgiving before it enveloped the country again. In New York, when the laundry workers at Bellevue, alarmed by the risk of contagion, walked out, instructors and students from Teachers College took over.[77]

Similar conditions prevailed at City Hospital and Training School on Blackwell's Island, where Carolyn Gray, one of the school's 1893 graduates and a former student of Teachers College, had been trying to bring order out of chaos for four years. Met by a penurious board, antiquated and unsanitary equipment, and understaffed facilities, the epidemic brought untold suffering there. Miss Gray appealed to Miss Nutting. What could be done to save and reform the old hospital? Its twenty-two Vassar Camp trainees, although serious and devoted to nursing, were nonetheless critical and outspoken about hospital conditions, particularly the prevalence of mice, rats, roaches, bedbugs, and lice. As an economy measure the hospital had been forced to abandon exterminator service.[78]

In her appeal for help, Miss Gray enclosed copies of students' observations written as a class assignment. One student wrote that she had expected to find many conditions not ideal, but that she was horrified at the deplorable lack of linens. She described patients from clean, respectable homes who had to lie on sheets soiled and damp for three or four days because no clean linen was available. Another student wrote that she had not seen a washcloth in the four weeks she

[76] Adelaide Nutting (New York) to Jane A. Delano (Washington, D.C.), February 20, 1918, MAN Papers.

[77] Clappison, *Vassar's Rainbow Division*, p. 97.

[78] (Copy) Carolyn Gray (New York) to Dr. Charles B. Bacon (New York), November 11, 1918; and Carolyn Gray (New York) to Adelaide Nutting (New York), November 11, 1918; MAN Papers.

had been on Blackwell's Island. Another Vassar girl wrote: "If I were a patient, I would be afraid to go to City Hospital for treatment. There is not enough equipment to insure proper care without danger of infection. If blankets are washed after a patient is discharged, the next patient to occupy the bed is cold." There was a shortage of diapers, and babies were often pinned up in pillow cases or sheets. New patients slept between sheets that former patients had used. "The shortage of blankets seemed to lead to more infection, for they are used over and over again on different patients until I hesitate to handle them," wrote one student nurse. "Nurses in baby wards often wash babies' clothes—doing laundry work when they should be nursing."[79]

The situation was appalling. Adelaide called Bird Coler, commissioner of the city's Department of Public Charities, and asked him to look into the matter at once and to see that something was done. He agreed, and the next day he appointed Adelaide to the newly created Advisory Board for the City Hospital, which was to formulate by-laws subject to the Commissioner's approval, and to hold office at his pleasure.[80] Under conditions such as these, Adelaide foresaw slight opportunity for the committee to achieve any significant and lasting reform in the city's hospitals, but she felt she could not honorably decline.

When a telegram arrived on December 11, 1918, advising that the campaign for nurses be ended on December 15, Miss Nutting's colleagues hoped she would begin to take life easier. She had celebrated her sixtieth birthday in November. She had never been strong, and Isabel Stewart was greatly concerned lest she become ill.

Adelaide's calendar reveals that she had no intention of slowing up. On December 2 she attended an executive meeting of the NLNE in Washington. On December 16 she sat in on a conference called by George Vincent, president of the Rockefeller Foundation, relative to courses of training for public health nursing. On December 18 she left for Chicago to attend a meeting of the Committee on Nursing, General Medical Board, Council of Defense, called at the request of representatives of state boards of nurse examiners and administrators who had served as assignors of the U.S. Student Reserves in Washington. On January 17 there was an important meeting of the direc-

[79] Carolyn Gray (New York) to Adelaide Nutting (New York), December 16, 1918, ibid.
[80] Bird S. Coler (New York) to Adelaide Nutting (New York), December 17, 1918, ibid.

tors of the ANA and the NLNE relative to the responsibilities those organizations would carry as a result of the cessation of war.

During the Christmas holidays Adelaide worked on papers summarizing the work of the General Medical Board's Committee on Nursing and preparing a letter to be sent to superintendents of training schools and presidents of boards of governors of hospitals. Isabel Stewart itemized the list of publications that had originated largely in the office of the Nursing Department at Teachers College and had been distributed by the three nursing organizations. In black and white the figures were stupendous: 70,000 copies of the pamphlet *Nursing*; 13,000 *Opportunities in the Field of Nursing*; 20,000 copies of *Bulletin of General Information for College Graduates*; 30,000 *Nursing: A National Service*; 55,000 *State Sources of Advice and Information on Nursing*; 5,000 *The Nation's Call for Nurses*; 15,000 *Message to School Principals*; and 2,000 *Preparatory Course for Nurses*. Of course, there had been additional publicity through magazine articles and the press.

Glancing over the committee's financial statement, Adelaide noted again that it had carried on its work through private donations. There was a cash balance of $1,699.99. Isabel Stewart had written most of the pamphlets and had balanced the budget, content to serve her adopted country quietly behind the scenes. The work of the Committee on Nursing was over, and its unfinished business was being turned over to other agencies; the most important project, the Student Nurse Reserve, was to be taken over by the Red Cross.

The committee's final letter of appreciation to superintendents of training schools and presidents of hospital boards would elucidate principles that Adelaide believed to be of great importance for the future of nursing. She submitted it to various members of the committee for approval, criticism, or suggestions. The copy that she retained for her personal file was the one returned by Dr. Welch. Across one corner he had written "Admirable. Heartily approve, W. H. Welch."

> As we bring our work to an end, we realize that while it is comparatively easy to transfer various activities in which we have been engaged to other bodies, there are certain intangible things, obligations and responsibilities of which we cannot divest ourselves, since they have arisen as a result directly or indirectly of measures instituted by us. We are particularly conscious of a sense of responsibility toward the young women who, through our instrumentality have been drawn into the training schools for nurses throughout the country. . . .
>
> Thousands have entered training schools, many highly qualified. Some might have chosen other professions if not for the war. It is our hope they will find in the various institutions which they enter not only

a spirit of equal generosity and patriotism but satisfying opportunities for the good instruction and training they have been led to expect.

And such good and wholesome conditions of life and work as would make them wish to continue their work in hospitals. . . . It seems to us most desirable that they should not only have no cause to regret their action, but that on the contrary, they would gladly recognize that has been opened up to them so vitally important and promising a field of women's work for which the training they are securing will adequately prepare them.

The war has revealed with striking clearness the great dependence of hospitals on the student nurses in their training schools. Of the many changes which are needed in our system of training, this question of hours is first and most fundamental. We believe once the situation is fully understood, there will be a movement toward shorter hours within the hospital, initiated by the governing bodies themselves, and not imposed from without. . . .

Our schools of nursing have come to take a vitally important place among our educational institutions, and with the progress of the public health movement, a whole new field is opened up to the nurses who are trained in these schools. . . . Our Committee would ill perform its obligations toward one of the nation's essential defenses if it passed out of existence silent on a matter which it believes to be of great moment.

Yours faithfully,

Adelaide Nutting, Chairman
Committee on Nursing[81]

A year later Miss Nutting received a formal, engraved certificate from Grosvenor B. Clarkson, director of the Council of Defense, in recognition of her services. She looked reverently at the impressive piece of parchment which bore the seal of the United States and the signatures of the secretaries of war, navy, interior, commerce, and labor. How much she owed America, for here she had found her life's work. She acknowledged the citation immediately, expressing "deep appreciation of sharing in the great work and purposes of the Council."

Too old for active service in the line of duty in my own field, that of nursing, yet desiring greatly to help in such ways as lay within power, the opportunity for needed service which was opened by the Council of National Defense was one for which I shall always feel deeply grateful.[82]

[81] M. Adelaide Nutting, "Final Message from Committee on Nursing, Council of National Defense," Department of Nursing Education Archives, Teachers College; Committee on Nursing, General Medical Board, Council of Defense, *Report of the Subcommittee on Public Health Nurse, Hygiene and Sanitation, Home Nursing, and Welfare, of the Committee on Labor, April 19, 1919* (Washington, D.C.: Council on Defense, 1919), pp. 20–24.

[82] M. Adelaide Nutting (New York) to G. B. Clarkson (Washington, D.C.), MAN Papers.

XIX

Honors from Yale, 1919–1922

Release from wartime responsibilities enabled Adelaide to devote more time to professional activities. She was in her sixteenth year as chairman of the NLNE's Committee on Education and her ninth year as chairman of the Isabel Hampton Robb Memorial Committee and of the Education Committee of the International Council of Nurses.[1] As a member of the Committee to Secure Rank for Army Nurses and chairman of the Endowment Fund Committee of The Johns Hopkins Hospital Nurses Alumnae Association, which had suspended its campaign for funds during the war years, her future promised to be a busy one.

Adelaide was well aware that American life had been vastly altered by the war, and she was quick to note the impact of these changes on nursing and public health. Smaller homes, fewer servants, and scientific advances in medicine and surgery increased the use of hospitals. There were fewer calls for private-duty nurses in homes, but there were more for hospital service, and it was imperative that nursing education be upgraded to meet these challenges.

Of the 1,500 training schools for nurses in 1918, almost 40 percent fell below the standards of the Red Cross Nursing Service. Given the increasing number of young people graduating from high school and college each year, the ANA in 1918 recommended the successful completion of one year of high school as a minimum requisite for admis-

---

[1] Miss Nutting was chairman of the Education Committee of the NLNE from 1903 through 1920 except for one year, June, 1909–May, 1910, when she served as president of the organization, and as chairman of the Isabel Hampton Robb Memorial Committee (1910). Mrs. Robb was elected chairman of the Education Committee of the International Council of Nurses in 1909. Upon Isabel Robb's death in 1910, Miss Nutting accepted the chairmanship, which she held until her retirement in 1925.

sion to nursing schools after January 1, 1919, two years of high school after January 1, 1920, and four years after January 1, 1922.[2]

To Adelaide, some of the problems facing the nursing profession could only be solved by the hospitals, some were the joint concern of the three national nursing organizations, and others required state and national legislation. On her own doorstep at Teachers College lay the responsibility for alerting the future leaders of nursing to the problems and for preparing them to meet the challenges by strengthening the curriculum, especially in the field of public health. The draft revealed that 29 percent of the youth called up for military service were physically unfit. Because many of the disabilities resulted from preventable conditions, there was a great upsurge in public health programs throughout the nation, and the unprecedented demand for public health nurses brought to the fore the matter of financing health projects and nursing education.

By 1920 a statewide health program was contemplated or in operation in twenty-eight states, although only five states maintained separate bureaus of public health nursing. Immediately after the war, the National Tuberculosis Association and the American Red Cross, with its extensive financial resources and a network of local branches, went into action, seeking to bring the gospel of health and prevention of disease to the most remote areas. Through state associations the National Tuberculosis Association attempted to eradicate that disease through its program of prevention. Studies by the Children's Bureau revealed the need for programs that would reduce infant and maternal mortality and promote child health.[3] Dr. Livingston Farrand of the Red Cross asked the Nursing Service Committee whether the head of the nursing program should be a public health nurse or a general nurse whose training was broad enough to handle the public health situation. Miss Nutting replied that the position called for leadership which would go beyond public health, and other nursing leaders concurred.[4]

The upsurge in public health programs imposed a demand on the nursing leadership. A few days after the armistice, Dr. George Vincent, president of the Rockefeller Foundation, invited Adelaide Nutting, Lillian Wald, Annie Goodrich, Dr. Herman Biggs (New York commissioner of health), Dr. C.-E. A. Winslow, and a few others to a luncheon at the Cosmopolitan Club to discuss informally public

[2] Mary M. Roberts, *American Nursing: History and Interpretation* (New York: Macmillan, 1954), p. 164.

[3] *Ibid.*, p. 165.

[4] Portia B. Kernodle, *The Red Cross in Action, 1882–1948* (New York: Harper & Bros., 1949), p. 245.

health nursing and the training of public health nurses.[5] The meeting produced sound discussion, and in January, 1919, the Rockefeller Foundation appointed a committee to investigate the proper training of public health nurses. Dr. Winslow, then of the Yale School of Medicine, was appointed chairman. Adelaide Nutting was invited to become a member of the committee, as was Dr. Welch of Johns Hopkins. The committee soon decided that both nursing and nursing education related to the care of the sick and the prevention of disease, and that they had to be considered as an entity if the committee's conclusions were to be considered valid. The membership of the committee was enlarged to include ten physicians, six nurses, one director of public health, and two laymen, in addition to Josephine Goldmark, who was to conduct the survey. The group was then renamed the Committee for the Study of Nursing Education.[6]

The Rockefeller Foundation agreed to allocate $20,000 for the project. Dr. Haven Emerson, who had directed the Cleveland survey with Miss Goldmark, was invited to become executive secretary. Miss Goldmark was a trained research worker who had served on the Henry Street visiting committee with Isabel Stewart. She was matter of fact and meticulous, yet could see the human and educational aspects of the problem.[7]

The committee's plan for the proposed study included an extensive survey of entrance requirements, curricula, hours, standards of schools for training public health nurses, and a similar study of nurses' training schools. The study was to be carried out extensively from a statistical standpoint and intensively in typical, selected institutions. The actual work of public health nurses and other public health educators would be observed, and the methods and results of typical state, municipal, and voluntary agencies that were doing effective work along public health lines would be investigated. Dr. Winslow also proposed that, for comparison, a study of the education and work of the public health nurse and health visitor in England be made by the executive secretary and one or two members of the committee.[8]

In the main the method of the Cleveland Survey would be used, but, instead of examining each of the 1,500 training schools in the

[5] George Vincent (New York) to Adelaide Nutting (New York), December 4, 1918, MAN Papers.
[6] C.-E. A. Winslow (New Haven, Conn.) to Adelaide Nutting (New York), June 27, 1919, ibid.
[7] Isabel M. Stewart, Oral History, 2 vols. (New York: Columbia University, Butler Library, 1958), 1:251–53.
[8] C.-E. A. Winslow (New Haven) to George Vincent (New York), March 11, 1919, MAN Papers.

United States, a generous sampling of various health agencies, hospitals, and training schools would be taken. Among these were (1) the larger training schools, such as Johns Hopkins, St. Luke's in New York, Presbyterian of Chicago, University of Minneapolis; (2) large municipal hospitals, such as Philadelphia General, Bellevue of New York, Boston City, Cook County of Chicago, Cincinnati General; (3) moderate-sized, endowed, or municipal or partly supported hospitals, such as Memorial of Richmond, Patterson General of Newton, Massachusetts, and Hackley of Muskegon, Michigan; (4) smaller hospitals, such as those of Englewood, New Jersey, Canandaigua, New York, and Bryn Mawr, Pennsylvania; (5) special hospitals, such as Children's of Boston, Columbia of New York, and Washington of Morristown, New Jersey, which had an accredited school for nurses; (6) Pacific Coast hospitals, such as California University or Lane Hospital of Stanford, Samuel Merritt, or Washington State University. Forty-nine public health nursing agencies and twenty-three training schools made up the final list.[9] It was three years before the final report was ready for release. In the interim, Adelaide kept in close touch with Miss Goldmark and attended meetings of the committee to hear preliminary reports.

Another of Miss Nutting's postwar concerns was the status of the city-owned and -managed Bellevue Hospital and Training School and the Training School on Blackwell's Island, where Carolyn Gray was struggling against vermin, contagion, an inadequate budget, lack of staff, vindictive students, and unsympathetic authorities. As a member of the Advisory Committee of the New York Charities Commission and as a friend of Carolyn Gray and the Vassar Camp trainees, Adelaide found herself deeply involved. A short time before she became a member of the Charities Commission, she received a letter from Carolyn, who wrote of one "knock-down blow after another."[10] It was largely Carolyn's predicament that influenced Adelaide to take a place on Bird Coler's committee. With the abatement of the influenza epidemic, Miss Gray found herself in greater straits. When she instituted the eight-hour day on January 1, 1919, the Board of Managers of the hospital refused to sustain her and referred the matter to the commissioner of charities, who asked her to resign. Mrs. Cadwalader Jones, a sympathetic member of the Advisory Committee of the Charities Commission, advised Miss Gray "to prepare a list of her

[9] "List of Training Schools to be Selected for Study, Winslow-Goldmark Survey," *ibid.*

[10] Carolyn E. Gray (Blackwell's Island, N.Y.) to M. A. Nutting (New York), December 7, 1918, *ibid.*

troubles"; if Coler wished her to resign, he should first prove her unfitness to head the school. In apprising Miss Nutting of the situation, Mrs. Jones said, "You were a tower of strength to me last time."[11]

Adelaide was concerned about the Vassar Camp trainees, fifty-seven college graduates who had entered Bellevue in September; three had died and half had gone home. Carolyn Gray feared for what might happen at City Hospital if all the unhappy students suddenly left. When trouble arose between the twenty remaining Vassar Protestants and the Roman Catholic students, it was more than Miss Gray could bear and on March 17 she resigned.[12] Adelaide feared she had been of little service to the Advisory Committee and wondered if she should resign, but Mrs. Jones prevailed upon her to remain at least for the present.[13] Both were greatly relieved when Carolyn Gray found employment as secretary of the Board of Nurse Examiners in Albany. Commissioner Coler was then faced with the problem of finding a successor.[14]

Adelaide admired Carolyn Gray for the stand she had taken on the eight-hour day. She herself had tried to set it up at Johns Hopkins and had never quite succeeded. When in May, 1919, Presbyterian Hospital shortened the working day for students, reducing night duty from seventy-seven hours to fifty-two, and day duty from fifty-seven hours to fifty-two, she wrote a warm letter of congratulations to Anna Maxwell, the hospital's superintendent.[15]

The NLNE was about to begin its campaign for the eight-hour day for all nurses, student and graduate. During the next few months two pamphlets, *The Case for Shorter Hours* and *Suggestions for Establishing Shorter Hours*, were prepared by the Education Committee of the League and circulated widely. Adelaide did not attend the organization's convention in Chicago in June, 1919, but Isabel Stewart went, well fortified with argument. From the convention Isabel wrote that the Education Committee's report had been well re-

[11] Mrs. Cadwalader Jones (New Haven) to M. Adelaide Nutting (New York), February 23, 1919, *ibid.*

[12] Carolyn Gray (Blackwell's Island) to M. A. Nutting (New York), March 18, 1919, *ibid.*

[13] Adelaide Nutting (New York) to Mrs. Cadwalader Jones (New Haven), March 22, 1919; Mrs. Cadwalader Jones (New Haven) to Adelaide Nutting (New York), April 6, 1919; and Adelaide Nutting (New York) to Mrs. Cadwalader Jones (New Haven), April 14, 1919; *ibid.*

[14] Carolyn Gray (Albany, N.Y.) to M. A. Nutting (New York), June 20, 1919, *ibid.*

[15] M. A. Nutting (New York) to Anna Maxwell (New York), May 7, 1919, *ibid.*

ceived, and that the committee had asked to have 5,000 copies of the hours pamphlets printed.

> Everybody asked for you and many felt the meeting lacked the force and impressiveness that you would have brought. But they were eager that you should be spared for the work's sake as well as your own. You need never have the slightest doubt of the feelings which your students and all the nurses have for you. They constantly express their great affection and admiration and they are so eager to consult you on all difficult problems because they respect your judgment and they want to do things you would approve of.[16]

Shorter hours would not come overnight. It would take much publicity, and many people would have to be convinced that student hours were unreasonably and inexcusably long and inconsistent with good educational theory. Long ago Florence Nightingale had said that hospitals should cure disease and not induce it. Adelaide believed that, if public hospitals could be made "to see the light," voluntary and private institutions could be brought into line.[17] It would be a long, hard battle.[18]

After a week at Montauk, Adelaide spent two weeks in New York, catching up on her correspondence at the college and completing committee work. Then, in August, she made the trip to Waterloo for a short visit with Charlie and Lizzie and on the way home stopped at her favorite vacation spot, Ogunquit, Maine.

Before leaving Canada she went to Ottawa to see Claire and Bruce, Keith, and Harold, who had returned safely from the war and were now back at work. Harold was planning to be married in December. Claire hoped Bruce would be able to enter McGill in the fall. Adelaide was especially happy to get better acquainted with Bruce. If he appeared to be a good student, she would help him.

Claire had written that Bruce's expenses at McGill would be $700 a year and that she would provide him with clothes and pocket money; if he got work during the summers, he should be able to earn from $250 to $300. Claire was grateful for Adelaide's offer to help, but she added: "If the expense is more than you can afford, for you must remember you have your old age to think of, he could take a surveyor's course here in Ottawa and work until he saves enough

---

[16] Isabel M. Stewart (Chicago) to M. A. Nutting (Montauk, Long Island), June 28, 1919, *ibid.*

[17] Committee on Education, National League of Nursing Education, "The Case for Shorter Hours in Hospital Schools of Nursing," Bulletin no. 1, n.d., *ibid.*

[18] Carolyn E. Gray, "Square Deal for the Pupil Nurse," *Modern Hospital*, February, 1919; also in the MAN Papers.

to take up engineering."[19] Adelaide promptly sent a check for $200 to start the college fund.[20] Jim would have been proud to have a son graduate from McGill. It made Adelaide sad when she thought of Charlie's law practice in Waterloo and the brilliant career he might have had in Ottawa, Montreal, or Toronto. Lizzie had been blamed for Charlie's blighted career, but the time to make changes was long past. Adelaide refused to let her mind dwell upon it; she would concentrate her efforts on young Bruce Nutting.

In September, Adelaide sent Claire a check for $150. It would help greatly, for Bruce's tuxedo would cost $75. "The thing that makes me happy," Claire wrote, "is that the hard feeling that used to exist between us all is, I hope, a thing of the past and that we may enjoy the feeling that we are welcome to the other's home whenever we are able to visit. Your coming to Ottawa was a great joy to me."[21]

Family had always meant much to Adelaide, and as she grew older it came to have even deeper meaning. Keith was well again and Harold had recovered from his wounds. Minnie and Gilbert's son, Ambrose, who had also served in Europe, and their daughter Armine, who had driven an ambulance for the British Red Cross, were home again. Adelaide shuddered when she thought of the young girl driving over rough terrain without lights, carrying the wounded from the front lines to the hospital and often having to take refuge in the trenches during bombing. Adelaide was proud of her nieces and nephews. Bruce would soon be off to McGill and Arthur to Cambridge. She hoped she was not expecting too much of them. Next year she hoped to spend her vacation in Newfoundland. She wanted to take a trip with her sister. In Europe she had always wished Armine were along to share the beautiful scenery, the historic spots, and the treasures of the great art galleries and museums.

In the late summer of 1919 Annie Goodrich turned over the Army School of Nursing to Julia C. Stimson, who had been chief nurse of the American Expeditionary Forces in France, and returned to New York to divide her time between Teachers College and the Henry Street Visiting Nurses Association.[22] Miss Goodrich had done an admirable job of organizing the Army School. By the date of the

[19] Claire Nutting (Ottawa) to Adelaide Nutting (New York), June 14, 1919, MAN Papers.

[20] Claire Nutting (Ottawa) to Adelaide Nutting (New York), July 4, 1919, ibid.

[21] Claire Nutting (Ottawa) to Adelaide Nutting (New York), September 10, 1919, ibid.

[22] M. Adelaide Nutting (Ogunquit, Maine) to Isabel M. Stewart, [New York], August 16, 1919, MAN–IMS Correspondence.

armistice 1,099 students were on duty in twenty-five military hospitals, 567 were awaiting assignment, and 10,689 applications had
been filed.[23] As the cantonment hospitals were closed, units were
combined. Many students left the Army School to marry, others to
return to their former positions. Eventually the units were reduced to
two, one at Walter Reed Hospital in Washington, the other at Letterman General Hospital in San Francisco.[24] From those who remained
would come some of nursing's most distinguished leaders of the next
generation.

Adelaide was pleased to have Annie Goodrich back in New York.
The two women did not always agree, but they were the best of
friends and stood shoulder to shoulder for the advancement of the
nursing profession. Just now they were particularly concerned about
proposed legislation to secure rank for army nurses.

Nurses overseas had reported difficulties in their relations with
army personnel which stemmed from their lack of authority, an
authority which Britain and Canada had conferred upon their nurses.
Early in the war, the Committee on Nursing of the Council of National Defense had sought congressional action, but had met stubborn
opposition.[25] A national committee to secure rank for nurses was
organized in June, 1918. It numbered among its members Mrs. White-
law Reid, Mrs. August P. Belmont, Mrs. H. H. Greeley, Mrs. Chester
Bolton, Mrs. Medill McCormick, Mrs. Caroline Hampton Halsted,
Miss Annie Goodrich, Miss Anna Maxwell, Miss Adelaide Nutting,
Miss Georgia Nevins, and other nursing leaders.[26] In July, 1919, a
circular letter was sent to all members of the NLNE, urging them to
push rank for nurses.[27]

After the armistice, the American Hospital Association and the
newly organized American Legion enthusiastically endorsed rank for
nurses, and a more responsive Congress incorporated the provision of
relative rank in the bill for reorganization of the army which it passed
in May, 1920. On June 4, 1920, President Wilson signed the bill, and
on August 10 the surgeon general of the army placed the gold oak

[23] Esther A. Werminghaus, *Annie W. Goodrich: Her Journey to Yale* (New
York: Macmillan, 1950), pp. 59–60.

[24] Roberts, *American Nursing*, p. 140.

[25] *Ibid.*, pp. 170–71.

[26] M. A. Nutting [Ogunquit, Maine] to Nathaniel Thayer (Newport, R.I.),
July 4, 1919; Caroline H. Halsted (Baltimore) to M. A. Nutting (New York),
[1918 or 1919]; and Exhibit A, "Testimonial Rank for Nurses"; MAN Papers.

[27] "Minutes of the National League of Nursing Education Board Meeting,
New York, October 15, 1919," *ibid.*

leaves of a major on the shoulders of Nurse Corps Superintendent Julia C. Stimson.[28]

Enrollment at Teachers College in September, 1919, was the largest in the school's history, and, of the 3,118 students registered, 250 were in the Department of Nursing and Health.[29] Hospitals, training schools, and public health agencies were now looking to Teachers College for nursing administrators, teachers of nursing, and public health workers. Adelaide's graduates were to be found in the large hospitals of the great cities and in public health service work in rural and urban areas. She kept the curriculum geared to the needs of the changing times. After World War I, courses in nursing venereal diseases and in new types of occupational therapy were offered. With the increased demand for school nurses, courses that were especially applicable were included in the curriculum. Although Adelaide heartily approved of physical training in the schools, she did not think it lay within the province of the school nurse.[30]

Adelaide continued her work as chairman of the NLNE's Committee on Education and as a member of the Rockefeller Committee for the Study of Training Schools, for which Miss Goldmark was making a survey. She read the preliminary reports and made extensive suggestions. In 1920 she joined the Hopkins Alumnae in their renewed drive for a $1,000,000 endowment. There were also other fund-raising activities in which she was interested. By 1920 the Robb Memorial Fund had reached $28,000, but it was not likely that the original goal of $50,000 would be reached; the hope for a chair of nursing was abandoned in favor of annual scholarships. Meanwhile, the NLNE and the ANA proposed that a memorial scholarship fund be established in honor of Jane Delano, who had died in France on April 15, 1919, while on an inspection of Red Cross hospitals. There were many calls for Adelaide's energies and funds. She pledged $100 to be applied to the expenses of the Hopkins endowment campaign, but on second thought decided to withdraw it and to give $1,000 to

[28] National Committee to Secure Rank for Nurses, "Victory," Bulletin no. 15, August 18, 1920, Department of Nursing Education Archives, Teachers College. The rank for a beginning nurse was second lieutenant; for a beginning doctor, it was first lieutenant.

[29] Lawrence Cremin et al., A History of Teachers College, Columbia University (New York: Columbia University Press, 1954), p. 15; Isabel M. Stewart, Twenty-five Years of Nursing Education in Teachers College, 1899–1925 (Teachers College Bulletin, 17th ser., no. 3, February, 1926), p. 16.

[30] M. Adelaide Nutting (Ogunquit, Maine) to Isabel M. Stewart (New York), July 31, 1918, MAN–IMS Correspondence.

the fund itself.[31] Like many other American nurses, Adelaide was interested in helping the Bordeaux School of Nursing.[32]

At the joint meeting of the ANA, NOPHN, and NLNE in Atlanta, Georgia, in April, 1920, Adelaide read a paper on the "Outlook in Nursing." In it she predicted:

> Prohibition and Woman Suffrage are two of the recent great social movements which will profoundly affect the future of nursing. The efforts of our fellow-workers in various branches of industry to secure an 8 hour day have undoubtedly strengthened our own attempts to secure shorter hours for both students and graduate nurses. On the other hand, our requirements for admission to schools of nursing must have a distinct effect upon the education of young women throughout the country (and, indeed, throughout other countries).

She noted considerable unrest, the shortage of applicants for training and of graduate nurses, and the estimated need for 50,000 public health nurses alone. In the face of these shortages she preferred to sacrifice numbers for quality. To make nursing attractive she asked for better and sounder training, high standards, a reduction of hours, increased wages, better living conditions, the elimination of apprenticeship methods, and training school funds that were free of hospital control. The hopeful signs were nursings' living memorials—the Isabel Hampton Robb fund, the Red Cross, the NOPHN, and the Nightingale School at Bordeaux, among others.[33]

At the Atlanta meeting Adelaide presented her resignation as chairman of the NLNE Committee on Education because she planned to go on sabbatical leave in 1921. She later agreed to serve as honorary chairman and to remain a member of the committee.[34]

After seeing the 1920 summer school launched with 192 students enrolled in nursing and health, Adelaide left for the long-anticipated vacation with her sister in Newfoundland. Min's children were now grown. Ambrose was in business, Frances Adelaide was married, Arthur was at Cambridge, and Armine was planning her wedding. As she had promised, Adelaide told Min and Gilbert all the details of the visits of the Baroness Mannerheim, leader of the Finnish Nurses, Miss

[31] M. Adelaide Nutting (New York) to Mrs. Thomas Cullen (Baltimore), December 2, 1920, MAN Papers.

[32] M. Adelaide Nutting (New York) to Lavinia Dock, [Fayetteville, Pa.], May, 1920, ibid.

[33] Adelaide Nutting, "Outlook in Nursing" (Address given in Atlanta, Ga., April 17, 1920), ibid., printed in The Public Health Nurse, September, 1920, pp. 1–5.

[34] Adelaide Nutting (New York) to Mrs. Flash (New York), May 20, 1920, MAN Papers.

Charlotte Munck of Denmark, and Miss Margaret Breay of England to Teachers College just before the ANA meeting in Atlanta. The baroness and Miss Munck had spoken before 100 students, and Adelaide had given a luncheon for them and a tea for forty afterward.[35] Min also wanted to hear about National Hospital Day, inaugurated on Florence Nightingale's 100th birthday, and the impressive service at the Cathedral of St. John the Divine, when she had marched with 2,000 other uniformed nurses.[36] She told her sister about the wonderful gift of $1,500 from students and alumnae at commencement to the Nutting Nightingale Collection, a gift which she had turned over to the Teachers College library to purchase history of nursing books.[37]

Adelaide read books and magazines that she had brought to share with Minnie and Gilbert, as well as her notes for articles she hoped to write, among them one for the first issue of the new scientific journal to be published by the Medical Department and Bureau of Public Health of the recently organized League of Red Cross Societies.[38]

While visiting in St. John's, news came that the Nineteenth Amendment to the U.S. Constitution had been ratified on August 26. Minnie and Adelaide rejoiced together. Minnie had worked hard to secure voting rights for women in Newfoundland. Like Lavinia Dock, she had been a great admirer of Mrs. Pankhurst and her daughters in their valiant campaign for woman suffrage in England. Adelaide told Minnie how Lavinia, staunch member of the Woman's party, had been arrested and sentenced to 30 days in the government workhouse at Oscoqua, Virginia, for picketing the White House, but had had five days taken off her sentence for good behavior. Adelaide had marched with other nurses in parades on Fifth Avenue, but she had never picketed.[39] She never urged nursing students to march in parades, but she told them that suffrage was very close to their work, and most of them marched.[40] Adelaide looked at woman suffrage not as an American, Canadian, or British cause but rather as a world

[35] Adelaide Nutting (New York) to Lavinia Dock, [Fayetteville, Pa.], May, 1920, ibid.
[36] Clippings from the Philadelphia Ledger, April 29, 1920, and the New York Times, May 18, 1920, MAN Papers.
[37] Stewart, Twenty-five Years of Nursing Education in Teachers College, p. 41.
[38] Thomas R. Brown (Geneva, Switzerland) to Adelaide Nutting (New York), January 28, 1920, MAN Papers.
[39] Editorial, British Journal of Nursing, November 24, 1917, clipping in the MAN Papers; The Johns Hopkins Nurses Alumnae Journal, November, 1917.
[40] Stewart, Oral History, 1:141–42.

movement. The enfranchisement of women meant liberation, the freedom to develop and to express.

Adelaide talked to Min about her sabbatical in the spring of 1921. Her plans were not definite, but she hoped to visit England, take another Mediterranean cruise, and visit Greece. Could Min and Gilbert join her? Gilbert often went to England on business. Why not take some time out for pleasure and see Italy and Greece? They promised to think it over.

Back in New York another record-breaking enrollment greeted Adelaide at registration. This year there were 342 students in the Nursing and Health Department, including students from Presbyterian Hospital, who were taking their theoretical work at Teachers College while working for their diplomas and bachelor of science degrees. In October good news came to the department when Helen Hartley Jenkins added $50,000 to the endowment. This would cover the salary of the assistant professor she had been providing for annually since 1914.

The Vassar Camp trainees held a reunion in November, and Miss Nutting was invited to make one of the principal addresses. Of the 399 girls who had entered nurses training schools, 174 had remained to graduate; 7 had died during the influenza epidemic. The sudden ending of the war before they were well into their training, marriage, sickness, and family responsibilities contributed to the high number of dropouts. Academically they were the best-educated group ever to enter nursing at one time. From them new leadership in nursing could be expected to emerge. Realizing their potential, Dean Mills and his staff had made plans for a reunion at Thanksgiving and had invited the graduates, their teachers, and the leaders in the various fields of nursing. Fresh from training school, the graduates would be alert to the faults of the present system; it was expected they would be frank and articulate.

Well aware of the unhappy and unpleasant experiences so many had encountered in their training, Dean Mills appealed to the young nurses:

> If you give up, you help to continue these unfortunate conditions; if you continue, you will help realize better conditions for yourselves and thousands of others in the future. You are one of the greatest, if not the greatest potential force in the country for bringing improvement.[41]

[41] Gladys Bonner Clappison, *Vassar's Rainbow Division, 1918* (Lake Mills, Iowa: Graphic Publishing Co., 1964), p. 126.

A large number of nursing leaders attended the reunion. Several were directors of the schools at which the nurses had trained, among them Carolyn Gray, Annie Goodrich, Anna Maxwell, Maude Landis, Nellie Hawkinson, Elsie Lawler, Isabel Stewart, Josephine Goldmark, and Martha Wilson. It was pleasant to greet old friends—Dr. Winslow, Dean Mills, Mrs. Blodgett, and President McCracken. They discussed topics varying from the apprenticeship system in schools of nursing, student government, and the separation of nursing schools and hospitals to what makes a successful nurse.[42] Adelaide spoke after the dinner on Friday night.

> It seems a far cry tonight from that hour two years ago when I stood here with other friends of the Vassar Training Camp to speed you on your way—not to the battlefields of France but to those other battlefields—our great hospitals where the never-ending warfare against disease goes steadily on as it has for centuries past. And there at Bellevue, at Philadelphia, at Boston City, you found your Argonne Forests, your St. Mihiel, your Belleau Wood. To no members of our Army Nursing Service in France or elsewhere was applied a test of courage or spirit more searching, more severe than that which you faced during those first awful weeks grappling with deadly pestilence.
>
> To us of the older generation, anxious watchers from without, the way in which you met that test, the quiet patriotism, the unfaltering devotion to the duty before you, can never be forgotten. But the real tests of life, I suppose, do not come to us in those great and stirring moments. Our actual characters, our genuine strength and worth are not shown in the ardour of our response to such appeals. They reveal themselves in the steadfastness with which we hold to a high purpose through the dull routine of daily duty, over long periods; in the fortitude and faith with which that purpose is pursued in the face of discouragement and sometimes defeat; in the dauntless spirit which holds "tasks in hours of insight willed can be through hours of gloom fulfilled."
>
> It is largely this spirit, this refusal to look upon the daily duty—made up of the necessary tasks of life—as a kind of slavery; this sense of responsibility for standing by our work as a captain stands by his ship, which forms the bone and marrow of nursing.[43]

Adelaide continued by recounting some of the heroisms and rewards of nursing—the desolate, dark, and doubtful hours that sometimes came to nurses, even to Florence Nightingale on the Crimean Heights. She asked that, if for any of the Vassar Camp trainees the bright vision of two summers ago had faded or vanished, they recapture it and grasp the fact that nurses everywhere are engaged in a

[42] *The Thermometer*, March, 1921, pp. 1, 4, 5, 6.
[43] *Ibid.*, pp. 1, 7, 8.

warfare which in one sense is even greater than that in which the world had recently been engulfed. She asked for improvements in nursing schools which would attract women of good potential and then draw forth and shape their highest powers. As she viewed the matter, the remedying of defects in the schools must come largely from within; those who would contribute toward the rebuilding of nursing's educational structure would have to bring not only knowledge, ability, and constructive imagination but much sympathy, patience, and affection. In conclusion she recalled her message to the trainees two year before: "In welcoming you . . . in giving you the hand of fellowship and affection, I find my last word to you is not unlike my first. It still breathes of *duty*. It points to what still remains to be done."[44]

As the winter of 1920 approached, Adelaide thought of all the things she wanted to accomplish before leaving at the end of the term for her sabbatical abroad. Uppermost in her mind was the Hopkins Training School Endowment Fund. It had been impossible to resume work in August because the Hopkins University and Medical School were campaigning for funds and did not want competition. The Rockefeller Foundation was not encouraging, so Adelaide's committee decided to study other ways and means of raising $1,000,000.[45]

After much hustle, bustle, and excitement, last-minute packing, and rushing about, Adelaide settled into her cabin aboard the S.S. *Cedric* on Friday, February 4, 1921. Isabel Stewart and Willystine Goodsell had helped her check her luggage and had carried aboard the sundry gifts of candy, books, and magazines sent by friends. The ship had scarcely cleared the Narrows when Adelaide began a note to Isabel. "More and more do I lean upon you, trust you, love you. Surely never were any more fortunate in having a friendship which stretches out into two ways, into work and into friendship."[46]

Adelaide was too tired to sleep for the first three days. After two rough and stormy days there were "marvelous seas," and she felt only the throbbing of the engine; she slept so well that she wished the voyage might last another week. She was refreshed by the eleven-day crossing, during which she did nothing but sleep and eat, read, and think of the loved ones she would meet in London. At last she

[44] *Ibid.*

[45] Amy P. Miller, "A Short History of the Endowment Fund of The Johns Hopkins Nurses Alumnae Association," n.d., MAN Papers.

[46] Adelaide Nutting (aboard the S.S. *Cedric*) to Isabel M. Stewart (New York), February 4, 1921, MAN–IMS Correspondence.

and her sister would be taking the trip of their childhood dreams, to England, France, Italy, Sicily, and Greece.

In London, Adelaide was met by Minnie and her daughter Armine, who was waiting to join her husband in Constantinople when he returned from India. Soon Adelaide and her sister were settled on Curzon Street and busy with plans. Frances Adelaide and the baby were coming over from Ireland, where her husband, Edward Haughton Nigel Kennedy, was an officer in the Royal Navy, and Arthur would come down from Cambridge for a weekend. Gilbert planned to come from Newfoundland and join them for part of the trip on the Continent. Adelaide's old nursing friends Mrs. Fenwick and Margaret Breay came for tea. Mrs. Fenwick was "exultant over her success in finally getting a registration bill passed by Parliament."[47]

On February 23, Adelaide and Armine, both in their sixties, set out to realize their youthful ambition. They stopped only briefly in Paris, since they planned to come back later, and then hurried on to Marseilles and two delightful weeks on the Riviera and in Nice, Genoa, Rome, and Naples. Adelaide thought France was "picking up at a wonderful rate" since the war, and that her people were showing great spirit and industry, but that Italy was very pathetic, "the war having brought a kind of deterioration and poverty which showed itself everywhere, in the hotels, in food, service, and equipment, on the railways, in the streets and shops." Italy's sheer physical beauty was "unsurpassed but the sordid and seamy side is constantly obtrusive."[48]

The two sisters spent three weeks in Siracusa, living in a hotel which had once been a Benedictine monastery and whose gardens looked out on Mt. Etna. Gilbert, who had expected to join them, cabled he could not get away, so they altered their itinerary and Minnie decided she should return home sooner that she had planned.[49]

Gilbert then decided that he must come, and the next thing Adelaide and Minnie heard was that he was in England trying to locate them. As soon as his message came, they packed up their belongings and started for Paris. Six days later they were in London, where Gilbert was planning a motor trip through southern England. As soon as Armine left for Constantinople, Gilbert, Minnie, and Adelaide

[47] Adelaide Nutting (London) to Isabel M. Stewart (New York), February 16, 1921, *ibid*.

[48] Adelaide Nutting (Siracusa, Italy) to Charles and Lizzie Nutting (Waterloo, Quebec), March 22, 1921, MAN Papers.

[49] *Ibid.*

set out, taking Arthur with them for the first few days. Adelaide
wrote Lizzie:

> Anything more enchanting than those days of rolling through Devon-
> shire, Cornwall, Hampshire and Sussex, in a luxurious Daimler car, with
> an experienced chauffeur to guide us, I can hardly imagine. We stopped
> at many lovely places on the coast and visited old cathedral towns,
> Winchester, Exeter, Wells, Salisbury. We saw Stonehenge, Bath, Clov-
> elly, St. Ives, and even spent a charming hour in Penzance. It seems too
> wonderful to be true; and when we got back to London I felt as if I
> had come to the end of a beautiful dream.[50]

After the motor trip and so many happy days together, Gilbert and
Minnie left for Liverpool, where Frances and the baby were to join
them on the voyage to St. John's, and a deep gloom settled over
Adelaide. At the Ruston platform she had broken down and cried.
"What on earth can I do to prevent becoming a tearful old lady?"
she asked Minnie in a letter begun before the Goslings had even
reached the Irish Sea. Adelaide hoped Minnie would not be too uncomfortable, but at least she had "good Gilbert and Frances and the
baby and friends about her." "Nothing," she wrote, "is unbearable if
there are loved ones to share it. Loneliness is the only truly awful
thing." Adelaide realized she and her sister would never have such
a holiday again. "I must console myself with all the lovely memories
which I am storing up—and all the trifling irritations and vexations
of the days are swiftly passing out of recollection."[51]

The fact that Adelaide's trunk had gone astray on the return from
Italy, while Minnie's had come straight through, contributed greatly
to her depressed state of mind. She could make no plans for returning
to France. "I can not stir without that trunk and so far there is not
a trace of it. I have done my utmost over the telephone with Cook's
squandering time, breath and money fruitlessly and really I don't
know what to do next."[52]

Somehow she felt better after committing her grievances and loneliness to paper, and she spent the afternoon at University College, attending a lecture on Egyptian excavations. On Sunday she went to
church and in the afternoon took a long bus ride into lovely rolling
country whose pretty settlements she identified with Ruskin and
Browning.

[50] Adelaide Nutting (London) to Lizzie H. Nutting (Waterloo), May 20, 1921,
ibid.
[51] Adelaide Nutting (London) to Armine N. Gosling (St. John's, Newfoundland), May 21, 1921, *ibid.*
[52] *Ibid.*

While Adelaide was abroad, Isabel Stewart kept her informed about the Nursing Department, conventions, faculty meetings, and matters of consequence to the profession. When Anna Maxwell's retirement as superintendent of Presbyterian Hospital was announced, and the possibility of an endowed training school appeared in the offing, Isabel relayed the exciting news to Adelaide, suggesting that this might be an appropriate time to approach the Rockefeller Foundation for a grant to launch the new school as an experiment in nursing education under the auspices of the Teachers College Department of Nursing and Health, on the condition that it should have a perfectly free hand in all school appointments. This Isabel wrote, would provide the necessary financial backing for the first two or three years and would allow time for raising the endowment necessary for buildings when the hospital was moved and the new medical school of Columbia University was constructed. Dean William Darrach of Columbia University Medical School had come to consult Adelaide and found she was away. Isabel Stewart assured him that Miss Nutting would be interested and gave him a copy of her pamphlet *Sounder Economic Basis for Training Schools*.

Later Isabel was invited to a conference to discuss a university school. The meeting was attended by Anna Maxwell and two physicians from Presbyterian Hospital, Dean Darrach and two other members of the staff of the College of Physicians and Surgeons, Dean James E. Russell, Maurice Bigelow and Annie Goodrich of Teachers College. Isabel reported to Adelaide that Dean Russell "did not warm up much." He had no desire for Teachers College to undertake any responsibility other than that of an advisor, and he refused to commit himself further without consulting Miss Nutting. At a small dinner party in her apartment, Anna Maxwell told Isabel Stewart and Annie Goodrich that she favored a university school, that fund raising would be no problem, and that President Nicholas Murray Butler had said he would support the school.[53]

Adelaide hastened to reply to Isabel's news:

> The situation at the Presbyterian is breath-taking and as you would probably guess my one burning desire is to take the first steamer home. My family here . . . think it unwise so I shall think the whole matter over carefully before deciding. . . . I approve heartily of the idea of bringing the Presbyterian School of Nursing up to a University basis and would urge the College to cooperate to the fullest of its resources in

[53] Isabel Stewart (New York) to Adelaide Nutting, [in Europe], April 8, 1921; and Isabel Stewart (New York) to Adelaide Nutting (London), April 21, 1921; MAN–IMS Correspondence.

any effort in that direction. To fail to do so would be to lose one of the most important opportunities for the advancement of nursing education that could possibly come to us. . . . I am eager to get back and go to work on the problem.[54]

Under the current five-year experiment, students from Presbyterian Hospital took theory and academic courses at Teachers College and did their clinical work at Presbyterian Hospital. Upon completing their studies they received a diploma in nursing from the Presbyterian Training School and a bachelor of science degree in nursing or public health from Teachers College. Relations between the Department of Nursing at the college and a new university school would be delicate, fraught with dangers as well as magnificent possibilities. The matter seemed to hinge on the selection of the school's director. Adelaide hoped it might be someone from her own staff who would be thoroughly familiar with the problem, and with the organization and philosophy behind a university school.[55] She was willing to cut short her holiday if necessary, and she eagerly awaited word from Isabel. After conferring with Dean Russell, Miss Stewart cabled Miss Nutting not to hurry home.[56] Meanwhile, Isabel had written Adelaide that there would be ample time to discuss matters on her return, and that, because Dr. Darrach and Anna Maxwell were soon to be in France, it might be possible to arrange a conference in Le Harvre, Étretat, or Paris.[57]

Adelaide concluded her professional visits at Oxford and in London and left for Paris early Saturday, May 28. She had written to Helen Hay, director of nursing for the Red Cross in Paris, who had secured a room for her at Hotel Letutia in the Latin Quarter which she hoped would not cost more than $2.00 a day. She was met at the station by Miss Hay, Alice Fitzgerald, Mary Gardner, and Lyda Anderson, four "noble professional colleagues" who were eager to help her "through the ever troublesome vexations, the wearisome job of getting baggage off trains, through customs, into a cab, out of a cab, upstairs and settled." To Adelaide's horror, the room reserved for her, the only vacant one in the house, cost 40 francs. Board was 30 francs a day. The next morning she was at the hotel desk early and switched to a

[54] Adelaide Nutting (London) to Isabel M. Stewart (New York), April 30, 1921, ibid.

[55] Ibid.

[56] Cablegram, Isabel Stewart (New York) to M. A. Nutting (London), May 16, 1921, ibid.

[57] Isabel Stewart (New York) to Adelaide Nutting (London), April 29, 1921, ibid.

cubbyhole of a room for $2.00 a day. She resolved to take her meals on the boulevards.[58]

It was warm in Paris, and Adelaide did not have the energy to do many of the things she had promised herself—"a visit to Fountainbleau and to Versailles to refresh fading memories of the historic spot, a visit to the devastated regions to visualize more sharply the horror of war." She "put them off for some time in the dim and distant future" and wandered aimlessly in the gardens, the Tuileries, the Place du Carrousel, the Concorde, the Luxembourg, the Champs-Elysées, with "one day in the Louvre revelling in its beauties, its Corots, Rousseaus, Millets," and other rare and beautiful pictures. With some of her nursing friends she went out to St. Germain and had tea on the terrace of the famous Hotel Henri Quatre. She also had tea with old acquaintances at the "sumptuous" Hotel Plaza Athene off the Champs-Elysées and with another friend at the very nice Columbine. She concluded that she was "acquiring an invaluable working directory of tea rooms, lunch rooms and hotels, etc." As the guest of Gay Rawlins, a Hopkins graduate of 1895, she spent two days in Chartres, whose beauty she thought paled in the light of memories of Wells, Exeter, Salisbury.[59]

While in Paris, Adelaide wrote to her old friend Mrs. Edith Kelly, now living in Switzerland, where she was educating her young son, asking if she would find her a quiet place in which to spend about three weeks. After an exchange of letters and telegrams, Adelaide duly arrived at the Hotel Byron, Villeneuve, about a mile from the Castle of Chillon, which was visible from her window. The blue of the water and the high surrounding mountains reminded her of Taormina. A tramway connected Villeneuve with Montreux, Vevey, Lausanne, and other resorts around the lake, and small steamers made the rounds every few hours. The hotel commemorated Byron, who, while staying in a smaller, earlier structure on the same site, had written parts not only of the *Prisoner of Chillon* but of *Childe Harold, Siege of Corinth,* and *Manfred.* A bust of Byron stood in the lobby. Shelley and Milton, Thomas Gray, John Evelyn, Horace Walpole, Jean Jacques Rousseau, and Edward Gibbon had all visited the hotel. "One treads sacred dust," Adelaide wrote her sister.[60]

The "fortnight on Lake Geneva" had been tranquillity itself, for

[58] Adelaide Nutting (Paris) to Armine N. Gosling (St. John's), May 29, 1921, MAN Papers.
[59] *Ibid.*
[60] Adelaide Nutting (Villeneuve, Switzerland) to Armine N. Gosling (St. John's), June 16, 1921, *ibid.*

"eye and soul were steeped in beauty." Adelaide next crossed the lake to Geneva with Edith Kelly and spent a few days "loitering about the older part of the city so eloquent of Rousseau and of Calvin, and then up into the mountains to Aix-les-Baines in the Haute Savoie where they stayed several days and had several lovely drives, drank the waters and then took a five-hour motor drive over motor passes of wild splendor and through green valleys of tenderest beauty arriving at Chamonix."[61] Mrs. Kelly then returned to her son, and Adelaide was left alone in the little hotel where she had stayed twenty years before. Everything except the prices had remained unchanged. From her window she could see Mt. Blanc, and in every direction she "beheld the superb heights of the great Alps." Adelaide had secured passage to Montreal on the White Star Line's *Megantic*, which would sail from Liverpool on July 30, and, after two weeks at the cool mountain retreat, she hurried on to Paris.[62]

In contrast to Chamonix, Paris seemed "a noisy inferno." Adelaide had, however, recovered sufficient energy to make the trip to Fountainbleau.

> When we went through Barbizon, and passed the very fields where Millet painted his Angelus and Gleaners—with the harvest spread out golden before us, and the low-lying, red-roofed village in the background I could have cried with the aching beauty of it all. The little houses in Barbizon in which Millet lived and Rousseau and Corot and others are all tenderly protected and tablets are on all of them. We drove through superb stretches of forest, and then we toured the palace. Endless rooms, gorgeous rooms, intimate and personal, state and official. Napoleon dominated the scene. One could not escape him.[63]

On another day when it was pleasant, Adelaide drove to Versailles and visited Malmaison on the way.

> Well, Versailles was worth the second visit. It all seemed new and in a way very thrilling. To stand in the Hall of Mirrors made one look back to the day in 1871 . . . when the German Emperor was crowned there— and contrast it with the day not long since which took away virtually the German Empire in the Treaty of Versailles signed in that very room.[64]

[61] Adelaide Nutting (Chamonix, France) to Isabel M. Stewart (New York), July 7, 1921, MAN–IMS Correspondence.
[62] *Ibid.*
[63] Adelaide Nutting (Paris) to Armine N. Gosling (St. John's), July 16–23, 1921, MAN Papers.
[64] *Ibid.*

In her letter to Minnie she confessed she had come down to her last coppers. Later, when she discovered the Rodin museum and bought some photographs, she walked home to offset her extravagance.

Dean Darrach and Anna Maxwell arrived in Paris on Sunday. The heat was oppressive, and, after the three had dinner together, they went into the garden on the Champs-Elysées to discuss the situation at the Presbyterian Training School and the matter of Miss Maxwell's successor. Adelaide appreciated Anna Maxwell's deep concern for the school she had built up, and she was glad to have the opportunity to talk over the whole situation with Dean Darrach and to hear his point of view. Adelaide appealed for a true university school, one distinctly apart from both the hospital services and the medical school, one which would be able to stand on its own financially. She recommended Annie Goodrich as the person best qualified to develop such a school.[65]

The next day Adelaide left for London to pick up her trunks and make some professional visits before sailing from Liverpool on July 30. It was cooler in London, and, after getting her trunks from Cook's and packing, she looked up some of her nursing friends. Then, "the inevitable thing happened."

> I struck a dinner being given to the Superintendent of Nurses of a London Hospital on the occasion of her departure for a new position at the Glasgow Infirmary—one of the most important positions in Great Britain. Of course I had to speak and that was almost superhuman effort—after all these months of silence and irresponsibility. But I had one delightful moment when I found that the nurse whom they were honouring with a dinner is an Oxford woman, had several years of training there, a full classical course and holds a degree. I think she is the only nurse in England with just that background and you know what grist that is to my mill.[66]

The *Megantic* was a "good little ship, clean, comfortable with excellent table and courteous service." The weather was foggy and rainy, so, despite the "feeble" ventilation of her inexpensive inside cabin, Adelaide spent most of her time inside, reading and resting. The ship docked at Montreal on Sunday, August 7. Because there were no trains on Sunday, she did not get to Waterloo until the next day.

[65] Adelaide Nutting (London) to Isabel Stewart (New York), July 26, 1921; and Adelaide Nutting (aboard the S.S. *Megantic*) to Isabel Stewart (New York), August 4, 1921; MAN–IMS Correspondence.

[66] Adelaide Nutting (aboard the S.S. *Megantic*) to Armine N. Gosling (St. John's), August 4, 1921, MAN Papers.

Adelaide found Charlie and Lizzie much the same although both were beginning to show the inroads of time. Charlie looked a little "less gaunt and shadowy" than he had the year before; Lizzie seemed tired and listless, but "plucks up and tries to make everbody happy." With an excellent, well-trained French girl and a man of all work, they seemed to be doing very well. Bruce Nutting was also visiting at Charlie's and Adelaide had an opportunity to size up her young protégé. He was nice looking, quiet, gentle, and easy going, but his academic record at McGill was not encouraging.

On her last day in Waterloo, Adelaide took a bouquet of sweet peas to lay on her mother's grave. As she placed them there, she noticed how lonely the small stones of her father's and Arthur's graves looked and she hurried back to get more flowers, phlox and larkspur, violets and mignonette, so that they too would be covered with fresh flowers. On the return visit she took Bruce along and gave him a lesson in family history. Later she wrote her sister:

> There is good stuff in the Nutting traits or we would not be the decent intelligent creatures we are. And I do not propose to see that side of the family history relegated to obscurity or oblivion. The dark pages of which we have our share are in the annals of about every family I know anything about. Ours are simply more conspicuous, everybody knew them all, and more than all. But we seem to have no skeletons hidden away.[67]

On the way back to New York, Adelaide met Isabel Stewart in Montreal and they visited between trains. Isabel, who was on her way to Quebec, had brought a packet of mail and the latest reports on the Department of Nursing.

With everyone at the Emerson away on vacation, it was quiet and lonely when Adelaide arrived. Within the week she finally pinned the manager down to a date for painters and paperhangers to take over. By the time the fall term opened, her apartment had been fully redecorated and cleaned. Every cupboard and closet had been painted, every dish, pot, and pan had been washed, fresh paper had been put on the shelves, pictures were back on the walls, and clean curtains hung at the windows.[68]

Adelaide soon found herself getting back into the swing of things. She had lunch with friends at the Cosmopolitan Club, and Annie

[67] Adelaide Nutting (Waterloo) to Armine N. Gosling (St. John's), August 21, 1921, *ibid.*
[68] Adelaide Nutting (New York) to Isabel Stewart (Ogunquit, Maine), August 28, 1921, MAN–IMS Correspondence.

Goodrich came over for a long talk. In June the first class of the Army School of Nursing had graduated in two widely separated hospitals, one from the Walter Reed Hospital in Washington, the other from Letterman General Hospital in San Francisco. Miss Goodrich had taken her uniform down to Washington for the occasion. She had been proud to stand by Julia Stimson, the first woman in America to hold the rank of major, and General Merritte W. Ireland as the graduates passed in review. Later the army recalled Miss Goodrich for two weeks and gave her the rank of second lieutenant so that she might go to San Francisco to deliver the graduating address at Letterman General. She was now back at Henry Street, but she felt restive.

The conversation then turned to Presbyterian Hospital, the future of the training school there, and Anna Maxwell's successor. Although the two women saw eye to eye on collegiate schools, Annie was quite surprised when Adelaide said she had recommended her to Dean Darrach to head the Presbyterian school, and she revealed a deeper humility than Adelaide had ever suspected she possessed. Adelaide promised to have a long talk with Dean Russell about the Presbyterian school.

The fall term opened with only 295 students in the Department of Nursing and Health. It was a decline from the 342 of the previous year, but the summer school of 254 had been the largest summer session in the history of the department. The Institute for State Inspectors had been highly successful. As soon as Isabel Stewart had time, plans would be drawn up for a similar institute and would thereby justify the role of the department as a service institution.

There was so much Adelaide wanted to do. It was time to revise the *Educational Status* volume. Some day soon she would have to take up with the U.S. Commissioner of Education the matter of re-issuing the book. Years before, she had promised D. Appleton Company that she would write a book on nursing. She had been young and eager in 1905, and before she went abroad in 1907 she had asked for an extension. She wondered if Appleton had forgotten.

For the moment, however, her thoughts were occupied with the Hopkins endowment. The drive had been launched in late February by a paid publicity worker, and thousands of pamphlets had been distributed, but by December, 1921, only $69,059.13 had been pledged. Adelaide refused to recognize the drive as a failure; rather, she analyzed the reasons for its lack of success. Could it have been that, with the hospital and the university asking for funds, it was not the opportune time for the nursing school to solicit funds? Would it

not be best for the alumnae to conserve their efforts until the Rockefeller Foundation published its report on nursing education? Adelaide
was confident the report would recommend university schools of
nursing. If the Hopkins School of Nursing were reorganized along
the lines of the report's recommendations, would the Rockefeller
Foundation contribute to its support on an experimental basis, perhaps even to the permanent endowment? It was an idea worthy of
further exploration. On January 27, 1922, Adelaide mailed a check
for $200 as another installment on her pledge of $1,000.[69]

In the late spring Isabel Stewart, her face aglow, handed Adelaide
a letter bearing the return address of President James R. Angell, Yale
University, and waited for her to open it. Adelaide read it, paused,
read it again, and passed it to Isabel. In recognition of her thirty
years of service to nursing, Yale University desired to confer upon
Miss Nutting the honorary degree of master of arts at its two hundred twenty-first commencement on June 21, 1922. Isabel congratu-
lated Adelaide, reminding her that last year Yale had conferred
honorary degrees on Madame Curie and Julia Lathrop. Adelaide recalled that Yale had similarly honored Jane Addams and Cecelia
Beaux. Isabel could have given the entire list of the seven women on
whom Yale had previously conferred honorary degrees, but she did
not want her remarkable knowledge of Yale's honors to women to
excite suspicion.[70]

While Adelaide was in Europe, Isabel had had correspondence with
Minnie Blodgett, Vassar alumna and patron, and wife of John Woods
Blodgett, Michigan philanthropist, relative to an honorary degree
from Yale. Since honorary degrees were not conferred in absentia,
Mrs. Blodgett advised Miss Stewart that it would be a strong point
in their favor to notify President Hadley and the committee on honorary degrees of Miss Nutting's probable absence and to ascertain if the
degree might be recommended this year and granted the next. President Hadley was heartily in favor of Miss Nutting; if he added his
endorsement to those they already had and recommended it to President Angell, the degree might be granted.[71] Even before public an-

[69] M. Adelaide Nutting (New York) to Mrs. Agnes Hartridge (Baltimore),
January 27, 1922, MAN Papers.

[70] Women recipients of honorary degrees from Yale prior to 1922 were: 1910,
Jane Addams; 1911, Mabel Boardman; 1912, Cecelia Beaux; 1914, Mary E.
Wooley; 1915, Katherine B. Davis; 1921, Julia Lathrop and Marie S. Curie. See
Lottie G. Bishop (New Haven) to Ysabella Waters (New York), July 20, 1922,
ibid.

[71] Minnie C. Blodgett (East Grand Rapids, Mich.), to Isabel M. Stewart (New
York), April 22, 1921, ibid.

nouncement of the degree, there were confidential whispers and buz-
zing among members of Adelaide's staff and her professional friends.
Isabel Stewart obtained the proper academic gown for her to wear
and hoped she would not be too tired to enjoy the ceremonies, for,
only a short time before, she had returned from Baltimore with another siege of the throat infection that always left her debilitated.[72]
On Friday before the Yale commencement, Isabel wrote from Teachers College Country Club, Ossining, where she had gone for a brief
holiday, that she would like to accompany Miss Nutting and be
present at the ceremonies.[73]

A heavy rain in the early morning of June 21 robbed the Yale
commencement of the colorful academic pocession of graduates,
faculty, fellows, alumni, and recipients of honorary degrees across the
campus to Woolsey Hall, where the ceremonies took place, but Miss
Stewart, for whom the bright parades were no novelty, rejoiced that
Miss Nutting would have only a short walk. Sitting in the seat that
had been reserved for her in the chapel, Isabel glanced at her program.

Soon the great organ would be playing Beethoven's Overture to
Goethe's *Egmont* and the graduates would enter. Five hundred sixty-
three students would be receiving various bachelors, masters, and
doctoral degrees, and fourteen persons would receive honorary degrees. Adelaide Nutting was the only woman receiving an honorary
degree. Isabel scanned the list. Miss Nutting was in good company:
Sir Robert Alexander Falconer, president of the University of Toronto; Adolph Simon Ochs, publisher of the *New York Times*; Francis
Patrick Garman, U.S. Assistant Attorney General; Lloyd Warren,
founder and director of the Beaux Arts Institute of Design; Edwin
Arlington Robinson, poet and playwright; Clifford Beers, a Yale
graduate of 1897 and author of *A Mind That Found Itself*; John
Joseph McCarty, vice-president of American Telephone and Tele-
graph; and Dr. Fu Chun Yen, Yale graduate of 1897, principal of the
Medical College of Yale in China.

The audience rose as the procession entered, the graduates in their
dark robes, the faculty with brilliant hoods, rich satins, velvets, gold
tassels, and here and there a scarlet gown from a foreign university.
With head erect and measured step, Adelaide took her place on the
platform in the front row next to Clifford Beers. There was a brief
pause, then the invocation, followed by the singing of the Sixty-fifth

[72] Adelaide Nutting (New York) to Elsie M. Lawler (Baltimore), May 6, 1922,
ibid.
[73] Isabel M. Stewart (Ossining, N.Y.) to Adelaide Nutting (New York), June
16, 1922, MAN–IMS Correspondence.

Psalm, which had been sung at the opening of Yale's first college building in 1718.

The dean of each faculty presented the respective candidates for the various degrees; then the "Slow Movement for Orchestra and Organ" from the Third Symphony by Saint-Saens was played. Isabel glanced at her program. The music stopped. Professor William Lyon Phelps stepped forward to present the candidates for honorary degrees to President Angell.

When it came Miss Nutting's turn to receive the scroll and hood, there was thunderous applause. Isabel leaned forward to catch every word as Dr. Phelps read the citation.

> Mary Adelaide Nutting. Born in Quebec, her original impulse was toward the arts and she studied painting in Canadian and American schools. She gave up that career to become a member of the first class of the Johns Hopkins Training School for Nurses. Later she became superintendent, and initiated most of the progressive policies that made that pioneer school preeminent. She was the first nurse to receive a chair in institutional administration in Teachers College where she organized a large department, training hundreds every year. Her zeal and knowledge made her conspicuous during the war when she was appointed by President Wilson, chairman of the Committee on Nursing in the Council of National Defense. She was awarded the Liberty Service medal of the National Institute of Social Sciences. She is joint author of an authoritative History of Nursing. Her devotion, courage, faith, skill, and magnificent perseverance have made her today one of the most useful women in the world.[74]

In the twinkling of an eye the hood of Yale blue satin was about Adelaide's shoulders and President Angell had clasped her hand and presented the Latin scroll.

As Isabel stood for the closing hymn, "God, Beneath Thy Guiding Hand," the benediction, and the recessional, the last words of the accolade resounded in her heart, high above the music of Elgar's "Pomp and Circumstance": "Her devotion, courage, faith, skill and magnificent perseverance have made her today one of the most useful women in the world."

[74] "Program of the Two Hundred Twenty-first Commencement, Yale University, June 21, 1922"; and clippings from New Haven Evening Register (June 21, 1922), New York Evening Post (June 21, 1922), New York Times (June 21 and 22, 1922), New York News (June 23, 1922), and New Haven Times-Leader (June 21, 1922); MAN Papers.

XX

The Last Years at Teachers College, 1922–1925

Letters and telegrams of congratulation started pouring in as soon as the press announced that Yale was conferring an honorary master of arts degree upon Miss Nutting. Among the very first was a joyous note from Lillian Wald at Henry Street.[1] Dr. C.-E. A. Winslow and his wife sent congratulations and invited Adelaide to be their guest while in New Haven.[2] Willystine Goodsell sent a note from Naugatuck, Connecticut, rejoicing that the honor had come to her and saying that it honored all women.[3] Dean William Darrach, College of Physicians and Surgeons, Columbia University, wrote that he was delighted his alma mater was conferring the degree and that Adelaide's faithful and successful work had been recognized outside the university and city. Letters continued to come in long after Miss Nutting had left to spend the first part of her vacation with Willystine Goodsell at Rockport, Massachusetts. Knowing that Adelaide would want to answer each one, Isabel Stewart placed them in a large envelope and posted them, or she tucked them in with reports of the summer session and a personal note about the enrollment, the largest classes, and whether any new student showed promise of professional leadership. When a cablegram came from France, the old gray-haired messenger who brought it to Teachers College insisted on delivering it personally. He explained to Miss Stewart: "You see it's a cable from France congratulating her on that degree she got from Yale. I read all about it in the papers and I told my wife nobody deserved it better and so when I

---

[1] Lillian D. Wald (New York) to Adelaide Nutting (New York), June 10, 1922, MAN Papers.

[2] Anne R. Winslow (New Haven, Conn.) to Adelaide Nutting (New York), [1922], *ibid.*

[3] Willystine Goodsell (Naugatuck, Conn.) to Adelaide Nutting (New York), June 16, 1922, *ibid.*

279

saw this cable I just brought it up as quick as I could to give it to her."[4]

From Seattle, Washington, where the National League of Nursing Education and the American Nurses Association were holding their conventions, came resolutions of congratulation, appreciation, and affection. Fifty-three nursing graduates from Teachers College who were attending the meetings sent a wire. Carolyn Gray, now head of the Department of Nursing Education, Western Reserve, wrote: "I have had such joy over the eagerness of many prominent persons to do you honor. Ex-President Taft in particular grasped at the opportunity and was very eager about it."[5] Georgia Nevins, now superintendent of nurses, St. Luke's Hospital, New Bedford, Massachusetts, wrote that she "loved the citation," but that the picture in the rotogravure section of the *New York Times* was awful.[6] Canadian nurses, who always held Miss Nutting in great affection, regretted that the degree had not been conferred by a Canadian university.[7] The week before Adelaide arrived in Waterloo, the weekly *Advertiser* carried a garbled but nonetheless complimentary account of the honors conferred upon the town's "most distinguished daughter."[8] Lizzie obtained extra copies to send to the Peasley and Nutting cousins. Adelaide was careful to explain that, in honoring her, Yale had really been honoring the profession for which she had labored for more than thirty years and to which she would be deeply committed in the years ahead.

Lizzie was proud to tell Adelaide about the dinner given for Charlie on July 10 by the Bedford District Bar Association in honor of his fifty years of service as a lawyer and King's Councillor.[9]

Almost immediately after Adelaide arrived in Waterloo, she wrote Isabel Stewart, inquiring about matters on campus.

I am sure the School Nursing Conference will be well worth while, d hope that you and all the others of our staff will give every bit of

bel M. Stewart (New York) to Adelaide Nutting, [Rockport, Mass.], July 22; and cablegram, American Nurses (Soisson-Aisne, France) to Adelaide (New York), July 8, 1922; *ibid.*
yn Gray (Cleveland, Ohio) to Adelaide Nutting (New York), July 11,

ı Nevins (New Bedford, Mass.) to Adelaide Nutting (New York),

G. Flaws (Toronto) to Adelaide Nutting (New York), August 1,
M. Fairley (Hamilton, Ontrio) to Adelaide Nutting (New York),
1922; and Helen McMurchey (Ottawa) to Adelaide Nutting (New
), 1922; *ibid.*
m the *Waterloo Advertiser*, July 14, 1922, *ibid.*
m the *Waterloo Journal*, July 1, 1922, and the *Journal de Water-*
bid.

time to it that they can spare. We, all of us, Training School people, as well as actual workers in Public Schools, need to give attention to this greatest branch of our Public Health work if we are to hold it at its fullest potentialities.[10]

She believed that two or three of the present graduate students showed talent and interest and might become the nucleus of experts and specialists in that branch.

> Now that I have got nicely rested and thinking about the future of our blessed work I'm beginning to get up steam, plans and measures are beginning to take shape. It is curious how they begin, as it were, in a mist, out of which something teasing and insistent is struggling to take form and to say things, and now after months, and sometimes years, something begins to snap into place, it fits and you know it is something that ought to be tried.
>
> Just now I am in the toils over two aspects of our problem (1) is that *attendant* who appears always to have been with us and only partially replaced by the trained nurse, and (2) the other is the small hospital (about 75% of all hospitals, in fact). . . .[11]

At that moment Lizzie's carriage appeared at the door and Adelaide left for a drive through the lovely Shefford hills, but, reading the unfinished paragraph, Isabel Stewart could easily foresee which of the vulnerable spots in the nursing system Miss Nutting would attack next.

Despite Adelaide's affection for her brother and his wife, a long visit to the home of her childhood was depressing, and, after a week in Waterloo, she arranged to join Georgia Nevins at Forest Hills Hotel, Franconia, New Hampshire. The hotel was a "spacious well-conducted house, broad verandahs," with "a superb view of the distant mountains" and a "good dining room." Although it was August, it was cool enough for a bright and crackling fire in the big fireplace in the lounge.

It was good to see Georgia, with whom she had spent many happy vacations and read so many books. The next day they would begin reading Strachey's *Victoria*. Georgia was looking well and enjoying her work at the New Bedford Hospital. Undoubtedly she had many useful years of congenial work ahead of her.[12]

[10] Adelaide Nutting (Waterloo, Quebec) to Isabel M. Stewart (New York), July 29, 1922, MAN–IMS Correspondence.

[11] *Ibid.*

[12] Adelaide Nutting (Franconia, N.H.) to Isabel M. Stewart (Ossining, N.Y.), August 9, 1922, *ibid.*

The house is full of people, and they are all about at the moment, playing bridge, a dozen tables or so stretched down the lounge; knitting and embroidery for others, gossip for the older ones and dancing and music in an adjoining room for the flappers. It is all most cheerful, and though after reading the last *New Republic* I know that Rome is burning, I can't help enjoying the fiddling! The views are superb.[13]

Adelaide anxiously awaited the latest issue of *Survey*, which contained an article on Miss Goldmark's report, and the August issues of the *Journal of Nursing* and *Modern Hospital*. After three years of research and study, the Rockefeller report on nursing education had been released. It was a carefully executed piece of work. Its conclusions were presented before the NLNE in Seattle and were subsequently publicized in the press and professional journals. As a member of the report committee, Adelaide had read the separate sections and wanted to hear the reaction of others.[14]

The Rockefeller report reaffirmed much that Miss Nutting had been advocating for years. The answer to the original question of the training of the public health nurse was simple. Public health nurses should be graduates of a basic course in nursing before undertaking the special preparation in classroom and field work essential to the practice of public health nursing. The existing system needed strengthening so that graduate nurses could better combine health teaching with nursing service.

The report also recommended that, where a training school required a high-school diploma as a prerequisite for entrance, the basic preparation of nurses might be reduced from three years to twenty-eight months, with an eight-hour day and, at a maximum, a forty-eight-hour week, and that the additional period of eight months be provided for the special training of health nurses and head nurses. Advanced work was also prescribed for supervisors, instructors, and superintendents. The report further recommended the preparation and licensing of attendants, who were to have nine months of instruction and supervision and could be given some of the time-consuming and less-responsible duties of the nurse.

Most significant was the Rockefeller report's call for more university schools of nursing, which would afford broad general and cultural

[13] Adelaide Nutting (Franconia, N.H.) to Isabel M. Stewart (Ossining), August 17, 1922, *ibid.*

[14] The report on nursing education sponsored by the Rockefeller Foundation is sometimes referred to as the Winslow report and often as the Goldmark report. It was published under the title *Nursing and Nursing Education in the United States*, Report of the Committee for the Study of Nursing Education and Report of the Survey by Josephine Goldmark (New York: Macmillan, 1923).

education as well as professional preparation and would give more emphasis to the social, preventive, and curative aspects of nursing.[15]

As members of the Advisory Committee of the Rockefeller Foundation, Miss Nutting and Miss Goodrich signed the recommendations because they felt they were sound and because they were convinced that much precious training time was wasted in non-educational work and in repetitive tasks.[16] Unfortunately, no organized follow-up program was planned in connection with the report. Hospitals would undoubtedly object to the emphasis on university affiliation and to the reduced length of the basic course. Adelaide did not anticipate an immediate transformation in training schools for nurses and public health visitors, but the report offered a chart and compass to far-sighted administrators and hospital boards, and the NLNE would continue to agitate for higher standards of training and service.

Teachers College statistics for the fall term, 1922, showed an enrollment in nursing education of 252 students from 36 states and 15 foreign countries. The fact that 37 students came from England, Scotland, Canada, France, Germany, Austria, Switzerland, Denmark, Sweden, Russia, China, Japan, the Philippine Islands, Smyrna in Asia Minor, and Palestine indicated the role the department was playing in nursing education.[17] Most of these 37 students would return to their homes as directors of hospitals, teachers of nursing, or as administrators and workers in public health. Adelaide took a special interest in these students, regarding them as individuals who would bring something cultural to the department as well as take from it. She was concerned about their personal problems, their adjustment to life in a strange country, the barriers of language, customs, and traditions, and she tried to see that the shy and timid made friends and that holidays were not lonely. In turn her files held rich testimony of their gratitude.

Isabel Stewart and Adelaide were always concerned about the future leadership of nursing. After Isabel attended a mediocre meeting of nurses in Boston, she lamented:

> I don't know what we're going to do without big people. Oh, for a wind from the hills to breathe some life into the dry bones. The only

[15] "Final Report, Committee on Nursing Education," mimeographed, MAN Papers; Mary M. Roberts, *American Nursing: History and Interpretation* (New York: Macmillan, 1954), app. 2, pp. 653–55.

[16] In Europe, nursing leaders were apprehensive that Americans were lowering standards in cutting back the time of nursing education to twenty-eight months. Isabel M. Stewart, *Oral History*, 2 vols. (New York: Columbia University, Butler Library, 1958), 1:253.

[17] "Annual Report of the Department of Nursing and Health, 1922," Department of Nursing Education Archives, Teachers College.

evidence of life was a squabble for officers between the aggressive Red
Cross section and the respectable hard shell Puritan aristocracy of
Massachusetts General, Peter Bent Brigham, Childrens and other leading
institutions.[18]

When Adelaide found it impossible to address a national meeting of
the American Hospital Association, she counseled the chairman that
the group's speakers should come from the younger generation, particularly those engaged in training school work, and she cited Carolyn
Gray, Helen Wood, Lillian Clayton, Louise Powell, and Elizabeth
Burgess as examples.[19]

Adelaide and her department at Teachers College became interested
in the East Harlem Health Center, which was being initiated by the
Red Cross. The center's primary purpose was to promote the health
of the community by bringing together in one central building the
staffs and activities of voluntary and official health and welfare agencies operating in the district. These included the Henry Street Nursing Service, the Association for Improving the Condition of the Poor,
the Maternity Center Association, and St. Timothy's League, a group
of philanthropic-minded non-professional alumnae of St. Timothy's
School, Catonsville, Maryland. The area served by Harlem Center had
a population of 40,638 in 1920; 46 percent were foreign born, 50 percent were of foreign extraction, and only 4 percent had native-born
parents; 71 percent were Italian; 23 percent were Russian, Polish,
German, or Austrian; 15 percent of the population was under five
years of age and only 59 percent was adult. These people lived in two-
to five-room apartments and depended on direct gas for heating. Because of low water pressure they were beset by water shortages and
plumbing problems. Stairs, roofs, and courts did not afford adequate
play areas, and the rate of sickness, tuberculosis, and infectious diseases was high.

Grace Anderson and Mabelle Welch were in charge of the East
Harlem Center, and Homer Folks, prime mover in the project, was
chairman of the center's governing board. Lillian Hudson of Miss
Nutting's staff, Dr. Thomas Briggs of the Teachers College staff, and
Alta Dines, an alumnus, all friends of Miss Nutting, were members of
the board. Funds were donated by the Red Cross, the Association for
Improving the Condition of the Poor, the Maternity Center Associa-
tion, and the Laura Spelman Rockefeller Fund. For the first three years

[18] Isabel M. Stewart (New York) to Adelaide Nutting [in Europe], July 17,
1921, MAN–IMS Correspondence.
[19] M. Adelaide Nutting (New York) to Laura C. Logan (Cincinnati, Ohio),
June 5, 1922, MAN Papers.

Harlem Center had an operating budget of $64,000. In December, 1923, certain of the voluntary agencies organized a health unit known as the East Harlem Nursing and Health Demonstration. These agencies participated autonomously in the coordination of health center services and in fulfilling their special functions, but merged their identity in the nursing and health demonstrations. Mothers were urged to come to the center to attend demonstrations in the care and feeding of infants and lessons in health protection. Obstetrical service was provided through the Henry Street Nursing Service, and weekly medical conferences were provided for the examination of midwives' cases and those not registered with physicians for home delivery or hospital care. A weekly class for expectant mothers took up one-fourth of the time and funds of the center. The Infant Health Service was set up largely to handle home visiting and two weekly medical conferences. Nursing and nutrition classes were offered for mothers. Immunization against diphtheria and smallpox was begun. In March, 1925, special mental hygiene was added to the demonstration program. Between 1922 and 1927, 31 percent of the residents of the area had been vaccinated through the Harlem Center; nursing and health services were rendered in 4,311 homes, and 171,110 home visits were made. Students from the Teachers College Department of Health and Nursing were afforded an opportunity to work with the center, giving either two months' service or the equivalent in two full days of work each week.

Reprints of East Harlem studies and outlines were invaluable to public health workers in New York and other cities. In 1928 the size of the area was enlarged to include 99,033 persons. During the Depression, however, less money was available to carry on the extension program. Foundations declined support after the federal government began its welfare program, and eventually the center was closed.[20]

The Winslow-Goldmark report favoring university schools of nursing raised Adelaide's hope that the Rockefeller Foundation might assist The Johns Hopkins School of Nursing in becoming an endowed school offering a collegiate program. Three months before the report was printed, she asked Dr. George Vincent, president of the foundation, if an appeal was in order for the Hopkins School of Nursing. The secretary of the foundation replied somewhat ambiguously that

[20] In 1941 the East Harlem Health Center ceased operation, and in 1944 the furnishings were brought to Dodge Hall, Teachers College, for use in a seminar room; Isabel M. Stewart, "Remarks at Opening of Seminar Room 107, Dodge Hall, May 22, 1944," Department of Nursing Education Archives, Teachers College.

the trustees were not unhopeful that the time might come when the foundation would feel it desirable to aid in developing some of the new programs and proposals in nurses' training.[21]

A few months later it was announced that the Rockefeller Foundation had negotiated a plan with Yale University whereby it would finance a five-year experiment to determine whether it would later permanently endow the Connecticut Training School for Nurses and make it a university school, with special emphasis on public health.[22] Almost immediately the announcement was made that Mrs. Chester Bolton of Cleveland had given $500,000 to Western Reserve University to start a school of nursing. Adelaide sent a telegram of appreciation to Mrs. Bolton, who replied that she felt quite unworthy because she had scraped together only half of what was needed.

> It is such a joy to be able to do it. The truth is, you and Miss Goodrich have filled me so full of your dreams for the profession and you have shown me so much personal consecration of life that I feel I am privileged beyond most to be able to be one of the builders of the temple.

She felt she must have Miss Nutting's and Miss Goodrich's help in organizing the school. Inviting them to come to Cleveland as her guests, as well as offering to go to New York, she concluded, "This isn't just for Cleveland, this is for nursing."[23]

Many of Adelaide's friends and former students wrote to her as soon as the announcements of the new schools were made. A letter from Laura Logan of Cincinnati General Hospital was typical:

> My dear Miss Nutting, I find myself wishing to write to you to congratulate you upon the founding of the school at Yale and to rejoice with you over the gift to Western Reserve. But [not] for you and your untiring perseverance would nursing have gone so far ahead, would so many have caught your faith.[24]

Before Adelaide had time to answer, word came that the deanship of the School of Nursing at Western Reserve had been offered to Carolyn Gray[25] and that Annie Goodrich would be dean of the new Yale

---

[21] Ethel Johns and Blanche Pfefferkorn, *The Johns Hopkins Hospital School of Nursing* (Baltimore: The Johns Hopkins Press, 1954), p. 346.

[22] James Rowland Angell, *Report of the President of Yale University, 1922–23*, 19th ser., no. 24, September 1, 1923.

[23] Frances Payne Bolton (Cleveland) to Adelaide Nutting (New York), April 11, 1923, MAN Papers.

[24] Laura R. Logan (Cincinnati) to Adelaide Nutting (New York), May 11, 1923, *ibid.*

[25] Helen M. Smith (Cleveland) to Adelaide Nutting (New York), May 25, 1923, *ibid.*

school. In thanking Miss Logan for her "kind and generous note," Adelaide concluded: "These are indeed stirring and eventful days in the history of nursing and I am glad to have lived to have had some little share in them."[26]

The announcement of the Rockefeller grant to Yale and Mrs. Bolton's gift of $500,000 to Western Reserve inspired Adelaide to write an editorial for *The Johns Hopkins Nurses Alumnae Magazine.* Entitled "New Era in Nursing Education," it began:

> The education of nurses passes over into a new era. It is because for the first time in history the education of nurses is accorded the status and the powers which are recognized in the conduct and development of other forms of professional education.[27]

With their own deans, governing boards, faculty classrooms, and budgets—the commonplaces of other professional, technical, and vocational schools—these schools would open a new era in nursing education.

In posting the editorial to Mary Dixon Cullen (Hopkins class of 1903), editor of the *Alumnae Magazine* and chairman of the Finance Committee of the Endowment Fund, Adelaide added a personal note. "While these great gifts have not come to us, they have come to *nursing,* and that is after all what we are working for, and for the fruits of good nursing. And envy is a base thing anyway, isn't it?"[28]

Adelaide remained optimistic. The fact that Yale had received a Rockefeller endowment did not mean that Hopkins would not get one.

Although Adelaide had been quite ill during the winter, in March she signed a contract with the U.S. Commissioner of Education, J. J. Tigert, to provide a typed report on the educational status of nursing by December 1, 1923.[29] Her health was quite improved by the time Isabel Stewart left for Europe on her sabbatical, which would terminate at the interim meeting of the International Council of Nurses in Copenhagen. By April, Adelaide concluded she would be well enough to address the ANA on June 19 on the topic "Thirty Years of Progress in Nursing."[30] On April 26 she spoke before the Hospital Association

---

[26] Adelaide Nutting (New York) to Laura R. Logan (Cincinnati), June 6, 1923, *ibid.*

[27] A copy of the editorial is on file among the MAN Papers.

[28] Adelaide Nutting (New York) to Mrs. Thomas Cullen (Baltimore), May 3, 1923, *ibid.*

[29] "Contract between M. A. Nutting, New York, and J. J. Tigert, U.S. Commissioner of Education, Washington, D.C., March 5, 1923," *ibid.*

[30] M. A. Nutting (New York) to Sally Johnson (Boston), April 24, 1923, *ibid.*

of Pennsylvania at its second annual meeting in Philadelphia, tactfully titling her address "How to Educate the Nurse and at the Same Time Properly Care for the Patient."[31]

In this address Adelaide presented some startling facts: 80 percent of the nursing care in 1,755 hospitals in the United States was being done by 55,000 students. Between 1910 and 1920, more than 630 new schools of nursing had been established, many of them in small hospitals that depended almost entirely on students for nursing care. According to the Rockefeller report, one-fifth of the students' time was spent in routine, unskilled work. Adelaide said that she had often thought how little understood and appreciated the contributions to public welfare made by students in schools of nursing were as they cared for the sick in the great hospitals. "For the past fifty years, in succeeding generations, they have unstintingly given day and night of their youth and strength, and sometimes their health." She referred to Dr. Hurd's famous analogy of a student nurse to the missionary who, invited by a primitive tribe to a banquet, found that he himself was expected to form the banquet. She also quoted the statement of Dr. Dock of Washington University, St. Louis, that many training schools were managed chiefly for the benefit of the hospital and that "pupils have gone on, for months or years, repeating a routine no longer educative."[32] Teaching was too often secondary to the exigencies of the hospital.

Throughout the spring and summer of 1923, Adelaide kept Isabel Stewart closely informed of the work within the department, progress in the construction of Russell Hall, which would house the library and administrative offices of Teachers College, and of the new addition to Dodge Hall, which would allow for expansion of the Nursing Department. She also briefed Isabel on matters that would probably come up before the International Council of Nurses in Copenhagen, indicating those which would be especially tricky, such as membership in the council. She warned her of the danger that management of nursing affairs might fall into the hands of non-professional persons. She also

[31] M. A. Nutting, "How to Educate the Nurse and at the Same Time Properly Care for the Patient," *Modern Hospital*, September, 1923; M. Adelaide Nutting, "How Can We Care for the Patient and Educate the Nurse," *"A Sound Economic Basis for Schools of Nursing" and Other Addresses* (New York: G. P. Putnam's, 1926), pp. 306–24.

[32] George Dock, "Essentials of Professional Education," *Proceedings of the Twentieth Annual Meeting of the National League of Nursing Education*, April, 1914, pp. 81–82, quoted in Nutting, *A Sound Economic Basis for Schools of Nursing*, p. 313.

reminded Isabel that there was a great difference between the American Red Cross and the Red Cross Societies in Europe.[33]

For the past year Adelaide had been an active member of Anne Morgan's Committee on Devastated France, and chairman of a special committee to draft a plan for establishing in Paris a school of nursing which would embody the ideals for which the members would wish to stand before the American public. The assignment included plans for the government of the school, organization and functions, administration, faculty, curriculum, admission requirements, length of term, and budget. Annie Goodrich, Anna Maxwell, and other members of the committee began their work with high hopes.[34] The Rockefeller report became their guideline, and they dared to propose a university school as their eventual goal. American funds would support the school for the first year. If the plan went into operation in 1924, as scheduled, Adelaide was confident it would be one of the great forward steps in the history of French nursing.

While Isabel Stewart was in London, Adelaide wanted her to learn all she could about the international public health course that the League of Red Cross Societies was sponsoring at Bedford College for Women. The College of Nursing cooperated in instructions and field work, and the British Red Cross provided an attractive residence for the students. The College of Nursing claimed among its members many "do-gooders," while Mrs. Fenwick's group was professional. Isabel was graciously received by the British leaders, feted and dined by Mrs. Fenwick and Miss Breay, and given insight into English nursing problems and the rivalry between the College of Nursing, dominated by Sir Arthur Stanley, and the older, British Nurses Association, founded by Mrs. Fenwick. Isabel wrote of international nursing affairs in the same chatty way that Lavinia Dock had kept Adelaide informed prior to her resignation as secretary of the International Council of Nurses in 1922. Lavinia believed intensely in the International Council, and had worked hard to hold it together through the years. It had been a true labor of love, for she had not accepted a cent in payment. She had even assigned the royalties on Volumes III and IV of the Nutting–Dock History of Nursing to the council.[35]

In turn Adelaide wrote to Isabel about the NLNE convention in

[33] Adelaide Nutting (aboard the R.M.S. Silvia, en route to Halifax) to Isabel Stewart, [in Europe], July 8, 1923, MAN–IMS Correspondence.

[34] "Report of the Sub-Committee on Nursing for Devastated France, December 4, 1922"; and "Minutes of the Third Meeting of the Sub-Committee, Teachers College, May 14, 1922"; MAN Papers.

[35] Isabel Stewart (London) to Adelaide Nutting (St. John's, Newfoundland), July 14, 1923, MAN–IMS Correspondence.

Swampscott, Massachusetts. She had missed the business meeting because her paper was not finished, and the last word had not been written until Monday afternoon, only a few hours before she took the
night train to Boston. Of her paper she modestly reported:

> "Thirty Years of Progress" was amicably spoken of and did not I be-
> lieve wholly discredit your chief. The other speaker of the evening
> turned out to be Mr. Embree [Rockefeller Foundation] who called me up
> to know what I was going to talk about, and Miss Logan . . . made a
> rather lengthy address going over the same ground that I had of neces-
> sity to cover. I warned all and sundry that it wouldn't do to relegate me
> wholly to the historical aspects of affairs. I might break out in other
> directions at any moment. . . . One thing emerges sharply to me and
> that is the slowness with which any effort is made to reduce the three
> years in any of our more important schools. They simply cannot bring
> their minds to grapple with it, and the ever present nightmare of pos-
> sible lack of students to form a decent incoming class, with no funds to
> pay graduates or helpers and the very greatest difficulty in securing
> enough [students] of good quality even when there are funds. I don't
> wonder at their hesitation and yet that reform simply has to come, and
> the sooner the two years is taken hold of, developed to the very highest
> educational possibilities, the sooner we shall be able to determine just
> what it really can do. At the end of a few years of most intelligent and
> well-directed effort with the two years we shall be able to see where our
> next step lies. It is that "next step" that really interests me. And in view
> of everything isn't it interesting that Miss Goodrich should be devoting
> her best energies for the next five years to showing just what can be
> done to develop a two year course which shall include some preparation
> for public health nursing.[36]

In Copenhagen, Isabel addressed the representatives of the ten
nations present at the International Council of Nurses and told them
about the report of the Rockefeller Committee for the Study of Nursing Education, Miss Nutting's role in urging the investigation, the
method of Josephine Goldmark's research, the type of data gathered,
and the committee's findings and recommendations. Standards, Miss
Stewart insisted, should not be lowered. Training would be strengthened if hospitals eliminated non-essential routine tasks often performed by trainees and maintained better ward supervision. When
these two steps were accomplished, training courses might easily be
reduced in length. For providing leadership, university schools should
be developed.[37]

---

[36] Adelaide Nutting (aboard the R.M.S. *Silvia*, en route to Halifax) to Isabel
Stewart, [in Europe], July 8, 1923, *ibid.*

[37] Margaret Breay and Ethel Gordon Fenwick, *History of the International
Council of Nurses* (Geneva: International Council of Nurses, 1931), pp. 180–81.

As soon as registration for the 1923 Teachers College summer school was under way, Adelaide departed for Newfoundland, leaving Elizabeth Burgess in charge of department affairs. It was Adelaide's rule not to teach in the summer school. That was her time for getting away, taking an objective look at the department, and evaluating and assessing the work that had been done, as well as what needed to be done. She caught up on her reading, developed ideas, and built up her depleted energy. A cool summer at the seaside, a mountain resort, or any ocean voyage always renewed her spirit and vigor.

This year's visit to St. John's would be Adelaide's last vacation there with Minnie and Gilbert, for Gilbert was retiring and the family was moving to Bermuda to live in the old Gosling home, Strawberry Hill. In forty years Gilbert Gosling had progressed from a serious, boyish clerk to an officer in his firm and a substantial citizen twice elected mayor. Minnie, too, had been active in the cultural and social life of the town, and had worked in behalf of poor relief, education, and suffrage. Adelaide and Minnie would spend the summer reading and sewing and going on drives and picnics with Gilbert. Perhaps Dr. Grenfell would put in for supplies and visit his old friends. Adelaide would help Minnie decide which pieces of furniture to ship and which to dispose of. A trunk full of letters—letters from mother, father, Arthur, Jim, Charlie, and Adelaide when she was in training and later on her travels abroad—and photographs had to be sorted. These awakened precious memories—mother wearing her prized black lace stole and the beautiful bonnet she had made; Father in his choir robe with the dog, Mr. Pip, at his feet; a faded little picture of Addie and Minnie, aged eight and five; and another faded one of Addie and Jim double-dating in Ottawa. How amusing it was to see the boys with walrus moustaches and bowler hats, the girls with mutton-leg sleeves and long bustled skirts, and Adelaide holding up a ruffled parasol.

Usually Adelaide returned from a sea voyage invigorated in mind and body, but this time she soon became desperately ill and was taken to Presbyterian Hospital for surgery on October 5. Recovery was slow, and in December Georgia Nevins wrote, offering to take a two-week leave from her work and go with Adelaide to Atlantic City to care for her during her convalescence. She would see that Adelaide was established in a comfortable room in a hotel which provided the good, nourishing food and fresh air so essential to health.[38]

Within a few days they were on their way. Georgia was a delight-

[38] Georgia Nevins (New Bedford) to Adelaide Nutting (New York), December 3, 1923, MAN Papers.

ful companion and a splendid nurse. Soon Adelaide was writing Isabel Stewart almost daily, inquiring about affairs at the office, the staff for the coming year, the courses to be offered, and the schedule of lectures.[39] After Georgia left for New Bedford, Adelaide was very lonely and returned to New York to spend Christmas in her apartment. Members of her staff and friends who remained in the city made it a point to drop in, perform errands, and help with her mail, which was always voluminous at holiday time.

In January Adelaide went back to Atlantic City because she did not want to be a burden to Isabel Stewart and other friends. Her sister wrote, begging her to come to Strawberry Hill for the remainder of her convalescence. Without friends, Atlantic City was a lonely place, and Adelaide decided to yield to Minnie's pleas and the lure of warm sunshine, good food, and pleasant company.

Situated on a green, wooded hillside, Strawberry Hill was a spacious old two-story home with a broad, sunny, upstairs veranda which offered quiet and seclusion. There chairs, steamer rugs, books, and magazines awaited Adelaide. A substantial breakfast was brought to her room at about eight-thirty, and she seldom got up before eleven. During the afternoons, she and Minnie sat on the veranda sewing, reading, and visiting. Gilbert, who had taken up painting since his illness and retirement, often sat beside them and painted, occasionally joining briefly in the conversation.

"There could hardly be a more perfect place for a weary invalid," Adelaide wrote Isabel, "and the weeks here will, I am confident, push me forward at a good pace." The Goslings had a horse and carriage, and they often took drives over the palm- and palmetto-lined roads. Richly colored flowers bloomed everywhere.[40] Each of Adelaide's letters bore evidence that she was improving.

> The days grow warmer and sunnier and my out-of-door hours lengthen. I am undoubtedly progressing—though no scales are to support that assumption by impressive figures. I am lazier than any human being ought to be and that breakfast in bed, and late rising are quite the right thing. . . . The nights are the stillest things imaginable—not a sound except when the wind is very high.

More and more her thoughts turned toward the college. Isabel had written about the housewarming at Russell Hall. The offices on the

<hr>

[39] Adelaide Nutting (Atlantic City, N.J.) to Isabel Stewart (New York), December 11, 1923, MAN–IMS Correspondence.

[40] Adelaide Nutting (Paget, Bermuda) to Isabel M. Stewart (New York), February 15, 1924, ibid.

ground floor, with their Turkish rugs and Italian furniture, were not like the Teachers College they had known for so many years. The library was spacious and beautiful.[41]

To this Adelaide replied:

> Do go down on your knees and thank God . . . that there is this precious bit of beauty and dignity in our most unlovely habitation. We need that more than a good many other things and every classroom and corridor should be as beautiful as we know how to make them—a precious and constant refreshment to tired stale souls, and lovely haunting memory, and it easily might be.[42]

Through the years, Adelaide and her friends and students had been assembling rare materials relating to the history and practice of nursing, as well as the most remarkable collection of Nightingalia outside England. Making note of this, Adelaide continued.

> I do hope that a pleasant and suitably spacious alcove is awaiting our treasures and trust no one will try to jockey us out of it. As a matter of probability, I expect the attempt will be made, but with vigilance and resolution we can, I trust, hold the space so long and frequently promised.[43]

Bermuda and the companionship of Minnie, Gilbert, and Arthur seemed to be just what Adelaide needed. They pressed her to cancel her passage for March 11 and stay longer. A frantic appeal was sent to Isabel Stewart to send data for her income tax return, and, when the March 15 deadline was met, she settled back to luxuriate in the Bermuda sunshine for two more weeks.[44]

As Adelaide grew stronger she began to plan the work she would do upon returning to New York. She promised Minnie that she would give up some of the time-consuming board and committee work and concentrate her energies where they would be most effective. Her illness had prevented completion of the revision of *Educational Status of Nursing* for the U.S. Office of Education. In January she had resigned from the Committee on Maternal Welfare,[45] and in October she resigned from the Committee on Nursing of the Henry Street

[41] *Ibid.*; Isabel M. Stewart (New York) to Adelaide Nutting (Paget), February 3, 1924, *ibid.*

[42] Adelaide Nutting (Paget) to Isabel M. Stewart (New York), February 20, [1924], *ibid.*

[43] *Ibid.*

[44] *Ibid.*

[45] Robert L. Dickson (New York) to Isabel M. Stewart (New York), January 16, 1924, MAN Papers.

Settlement, suggesting that Lillian Hudson, who had just returned from an official visit to Soviet Russia with Lillian Wald, be appointed. She gave up her membership in the Teachers College Country Club, but retained membership in the Cosmopolitan Club, the Foreign Policy Association, the education committees of the NLNE and the International Council of Nurses, and a few lesser organizations. She wanted to give her best efforts to the department at Teachers College and to The Johns Hopkins Endowment Fund.

Meanwhile, the degree program instituted by the affiliation of Presbyterian Hospital with Teachers College was being terminated by mutual agreement. The arrangement with St. Luke's had been discontinued in the spring of 1923.[46] The five-year plan had been inaugurated in the hope that the proposed Columbia School of Nursing would go through and that the program and its affiliations would be absorbed.[47] Before relinquishing the affiliation, Adelaide carefully evaluated the program: forty-eight students had entered the course, thirteen had dropped out, thirteen had degrees, two more would receive their degrees in June, eight were doing their clinical work in the hospital, and eleven were taking their courses in nursing education. She wanted to see the program continued only if it could serve as a model for other schools. She was well aware of the shortcomings of the arrangement. The college group was not easily assimilated by the non-college students; two years under the conditions they had to meet did not allow enough time in the hospital for experience in various fields; there were gaps between college science courses and their application to hospital conditions; there had to be many special arrangements; hospital and campus seemed remote; most students were not ready for specialization by their fifth year. The age gap was another difficulty: Presbyterian insisted on students being twenty-one.[48]

Because Teachers College was in the process of becoming strictly a graduate school, entering students were expected to complete their undergraduate work within four years. Dean Russell raised the possibility of making exceptions in nursing education, although he realized it would be more difficult to accomplish in this department than

---

[46] George F. Clover (New York) to M. Adelaide Nutting (New York), February 26, 1923, Department of Nursing Education Archives, Teachers College, and MAN Papers.

[47] In 1935 the Presbyterian Hospital School of Nursing was accepted as a department of the Medical School of Columbia University. It has both diploma and degree programs in nursing. "Speech of Margaret Conrad at the Fortieth Anniversary of Teachers College, October 13–14, 1939," MAN Papers.

[48] M. A. Nutting, "Notes on Five Year Plan Affiliation with Presbyterian Hospital School of Nursing, 1924," Department of Nursing Education Archives, Teachers College.

in others. Adelaide's faith in the university school, however, did not waver. When Mary Roberts, who succeeded Sophia Palmer as editor of the *American Journal of Nursing*, became discouraged that none of her "progressive policies" had been accepted by the journal's board, and began to consider accepting the position of director of the School of Nursing and Health at the University of Cincinnati, Adelaide encouraged her.

> I believe this is the first example of a municipal School of Nursing conceived as an integral part of a great municipal University. "The very idea is enough to stir the imagination." . . .
> University Schools of Nursing form the only hope for any genuine educational development in our work and these schools are in a sense still on trial. There are many doubtless honestly unable to believe that nursing has any need which the University should be called upon to satisfy. And there is also a stalwart body of opponents, chiefly medical. I believe that the full weight of your intellectual power should go into the balance at this time. It would . . . be a serious blow to good growth and advancement of our work if the important School of the University of Cincinnati should drift into the hands of mediocrity.[49]

The long sojourn in Bermuda had been most beneficial to Adelaide's health. Before returning home she was able to walk half a mile without stopping to rest or feeling completely exhausted. Back in New York, she attended a Foreign Policy Association luncheon on April 5. Since she was not teaching, she had time to spend in organizing her files, catching up on her correspondence, talking with students, and doing what she called the sundry "odd jobs."

One of these pet projects was the NLNE calendar, an annual publication which had begun in 1922. The calendar consisted of photographs and short biographical sketches of nursing leaders and appropriate descriptive quotations from English and American authors. One folder in Adelaide's files bulged with "the gems" of her reading —excerpts from Carlyle, Shakespeare, Francis Bacon, James Shirley, John Milton, Emerson, and Wordsworth, on such subjects as habit and work, perseverance, courage, education, and fellowship.

Another of Adelaide's personal projects was collecting books and magazines to send to the Clinton State Prison at Dannemora, New York. Adelaide especially wanted to secure books in Italian for Italian prisoners who could not read English, and to see that each of the

[49] M. Adelaide Nutting (Ogunquit, Maine) to Mary Roberts [Cincinnati], July 20, 1924, MAN Papers.

prisoners had a calendar in his cell.[50] Upon the suggestion of Warden H. M. Kaiser, she solicited and obtained 1,400 calendars for the prisoners.

Also, for a number of years Adelaide invited friends to join her in contributing money so that $100 could be sent to Sister Agnes Karll, who was trying against desperate odds to build up nursing standards in Germany.[51]

Each year more foreign students came to Teachers College, and Dean Russell asked the Nursing Education Department to work out a plan whereby these students could become better acquainted and enjoy the cultural advantages that New York afforded. Confronted with a language handicap and differences in social customs, the foreign students were often reticent and hesitant. Dean Russell suggested paying a senior to take over the matter of arranging trips to museums, art galleries, and theaters. Isabel Stewart appointed one of her majors to give special attention to the ten foreign students currently enrolled in nursing education. Adelaide heartily approved the idea, hoping some of the world's future leadership in nursing might be among those gravitating to Teachers College. She tried to get to know the foreign students personally and she introduced them to faculty members who would extend hospitality. Already some distinguished leaders had attended Teachers College. Countess Louise d'Ursel of Brussels, Belgium, had studied in the department in 1920 and recently had accompanied Isabel Stewart to the International Council of Nurses in Copenhagen.[52] Currently, Christianne Reimann, a scholarly and financially independent Danish nurse who had succeeded Lavinia Dock as secretary of the International Council, was enrolled as a student in nursing education. Special efforts were made to see that she became acquainted with Lillian Wald and other nursing leaders in New York and to discuss the issues which might be brought before the council. Miss Reimann begged Miss Nutting to attend the council's forthcoming meeting in Finland and preside at at least one of the sessions, but Adelaide had no such plans. She tried to get off the council's Education Committee, but Baroness Mannerheim urged her

[50] M. A. Nutting (New York) to President, State Committee on Prisons, [Albany, N.Y.], May 31, 1922; M. A. Nutting (New York) to Rev. A. J. Hervieux (Dannemora, N.Y.), June 28, 1922; A. J. Hervieux (Dannemora) to M. A. Nutting (New York), December 29, 1922; M. A. Nutting (New York) to Warden H. M. Kaiser (Dannemora), December 29, 1922; and A. J. Hervieux (Dannemora) to M. A. Nutting (New York), February 10, 1925; ibid.

[51] M. A. Nutting (New York) to Agnes Karll (Berlin), November 21, [1922], ibid.

[52] Countess Louise d'Ursel (Brussels) to Adelaide Nutting (New York), September 21, 1921, ibid.

to stay on, and she remained only because she did not want the work to fall into the hands of those who might compromise standards.

Before Adelaide left for Ogunquit in 1924 to spend a large part of her vacation with Georgia Nevins, she went to Baltimore to attend The Johns Hopkins Nurses Alumnae meeting and to discuss plans for The Johns Hopkins Nurses School Endowment.[53]

A sad-faced Georgia greeted Adelaide at North Street Station in Boston on the way to Ogunquit. Georgia, who the year before had seemed so happy and secure in her position as superintendent of St. Luke's Hospital, New Bedford, Massachusetts, had been released from her job, and a man had been installed in her place. Adelaide confided to Isabel:

> The story as she tells it is astounding. The decision about her and supplanting her by a man was reached by the Executive Committee, almost all men (and a doctor is on that); and the rest of the Board . . . women who have given so much to the hospital and indeed created [it], were not even informed. It is the clearest case of medical domination that I have ever seen. . . . the end was clearly predictable once Miss Nevins opposed them about the twenty-four hour day.[54]

Georgia had sustained and cared for Adelaide in her illness. Now it was Adelaide's turn to help Georgia rid herself of the feeling that after more than thirty years of successful hospital work she was "a failure." They read, talked together, and played bridge. For a while Georgia appeared to be gaining her natural composure and charm, then suddenly she became depressed and burst into tears, and it was sometimes a day or two before she resumed a cheerful mien. Adelaide arranged for her to go on long drives and outings with Mrs. Jenkins, who was summering at a nearby resort, and used the precious hours alone for rest and correspondence.

As soon as Adelaide had shaken off the dust and weariness of the trip to Ogunquit, her thoughts turned to the department and the staff, which she affectionately called "the family." By 1924 everyone at Teachers College seemed to be immersed in research. "What is it that we ought to try to do?" she wrote Isabel Stewart. She then suggested that the staff get together, seriously consider the matter, and settle on some narrow phase of child life to study—for example, "sleep, . . . how it affects the child and the conditions affecting sleep, noise, lack

[53] "Alumnae Meeting, May 14, 1924," *The Johns Hopkins Nurses Alumnae Magazine*, August, 1924, p. 90.

[54] Adelaide Nutting (Ogunquit) to Isabel M. Stewart, [New York], July 4, 1924, MAN–IMS Correspondence.

of air, bedding, clothing, food eaten at supper, unhappy or exciting home life. Could these data be obtained through visiting nurses?" In the same letter she suggested that Carolyn Gray's services be used to help the department start its *Bulletin*: "let us see what can be done to build up a real educational journal."[55]

In the months that followed, Adelaide gave much thought to the future of the department and her role in it. The 1924 fall enrollment was 367, the largest in the history of the department. The staff now consisted of three full-time professors, three full-time and two part-time instructors, two secretaries, and a number of visiting lecturers. In the seventeen years since Adelaide began her work at Teachers College, the department had expanded from one small room in Thompson Building into eight offices, a staff library room, a conference room, and a nursing laboratory and classrooms. There had been only 4 students in nursing education in 1907. Gradually the nursing certificate had given way to bachelor of science and master's degrees; 54 students would receive the B.S. degree at the close of the academic year in June, 1925, and 8 would receive master's degrees. The early students had come from the United States and Canada, but now they came from all parts of the world, and the department was in a very real sense an international center of nursing education.[56]

In November Adelaide would be sixty-six. She hoped she did not look her age, but there were days when she felt much older. Her hair was gray and seemed to accent the blue-gray of her eyes, and there were tired lines about her face. She had begun to think seriously about retiring. Although frail, her general health was better than it had been for several months. Years before, she had written her sister that she wanted to go out while the flags were still flying and the band playing. She did not need to give Dean Russell her final word until February, so she went quietly about her work, telling only the dean and Isabel what she was considering. On November 14 she went to the Astor with Willystine Goodsell and Lillian Hudson to a dinner honoring her friend Mrs. Florence Kelly on the twenty-fifth anniversary of her work for women, children, and suffrage. She spent Thanksgiving with Lillian Wald, and in the quiet candlelight after dinner they talked of Henry Street, Lavinia Dock, Annie Goodrich, and the services that the visiting nurse service had rendered. Lillian had shared her joy in helping the unfortunate by enlisting the moral

---

[55] Adelaide Nutting (Ogunquit) to Isabel M. Stewart (New York), July 27, 28, and 29, 1924, *ibid.*

[56] Isabel M. Stewart, *Twenty-five Years of Nursing Education in Teachers College (Teachers College Bulletin*, 17th ser., no. 3, February, 1926), pp. 12–13.

and financial support of people like Jacob Schiff, Felix Warburg, and Helen Hartley Jenkins. Adelaide always returned refreshed and inspired after her visits with Lillian.

Holidays afforded time for catching up on personal correspondence. Sally Johnson of Massachusetts General Hospital wrote of the meeting of the Massachusetts State League of Nursing, at which one topic of discussion had been "Why TC, by Some of Us Who Have Been There." "I wish you could have heard the ten minute talks which these women gave. After the meeting Miss [Carrie] Hall said, 'Do you realize all this has been made possible by Miss Nutting?' "[57] To Miss Johnson Adelaide replied:

> Your letter came at a moment . . . when I was just a bit down, rather weary . . . and it was heartening to have your words of good cheer but please, dear Miss Johnson, don't make any mistake about my part in the work here and do not let others do so if you can help it. Miss Stewart, Miss Goodrich, Miss Hudson and Miss Strong, when she was with us, and more recently Miss [Elizabeth] Burgess as well as others—what is here is more truly theirs than mine. So I know you will forgive me for reading all but the personal part of your letter at our staff conference the other morning to pass on as it were to these dear colleagues a whiff of the fragrance of your flowers.[58]

In January, Adelaide attended the board meeting of the NLNE, and on February 9 she spoke at the dedication of the new Faculty Women's Club on West 117th Street. After several moves the club had at last obtained permanent rooms in a building adjacent to the Men's Faculty Club and the new Columbia University dormitory, Johnson Hall. As a founder of the club, Adelaide had been asked to light the fire in the beautiful marble fireplace. On neither occasion did her remarks betray the letter the trustees were to act upon the day following the club's reception. Perhaps no one but her closest associates in the department read any nuances of sadness into her charming speech. After telling something about the founding of the club, it was her "happy task to light the hearth fire."

> I light no new fire today, but I relight in a new shrine the fires of affection and friendship which alone have brought into being this beautiful home and which will make it meaningful and truly worthwhile in our lives.[59]

---

[57] Sally Johnson (Boston) to Adelaide Nutting (New York), November 17, 1924, MAN Papers.

[58] Adelaide Nutting (New York) to Sally Johnson (Boston), November 24, 1924, *ibid.*

[59] Adelaide Nutting, "Speech at New Faculty Women's Club, Columbia University, 410 West 117 Street, New York, February 9, 1925," *ibid.*

The next morning the Board of Trustees of Teachers College accepted Adelaide Nutting's resignation and appointed her professor emeritus. Dean Russell, who was himself approaching retirement, wrote to tell her personally how reluctantly he had presented the notice.

> We have worked together so long and had so much pleasure that I feel as if this break was the beginning of the end. . . . When I see what you have done and when the work was started, I can't be downhearted at anything that can happen. You have made a wonderful success and I am proud to have had some small part in it if only by . . . clearing the way for you. . . .
>
> The woman you are has made everything possible—it is itself sufficient reason to account for all that has happened. I am better for having been a friend.
>
> Faithfully yours,
> James E. Russell[60]

Although Adelaide had given the matter of retirement serious thought, the full impact of what it meant did not fully dawn on her until letters from friends and students began to pour in. Then it became a frightening thing. After the last lesson was taught, the last paper graded, the last class dismissed, "What?" she asked. Privately she cried, then pulled herself together to acknowledge the loving messages. To Edwin R. Embree of the Rockefeller Foundation she wrote:

> It is no small pleasure to have your friendly letter about my withdrawal from the College, and I must thank you for the kind things you say of my work here. . . .
>
> Just at this moment of laying down the absorbing task of years, the chief thing I have to struggle against is the conviction that the world has quietly come to an end. I suspect this is not an uncommon state of mind, given the conditions, and it will probably pass. At any rate I am holding fast to the idea that after some months of rest, and if possible of travel, I shall be again engaged in the useful work you are good enough to wish for me.[61]

There was little doubt who would succeed Miss Nutting. For fifteen years Isabel Stewart had been quietly and unobtrusively groomed for the position, although the matter was never discussed between the two women until just before Miss Stewart left for her sabbatical in

[60] James E. Russell (New York) to Adelaide Nutting (New York), February 10, 1925, ibid.

[61] Adelaide Nutting (New York) to Edwin R. Embree (New York), April 22, 1925. Ibid.

1923. Isabel Stewart had natural ability and had grown in the years she had been in the department, especially since learning of the impending responsibilities. Whatever reluctance Adelaide may have had in retiring was not motivated by doubt of the competence of her successor.

The weeks that followed the public announcement of Adelaide's retirement, which was made in a note to the Hopkins Alumnae dinner in New York on February 12, passed in a whirlwind of activity which was very taxing on her slender reserve of strength. There was so much she wanted to accomplish in those few remaining months. She went to Boston on February 27 to discuss nursing matters with Sally Johnson at Massachusetts General Hospital. While there, she went out to see Anne Strong, who had done such fine work in building up the courses in public health at Teachers College before joining the staff of the department of Nursing Education at Simmons College. Now Miss Strong was very ill. Adelaide "invited her to get well for the express purpose of joining in the proposed enterprise of a free and unfettered little publication on and for nursing. [Miss Strong] seemed greatly exhilarated by the idea and pledged herself unreservedly to it."[62] Aside from financial problems, Adelaide assured Isabel, "You begin to see a shadowy editorial Board of a mythical Journal on Nursing Education projecting itself in the dim future."

Later in the month Adelaide took up the matter of the reorganization of The Johns Hopkins Hospital School of Nursing and the endowment fund. Elsie Lawler, superintendent of nurses and principal of the school, had written that as far as she could gather there was no hope of any connection with the university.[63] Adelaide replied that she did not think it necessary to abandon all hope of connection with the university because it had decided not to give bachelor of science degrees in the future.

> It would seem that you have an excellent opportunity to create not the usual kind of a school perhaps, but an unusually important kind of graduate school, in that you have the resources of the School of Hygiene and the School of Education open to you.
>
> You are in a position to go far ahead of anything we have been able to do, I suppose, certainly in the training for public health work where we greatly need women of more liberal education than can now be secured, and as for teachers, we are simply swamped with requests we

---

[62] Adelaide Nutting (Boston) to Isabel Stewart (New York), March 2, 1925, ibid.

[63] Elsie M. Lawler (Baltimore) to M. Adelaide Nutting (New York), March 25, 1925, ibid.

can not fill. . . . Do not be discouraged because the first plan had to be abandoned and do not allow the door you have opened to be closed as yet.[64]

Adelaide further suggested that Miss Lawler talk things over informally with Dr. Frank Goodnow, president of The Johns Hopkins University, because she believed he had a sincere interest in nursing problems. Later, when it seemed expedient to postpone the Conference on the University and Nursing School until fall, Adelaide wrote to Miss Lawler again:

> You will be delighted, I know, to hear that the Yale School of Nursing has finally been able to arrange for the degree of B.N. and you will be interested too, because you have always liked the idea of a special degree. And you will also be glad because every step forward in other universities may be of help in strengthening your appeal.[65]

Elsie Lawler was an excellent administrator and a kindly sympathetic woman whose first thought was the comfort of the patient. She got along well with the Hopkins trustees, medical staff, and nurses and had great affection for her alma mater. Would she catch the torch and grasp the vision? Would she see nurses training as education, as scientific, as creative? Time alone would tell.

There were far more social and professional invitations than Adelaide's strength would permit her to accept. Since she would be returning to New York in September, the public dinner at which her friends at the university wished to honor her was postponed until then. On May 7 the twenty-fifth anniversary of nursing education at Teachers College was celebrated with a nurses banquet. There was a birthday cake, group singing, and amusing and affectionate speeches were made. Adelaide enjoyed the affair, later writing on her program in pencil, "Like a regular rollicking undergraduate boys' dinner."[66]

The Nursing Committee of the Henry Street Settlement Visiting Nurses Service gave a tea on May 22 at the central administration building in honor of Miss Nutting, Lady Aberdeen, and the foreign delegates attending the International Council of Women.[67]

Two days before, Adelaide had put on her academic gown with the

[64] Adelaide Nutting (New York) to Elsie M. Lawler (Baltimore), March 30, 1925, ibid.

[65] Adelaide Nutting (New York) to Elsie M. Lawler (Baltimore), April 16, 1925, ibid.

[66] "Program, Nurses Banquet, May 7, 1925," ibid.

[67] Frances Biggs (New York) to M. Adelaide Nutting (New York), May 16, 1925, ibid.

Yale hood for the last time and had proudly marched in the procession. Never again would "Pomp and Circumstance" have the same meaning for her. After the speeches, the conferring of degrees, the closing hymn, the benediction, and the recessional, the convocation ended. When the last graduate and the last staff member had shaken her hand, Adelaide walked slowly home. Except for the retirement check, her formal association with Teachers College was at an end. She could go on living in Emerson and take her meals in the college dining rooms, attending faculty teas and receptions, but being a professor emeritus would be different. There was unfinished business to be done. Not all her dreams for nursing education had been achieved. She wanted to continue her writing and correspondence. To escape the heat of New York she would spend a few weeks with Georgia Nevins at Hawthorne Inn, East Gloucester, Massachusetts, where she would catch up on sleep and reply to the many letters that had descended upon her following the announcement of her retirement. After that she would go to Waterloo.[68]

The last class had been taught, the last paper graded. The world seemed empty for the moment, yet Adelaide felt somehow she should pull herself together and get busy. She read again Isabel Stewart's article about her retirement in the June issue of *American Journal of Nursing* and then wrote Isabel.

> This is a wonderful person, dear I.M.S., but she is not me, as I know her. She is however what I would like to be, and I must see if I can't live up to her in my remaining years. This glowing picture is just the challenge one sometimes needs—in order not to fall down in a heap and crumble away.
>
> Much love, much gratitude.
>
> A. N.[69]

[68] M. Adelaide Nutting (East Gloucester, Mass.) to Armine N. Gosling (Bermuda), July 25, 1925, *ibid.*
[69] Adelaide Nutting to Isabel Stewart, n.p., n.d., *ibid.*

XXI

Professor Emeritus, 1925–1932

East Gloucester, Massachusetts, held little enchantment for Adelaide the summer of 1925, but it did offer cool breezes and beautiful sunsets. To Adelaide, Hawthorne Inn was just "a great caravansary of a place feeding 450 persons at a meal . . . with verandahs and rocking chairs all over the place and noisy gabbling people filling them," although undoubtedly they were persons "of the very utmost and obvious respectability." She contented herself to stay in her room, rest, and attack the voluminous parcel of work that she always seemed to take on her vacations. The report of the International Committee on Education which Miss Stewart would present for her at the International Council of Nurses meeting in Helsinki had priority, and Adelaide began to work on it even before she unpacked her luggage.[1]

Adelaide was resigning from the chairmanship of the International Council's Committee on Education, which she had held since its creation in 1910. Little work had been done on the curriculum the council had hoped might lead to an international standard in nursing education since World War I had suspended all activities of the council. In the spring of 1925, however, a representative had been named to the committee from each of the fourteen member countries of the organization, and Miss Nutting and Miss Stewart as secretary had drafted a report to be acted upon by the committee, amended or approved, and then submitted to the delegate body for ratification or rejection. The report was in two parts: the first part set forth the requirements in hospital conditions, resources, and administrative policies necessary for the conduct of a satisfactory plan of education; the second part outlined a tentative curriculum. Copies of the report would be sent in advance to the committee, and, in Helsinki, Isabel Stewart would re-

[1] Adelaide Nutting (East Gloucester, Mass.) to Isabel Stewart (New York), July 3, 1925, MAN–IMS Correspondence.

ceive comments, suggestions, and amendments. After adoption by the council, implementation would be left up to the various countries.[2]

Adelaide warned the Education Committee that, because of the differences in systems of education, attitudes toward the education of women, and the problems peculiar to nursing in all countries, progress would be slow and often difficult. She hoped, however, that some of the standards set up could be universally accepted and improved upon year after year, and that all countries would be able to look to the International Council for expert help in establishing correct ideas and standards in the training of nurses. The report, she told Isabel, must embody the distilled wisdom of thirty years of nursing education, as well as a manifesto of principles applicable to nursing everywhere.[3]

When the report was finished, Adelaide's thoughts turned to the reorganization of the Hopkins School and its endowment fund. Elsie Lawler and Isabel were traveling to the International Council in Helsinki on the same ship, and Adelaide jotted down some approaches Isabel might use in conversation.[4] She was delighted when Isabel wrote from the first port of call that she had talked with Miss Lawler and believed that "the university idea was beginning to take hold there."[5]

Isabel had no time to write from Helsinki, so crowded were the days and nights with receptions, banquets, and sightseeing, but from Stockholm she sent a detailed and intimate account of the meetings, from the grand convocations to the behind-the-scenes political maneuvers, personal foibles, and national rivalries. Eleven hundred nurses had attended the congress; seven hundred were Finnish, and the remainder came from thirty-two other countries. Forty nurses from eleven countries had attended the Teachers College luncheon. The Education Committee had approved Miss Nutting's letter and her part of the report unanimously, but no decisive action was taken relative to the Nightingale memorial.

The climax of the congress came when honorary membership in the Association of Nurses of Finland was conferred upon Adelaide Nutting, Anna Maxwell, Clara Noyes, Mary Agnes Snively, and several others. The Baroness Sophia Mannerheim made the presenta-

---

[2] Adelaide Nutting (New York) to Countess d'Ursel (Brussels), June 9, 1925, MAN Papers.

[3] Adelaide Nutting (East Gloucester) to Isabel Stewart (New York), July 3, 1925, MAN–IMS Correspondence.

[4] Adelaide Nutting (East Gloucester) to Isabel Stewart (New York), July 5–6, 1925, ibid.

[5] Isabel M. Stewart (aboard the Swedish-American Line's Drottingholm) to Adelaide Nutting (East Gloucester), July 16, 1925, ibid.

tions, and Isabel Stewart accepted the pin and certificate in behalf of Miss Nutting.[6]

Meanwhile, Adelaide was joined at East Gloucester by Elizabeth Christine Cook of the Teachers College English Department. They planned a schedule of work, rest, and recreation. In the mornings Elizabeth worked on her next novel, and Adelaide wrote replies to the hundred or more letters she had brought along and the letters that continued to come. Following lunch they rested, then walked for an hour, and after dinner they sat on the "endless verandahs with a horde of people" and watched indescribably beautiful sunsets. Always a rapid reader, Adelaide finished *Passage to India*, *The Constant Nymph*, *The Old Ladies*, *The House of the Arrow*, *God's Step-Children*, and *The Life of Olive Schreiner*. She then resolved to concentrate on Greek history. Friends had advised her to take a year off from all work, and she had half made up her mind to go to Europe if Georgia Nevins could accompany her.[7] After four weeks, however, she had reached "the limit to the pleasures to be obtained from watching sunsets" and was quite ready to go on to Waterloo. She would leave Gloucester in "the gray of the morning" and take the nine o'clock train from Boston; this would stop at a queer little junction among the hills, where Charlie and Lizzie would be waiting for her.

One of the sundry tasks that Adelaide agreed to do during her vacation, and the first to which she affixed the title "professor emeritus," was a greeting or preface for the souvenir program of the annual convention of the New York State Nurses Association, the New York State League for Nursing Education, and the New York State Organization for Public Health Nursing, which was to be held at the Hotel TenEyck, October 27–29, 1925.

My friends:

The nurses of this state have been engaged for nearly twenty-five years in continuous efforts to improve the quality of nursing through improving the schools in which nurses are trained. It has been particularly difficult work—uphill, costly and precarious but there can be no doubt that because of their efforts the sick in this state are very much better cared for than ever before, standards of living are better safeguarded, and the work of physicians has been strengthened. This is a good record, but it must be evident to all of us that there can be no slackening of efforts, and that our great first task still lies in our Schools

[6] Isabel M. Stewart (Stockholm) to Adelaide Nutting (Waterloo, Quebec), July 28, 1925, *ibid.*

[7] Adelaide Nutting (East Gloucester) to Armine N. Gosling (St. John's, Newfoundland), July 25, 1925, MAN Papers.

of Nursing. As a profession we shall go no further than they enable us to go. . . . At the moment I am concerned with another and little discussed aspect of the situation, and that is the way in which the body of graduate nurses in their several fields react upon our schools. . . .

Public opinion of any profession will be formed not by a few conspicuous representatives, but by the large body of persons practicing. Now private nurses outnumber others in the proportion of four or five to one. Their well being and happiness, their ability to give satisfactory service in their work, their capacity to develop into something better, the public esteem in which they are held, all are matters which obviously affect the number and quality of applicants to our schools of nursing. For our schools, then, the conditions under which these least protected of our members are living and working are really vital issues. Clearly our private nurses must not be left to struggle unaided with distracting problems for which they alone are not responsible, and which concern all of us. These problems are bound up with economic facts and they demand the serious study of experts. It is encouraging to note that one of the various committees of medical men who have been struggling with the nursing problem suggests cooperation with a Committee on Economics. Encouraging too are the efforts of certain alumnae associations to establish the right of their members to share in determining the conditions under which they can do their best work and live the right kind of lives. That spirit is sound and wholesome.

We need to realize and to affirm anew that nursing is one of the most difficult of arts. Compassion may provide the motive but knowledge is our only working power. Perhaps, too, we need to remember that growth in our work must be preceded by ideas, and that any conditions which suppress thought must retard growth. Surely we will not be satisfied in perpetuating methods and traditions. Surely we shall wish to be more and more occupied with creating them.

Yours faithfully,

M. Adelaide Nutting
Professor Emeritus of
Teachers College, Columbia[8]

In these few paragraphs she crystallized the wisdom gleaned from forty-five years of nursing experience in the ward and classroom. One sentence, "Compassion may provide the motive but knowledge is our only working power," would be quoted and paraphrased again and again.

Late in August Adelaide returned to New York from Waterloo, and after three weeks of renovating, refurbishing, and finally renting the apartment she took some rooms in Butler Hall, a new apartment hotel

[8] Adelaide Nutting, "Greeting at the Annual Convention of the New York State Nurses Association, New York State League for Nursing Education and New York State Organization for Public Health Nursing, New York, October 27, 28, 29, 1925," *ibid.*

on 119th Street and Morningside Drive, and remained there until she and Georgia were ready to leave for Europe. Meanwhile, she signed a contract with G. P. Putnam's Sons to publish a volume of addresses and papers she had written through the years. This would require endless sorting and selecting before the editing could begin. She planned to edit the papers during the winter, for neither she nor Georgia felt equal to rushing from gallery to gallery, concert to concert, as they had done in 1914.

The Faber Line's S.S. *Providence* was scheduled to sail on December 5. Adelaide had neither time nor inclination to shop for traveling. The trip would be expensive, and she resolved to make her old clothes do. In November she visited Hopkins in the interest of the Endowment Fund and the future development of the School of Nursing.[9] The campaign launched ten years before had met with numerous setbacks; only $87,742 of the $1,000,000 originally sought had been pledged, and of that amount $1,200 had been expended on the second drive.

Following the publication of Miss Goldmark's *Nursing and Nursing Education in the United States*, the trustees of The Johns Hopkins Hospital asked Carolyn Gray to survey the school and explore the untapped resources for nursing education in Baltimore. After six weeks' intensive research, Miss Gray recommended that the School of Nursing be affiliated with The Johns Hopkins University and offer five-year and three-year programs. The five-year plan provided for two years of study at the university and two years of work in the hospital, where students would deal specifically with the principles and practice of clinical nursing. During the fifth year, provision was made for four months' training in public health and four months in an elective field, with courses given coordinately at the university. The public health program would be worked out with the university's School of Hygiene and Health. At the conclusion of the five-year program the hospital would grant a nursing diploma, and the university would confer the bachelor of science degree. The three-year program would be given entirely in the School of Nursing and would include four months of field work in public health nursing. Miss Gray recommended that students enrolling in either program qualify for entrance to the university.[10]

The Hopkins Training School Committee acted favorably on the five-year program but hesitated to endorse the recommendation that

[9] Adelaide Nutting (New York) to Armine N. Gosling (St. John's), September 17, 1925, *ibid.*

[10] Ethel Johns and Blanche Pfefferkorn, *The Johns Hopkins Hospital School of Nursing* (Baltimore: The Johns Hopkins Press, 1954), pp. 202–3.

all students qualify for university entrance. Both programs advanced to the University Advisory Committee. The Advisory Committee on the Bachelor of Science Degree acted favorably on the five-year plan, but action on the three-year plan was held up, pending the submission of a detailed plan. At this point President Frank J. Goodnow proposed radical changes in the educational policy of the university, and the nursing proposals were held in abeyance.[11] Miss Nutting, Miss Gray, and others who were committed to the idea of an autonomous school of nursing within the structure of the university and not subservient to the nursing service of the hospital, began to look for ways of bringing up the matter again.

The launching of the Half-Century Campaign by the university and hospital to obtain $50,000,000 over a ten-year period offered the opportunity of at least "half a loaf," inasmuch as $500,000 of the first $11,000,000 raised would be allocated to the School of Nursing. Later, $50,000 would be set aside for the greatly needed Nurses' Home. Before accepting the invitation to assist in the fund raising, the Alumnae Committee wanted to know how the $500,000 would be spent for the school, and it asked that the committee be enlarged.[12]

To inform the public and to interest important groups in Baltimore in the Greater Endowment Fund, Mrs. John S. Gibbs, Sr., daughter of a former hospital trustee, opened her spacious country home for a public meeting on November 16. It was here that Adelaide pleaded the cause of an endowed and autonomous training school. She declared that the weakest link in the nursing profession was its system of education.[13] She was not willing to accept minimums for Hopkins.[14] Delighted by the warmth and enthusiasm of the people she met, she returned to New York with high hopes that her dreams for Hopkins would finally be realized.

On November 30, at the Men's Faculty Club, a dinner was given for Miss Nutting by her former colleagues. Her nephew, Arthur Gosling, accompanied her. She wrote her sister that the affair was "the sweetest and friendliest thing imaginable." There were about eighty people there, and the speeches were "kindly and generous."[15]

---

[11] Amy P. Miller, "A Short History of the Endowment Fund of The Johns Hopkins Nurses Alumnae Association," n.d., MAN Papers.

[12] Johns and Pfefferkorn, *The Johns Hopkins Hospital School of Nursing*, pp. 348–49.

[13] Clipping from the *Baltimore Sun*, November 17, 1925, MAN Papers.

[14] M. A. Nutting (New York) to Mary Beard, [New York], October 24, 1926, *ibid.*

[15] Adelaide Nutting (aboard the S.S. *Providence*, en route to Boston) to Armine N. Gosling (Bermuda), December 3, 1925, *ibid.*

Among those who spoke were Dean Russell, Patty Hill, Willystine Goodsell, who lauded her work as an education co-worker and founder of the Faculty Women's Club, and Isabel Stewart, who spoke on behalf of the department. Then it was Adelaide's turn to express her gratitude and affection to Dean Russell, President Butler, the trustees of Teachers College, and her friends and colleagues in nursing education, to tell of her confidence in Isabel Stewart, who would succeed her, and lastly to express her belief in Teachers College and the future.[16] She found it hard to say the words she had so carefully thought out. Then came the bon voyage gift, a beautifully illuminated citation from her colleagues which was bound in blue leather and bore her monogram in sterling silver.

> Mary Adelaide Nutting, pioneer in the University training of nurses, the first nurse to hold professional rank in any University, honored by the Government of the Learned World and by all who have an intelligent interest in the welfare of the community.
> We, your colleagues, send to you upon your retirement from active professorial scene, these few words of formal but very sincere appreciation of the great work done by you in Teachers College, Columbia University.
> We honor you for what you have done in elevating the profession of nursing; we respect you for your zeal in a cause so vital to the welfare of the race; we admire your cordial spirit of co-operation in all genuine educational movements; and we assure you not merely of our friendship and esteem, but also of an affection which is as genuine as your life has been in our midst.[17]

Adelaide then rose to acknowledge the gift and to say "thank you" for the years of kindness and friendship she had enjoyed at Teachers College.

Back at her apartment, Adelaide read the signatures on the citation: Nicholas Murray Butler, who had had faith in the enterprise of graduate study for nurses; James E. Russell, the dean who had made it possible; Paul Monroe, John Dewey, Edward Thorndike, David Snedden, George Strayer, William H. Kilpatrick, Frank McMurray, and Thomas Briggs, her mentors in the study of education; Henry Johnson and Mary Townsend, the history teachers with whom she loved to talk and from whom she had learned so much; Elizabeth Christine Cook; Willystine Goodsell; Thomas D. Wood and David Eugene Smith, colleagues and neighbors with whom she had taken so many meals in the Lowell dining room; Emma Gunther, Ray Balderston, and May B.

[16] *Ibid.*
[17] "The Citation Given at the Dinner, November 30, 1925," *ibid.*

Van Arsdale, whom she first came to know when nursing education was an adjunct of the Household Economics Department; C.-E. A. Winslow, Haven Emerson, Josephine Kenyon, and Robert Chaddock, who had lectured on public health in the early years; then the nursing education staff, Isabel Stewart, Lillian Hudson, Maud Muse, Mary Hulsizer, and so many more. There were sixty-two signers in all.

After Adelaide's plans became known, Anna Wolf wrote to all graduates of Johns Hopkins and to those who had taken work in nursing education at Teachers College for a year or more, inviting them to contribute to a gift to be presented to Miss Nutting before she sailed for a few months' rest in Italy. By the Wednesday before she sailed, $3,000 had been received, and Anna Wolf, Isabel Stewart, Mary Roberts, and Alta Dines called at Adelaide's apartment to make the presentation. Miss Wolf had cut excerpts from the letters of love and appreciation which accompanied the contributions and had pasted them in a parchment notebook bound in handsome, tooled Venetian leather. To Adelaide the gift was almost unbelievable; at once she began to think of how the money might be used to advance nursing.[18]

That same morning she received a letter from Dean Russell, advising her that the Board of Trustees had voted to take similar cognizance of her years of service.

Dear Miss Nutting,

The enclosed check for $3,000 brings to you the best wishes of the entire college for freedom to enjoy during your stay abroad the leisure which has been denied you in your years of service with us.

In the minds of the Trustees it is a substitute for the half salary which would have been yours had you waited for your next leave of absence but to me it is a testimonial of the love and affection which we have for you. Please accept it in the spirit in which it is offered and use it to recover the health and strength which will permit you again to exercise the influence which has been so beneficial to the whole world. With it goes my own personal gratitude to you for the years of delightful cooperation in a great cause. God bless you. I am

Faithfully yours,

James E. Russell[19]

---

[18] Anna D. Wolf (New York) to Nurses Alumnae, Teachers College and Johns Hopkins (New York and Baltimore), November 7, 1925, and [December], 1925, Department of Nursing Education Archives, Teachers College.

[19] James E. Russell (New York) to Mary Adelaide Nutting (New York), December 2, 1925, MAN Papers.

Adelaide's cup seemed to be running over. The next day she attended an informal luncheon with twenty-five friends at the Cosmopolitan Club. Adelaide thought the speakers were overgenerous about her achievements, so much so that it made things seem "a bit forced and unreal," but of their genuine friendliness she had no doubt.[20]

Saturday was sailing day. There was a frenzy of goodbyes at the pier, and a multitude of parcels, gifts, flowers, and candy was sent to her stateroom. As soon as the S.S. *Providence* cleared the harbor, Adelaide settled down to write various notes which she would post at the first port of call. "The past week has been little short of a cyclone," she wrote her sister. "It took the strenuous efforts of Miss Hudson, Miss Stewart, Mrs. Braddon, a laundress and sundry other aides to get my belongings sorted out and packed up and my tired and bewildered self finally on board this ship." Georgia Nevins joined Adelaide in Boston, where the ship docked to take on passengers.[21]

The *Providence* was not a large vessel, weighing only about 16,000 tons, but it had scarcely any roll, and Adelaide averred that "it would take a lively imagination for anyone to be seasick." The captain was a Sardinian, a sturdy, cheerful, and confident man. Twelve passengers sat at his table. Opposite Adelaide and Georgia were the parents of Allan Seeger, the young poet who had written "I have a rendezvous with Death," and had died early in World War I. Also, opposite them was a young Italian aristocrat who had been in the diplomatic service in Philadelphia, was a devotee of Mussolini, and believed dictatorship to be the only possible form of government for Italy. Beside him was a good-looking, well-bred, French-Canadian woman, a descendant "one would suppose of one of those very good French families who established the seigniories in Canada hundreds of years ago." Everyone on board spoke French rapidly except Adelaide and Georgia, who felt "genuinely humiliated . . . to be so ignorant and fumbling in trying to handle affairs on a French boat." Adelaide resolved to study the language again while in Europe.[22]

During the thirteen-day voyage to Palermo, Adelaide had written dozens of notes acknowledging gifts and courtesies and had spent some time working on the *Introduction to the Curriculum*, which she had promised to send Isabel Stewart at the earliest possible moment. As soon as she was settled at a desk she would begin revising the articles that were to appear in the book for Putnam's.

[20] Adelaide Nutting (aboard the S.S. *Providence*, en route to Boston) to Armine N. Gosling (Bermuda), *ibid.*
[21] *Ibid.*
[22] *Ibid.*

Looking forward to the quiet peace and beauty of Sicily, Adelaide recalled with nostalgia her visit there with her sister. The *Providence* reached Sicily at about five o'clock in the afternoon, and it was quite late before Adelaide and Georgia were established in the Hotel des Palmes. When they went for a walk the next morning, they came upon an acquaintance Adelaide and her sister had made four years before. She said that the Society for Prevention of Cruelty to Animals had taken on new life through a gift from an American woman, that it now had an office and agents, and that conditions were improving. Adelaide thought the horses really looked better, but there was still work to be done. When she learned that a dance for the benefit of the society was to be held that afternoon, she took Georgia. They watched the dancing, commenting that "some mites had been contributed to a good cause." Adelaide decided to go to the offices of the SPCA and make a small donation as her Christmas gift to her absent sister. On Sunday they attended a Palermo Symphony concert. Among the eighty or more players were eleven women. It delighted Adelaide to see how competently these fine-looking young women played the violin, viola, and harp.[23]

After breakfast on Christmas Day, Adelaide and Georgia ceremoniously opened the packages so carefully labeled, "Do not open until December 25." Georgia set up a foot-and-a-half collapsible Christmas tree and decorated it with "all its shining treasures," they read Rachel Louise Metcalf's poem for the occasion, and then they sampled the sweets, nuts, cakes, and all the other things which friends had brought to the ship.[24] To her sister Adelaide wrote, "It all served to cheer two rather drab old persons who felt rather far away and lonely and without belongings in spite of the beauty of the country and the enchantments around us at every turn."[25]

The day after Christmas, Adelaide mailed to Isabel the corrected pages of the *Introduction to the Curriculum*, which was being reissued by the National League of Nursing Education. Adelaide was not satisfied with the result of her "spasmodic efforts" in the crowded writing room aboard ship and in the small room she shared at the hotel. She felt the manuscript needed much more careful and searching revision than she had been able to give at such a distance from persons and sources of exact information. In her letter to Isabel she wrote:

[23] Adelaide Nutting (Palermo, Sicily) to Armine N. Gosling (Bermuda), December 22, 1925, *ibid.*
[24] Adelaide Nutting (Palermo) to Isabel M. Stewart (New York), December 27, 1925, MAN–IMS Correspondence.
[25] Adelaide Nutting (Palermo) to Armine N. Gosling (Bermuda) December 27, 1925, MAN Papers.

I think we ought to bring in something about the use of attendants and helpers, and we ought perhaps to stress more that matter of funds, endowments or other contributions or state or city aid. . . . we ought not to leave the question of "correlation" hanging in mid-air but say something true and clear cut about it, showing [how] necessarily limited in actual working possibilities it is and must continue to be.[26]

Adelaide had wanted to go to Egypt, but the trip was far too expensive. Thinking that a glimpse of Africa would be better than nothing, she and Georgia decided to visit Tunis, which was only eighteen hours from Sicily by boat.

Adelaide was deeply impressed by what she saw in Tunis. The French sector, with its sidewalk cafés, was much like Paris except for the men in white burnous and red fez drinking coffee for hours at a stretch, a few obviously foreign women, and an occasional veiled Moorish or Arabian servant woman hurrying past on an errand. The large, walled, Arab quarter revealed mosques, minarets, palaces and homes, bazaars, and a caravan of camels in from the desert. From one of the bey's palaces, Adelaide viewed the city spread out below and the great mountains in the distance. She regarded the position of Arab women as generally "pitiable and degraded in the extreme—a toy in rich homes, a beast of burden in poor ones—a clue to my belief [that] the whole problem of this civilization lies in its attitude toward women."[27] At Carthage, Adelaide and Georgia walked among the ruins and thought of the Punic Wars, "the long struggle of Rome for supremacy, her failure and downfall." Back in Sicily they spent some time in Girgenti, Siracusa, and Taormina, where Adelaide reminisced about the days she and her sister had spent there.[28]

Adelaide and Georgia wandered among the sites of the ten Greek temples near Girgenti. The Temple of Concordia and the Temple of Juno were golden brown, and the vistas, in every direction defined by the great columns, were enchanting. The almond trees were just beginning to blossom and their delicate pink blossoms stood out among the scattered clumps of olive, pine, and palm trees. Georgia was satisfied to have seen Greek temples in Sicily and did not want to go on to Greece, but Adelaide was only the more desirous of going. "D.V.," she wrote her sister, "I shall go even if for only a week." Of Taormina, she wrote:

[26] Adelaide Nutting (Palermo) to Isabel M. Stewart (New York), December 27, 1925, MAN–IMS Correspondence.
[27] Adelaide Nutting (Tunis) to Arthur Gosling (St. John, New Brunswick), January 4, 1926, MAN Papers.
[28] Adelaide Nutting (Palermo) to Isabel M. Stewart (New York), January 11, 1926, MAN–IMS Correspondence.

The food everywhere is a good deal better than when you and I sojourned here. And I hardly need tell you that wine is on every table as common as the chairs we sit on, and that sometimes when I am too cold and tired to care, my principles on this matter do go "a glimmering." But that is not often.[29]

Adelaide encouraged Georgia to accompany other tourists at the hotel on trips about the countryside so that she herself might have uninterrupted time to work on her manuscript. Forwarded by Isabel, a note from Putnam's stimulated her to greater activity.

> I wonder if you women at Teachers College appreciate how much you have done in the past few years to make the School of Nursing Education of Teachers College a kind of guiding star for the nursing profession of the entire country. I do not believe you realize it as much as do those who are in the business of supplying training schools with whatever they may need. Certainly the record has been made, and the reputation which has been established by the school at Teachers College is an enviable one. You and Miss Nutting may rely upon our best efforts to secure proper distribution for the forthcoming volume.

Adelaide was grateful for Isabel, who would work as hard for the book as she would herself.[30]

The travelers spent a month in Sorrento, living in an old Jesuit rest house in a room whose large balcony overlooked the tops of orange and lemon groves and offered a view across the bay to the island of Ischia, Naples, and Mt. Vesuvius. In deference to Georgia, Adelaide gave up her plans to go to Greece, at least for this trip. In Sorrento she drove herself to work on the manuscript and urged Georgia to go sightseeing alone. The self-discipline and energy that writing demanded became very irksome, and at times Adelaide thought she had been foolish to go abroad before the book was finished.

At other times Adelaide pushed her work aside and entered into the spirit of Italy. Through a former student in Naples she managed to secure tickets to "Pagliacci" in the famous San Carlo Opera House built in 1737, and she planned to visit Milan before the season at La Scala ended.[31]

After a week in Naples, Adelaide and Georgia went on to Rome. Adelaide was delighted not only by the beauty of the Roman spring

[29] Adelaide Nutting (Girgenti, Sicily) to Armine N. Gosling (Bermuda), January 12, 1926, MAN Papers.

[30] Adelaide Nutting (Taormina, Sicily) to Armine N. Gosling (Bermuda), January 17, 1926, ibid.

[31] Adelaide Nutting (Naples) to Armine N. Gosling (Bermuda), March 2, 1926, ibid.

but also by the charm and vividness of life there. "Just think of going to hear Jascha Heifitz play to a Roman audience in a music hall which was once the mausoleum of Augustus, built in 28 B.C."[32] Adelaide was intrigued by the gardens, fountains, drives, and ruins. She and Georgia spent a morning with an archeologist going over the Colosseum and the Golden House of Nero. Adelaide then chided herself, "I ought to be reading Italian history now."[33]

Florence was not as appealing to Adelaide as Rome had been and she spent most of her time there working on the book. She appreciated the "beauty of many of its buildings, the splendor of its history. Savanarola thunders from San Marco, the magnificent Medici pervade the place—the Uffizi and the Pitti palace overwhelm me but somehow I left with no such vivid warm sense of the greatness and beauty of Italy as Rome gives."[34]

It was exhilarating to follow the spring northward to La Spezia, where poor Shelley washed ashore, then to Rapallo, Sta. Margherita Ligure, Genoa, and Menton. Everywhere flowers and shrubs were beginning to bloom, especially banksea, roses, and wisteria. Adelaide and Georgia regretted the end of their four-month stay there, but they made ready for Avignon and other old towns of Provence, once parts of the Roman Empire, whose ruins ought still "to shout a loud warning to our friend, Benito Mussolini."[35]

Nice was delightful. Three blocks from the sea, Adelaide found a quiet English hotel with small but sunny bedrooms and fairly good meals where she and Georgia could live "all told for $2.00 a day"—a boon to their dwindling purses.[36] Adelaide was determined not to spend any of the $3,000 that had come from her students at Johns Hopkins and Teachers College for "travel, study and research." She wanted to put it back into the hands of the nursing world as soon as she found the right way. "I wanted no gift from nurses, and though grateful for the generous impulse which prompted it, I feel embarrassed over the obligations it entails."[37]

[32] Adelaide Nutting (Rome) to Armine N. Gosling (Bermuda), March 21, 1926, ibid.
[33] Adelaide Nutting (Menton, France) to Armine N. Gosling (Bermuda), April 11, 1926, ibid.
[34] Adelaide Nutting (Sta. Margherita Ligure) to Armine N. Gosling (Bermuda), April 8, 1926, ibid.
[35] Adelaide Nutting (Menton) to Arthur Gosling (Bermuda), April 20, 1926, ibid.
[36] Adelaide Nutting (Avignon, France) to Armine N. Gosling (Bermuda), May 16, 1926, ibid.
[37] Adelaide Nutting (Rome) to Armine N. Gosling (Bermuda), March 21, 1926, ibid.

While in Nice, Adelaide and Georgia took the motor drive to Grasse, the city of perfume, which Adelaide had always longed to visit. She was delighted with "the pretty little town" on the hillside with the lovely stretch between it and the sea. The gardens about the town were breath-taking; 60,000 acres had been given only to flowers —roses of all varieties, violets, lilies, and others. On one mountaintop not far away there were great sweeps of wild lavender. Adelaide visited one of the thirty perfume factories and bought one small bottle for her sister.

The travelers planned to stay a week at Avignon, where they would visit papal palaces, the lovely old bridge, the cathedral, the Promenade des Doms, and the cemetery on the outskirts, where John Stuart Mill is buried, and take a short motor trip to Nîmes, Arles, Orange, St.-Rémy, and the Fountain of Vancluse, where Petrarch's Laura lies. The spring rains caught up with them, however, and they were unable to visit the nearby towns. Through a former student Adelaide had secured tickets to a concert by Fritz Kreisler in Paris; she was eager to hear him play before a French audience. She assured herself she would come to Europe again, alone if necessary, to see Greece and the other places missed on this trip. "But for the present," she wrote her sister, "I have had enough, quite enough in fact—six months of this kind of life is long enough for a person who likes to be doing something worth while. I can do nothing in the way of serious study . . . for there are no books."[38] She wanted to get back to New York, settle herself in a new apartment, and begin something worthwhile. She confided to Isabel that, above all other things, she wanted to get a periodical on nursing education started, a journal for which the need was imperative. She wanted the question raised at the NLNE meeting in 1927.

Adelaide had broached the question to the president of the league ten years before. If the league now thought well of setting up a committee to study the question, and, if she could do something on such a committee, she believed she could "face the coming year with her heart somewhere but in her boots." She was confident that, if a plan could be worked out and she were given an opportunity to struggle along with the idea for a few years, nursing education would eventually have a strong, courageous, helpful journal. One alternative would be to ask a few people to join her in experimenting with such a periodical, working it out carefully and collecting funds to support it. Adelaide would use her $3,000 cheerfully on that, and then, when the

[38] Adelaide Nutting (Avignon) to Armine N. Gosling (Bermuda), May 16, 1926, ibid.

magazine was a "well-established going concern," she would turn it over as a gift to the NLNE, free from any taint of politics.[39]

A letter from Dr. J. Norris Myers of Macmillan Company, inquiring about the possibility of Miss Nutting writing a book on Florence Nightingale, had been forwarded to Italy.[40] Adelaide had often thought of compiling a series of essays on Miss Nightingale's views on education and nursing administration, and she believed the subject was "fascinating," but for the present she did not feel "equal to any hornet's nest such as nursing matters were in England." The past three or four years of her life had been devastating to the point that everything had become an effort. Later on she would be glad to spend a year in England. At the moment her one thought was to get home. The last chapters for the book *A Sound Economic Basis for Schools of Nursing* were mailed from Nice on May 9. Only the Preface remained to be written.[41]

In Paris, Adelaide changed her sailing date from August 28 to August 7. She spent a few days sightseeing with Georgia, who was reticent about going places alone. Adelaide saw a great deal of the Baroness Sophia Mannerheim of Finland, who was visiting in Paris. They had lunch and dinner together and discussed international nursing affairs, the International Council, and the League of Red Cross Societies.[42] Adelaide felt she was returning to America with a better idea of the international scene insofar as nursing was concerned. As for politics, she was concerned about the vast amount of conservatism everywhere.

To escape the sweltering heat of Paris in July, Adelaide and Georgia went to Oberhofen on the Lake of Thun in the Bernese Alps, and the week before they sailed they motored to Vannes in Brittany. Each letter to Isabel Stewart revealed more of Adelaide's concern to get home, find new living quarters, finish the book, and begin to explore the possibilities of the nursing education journal. On August 7 Adelaide and Georgia sailed from Cherbourg on the S.S. *Antonia* bound for Montreal. From there Georgia would take the train to her home, and Adelaide would visit briefly with Charlie and Lizzie in Waterloo before going on to New York and apartment-hunting.

[39] Adelaide Nutting (Menton) to Isabel M. Stewart (New York), April 27, 1926, MAN–IMS Correspondence.

[40] J. Norris Myers (New York) to Adelaide Nutting (Palermo), January 5, 1926, MAN Papers.

[41] Adelaide Nutting (Nice, France) to Isabel M. Stewart, [New York], May 9, 1926, MAN–IMS Correspondence.

[42] Adelaide Nutting (Paris) to Isabel M. Stewart [New York], June 18, 1926, *ibid.*

Waiting on the dock when the S.S. *Antonia* arrived in Montreal was Lillian Hudson, who had come all the way from her home in Ontario. A few feet away stood Adelaide's nephew Bruce. It was quite late at night and because the customs officers would handle no trunks, only hand luggage, Adelaide and Georgia spent the night aboard ship. The next morning Bruce found rooms for them for the day, and in the afternoon Miss Hudson took them for a drive up the mountain, where there was a "superb" view of Montreal and of "the great sweep of the St. Lawrence with its miles of wharves and grain elevators."[43]

At Waterloo, proofs on the book awaited Adelaide and, as soon as she had a good night's rest, she set herself to reading; soon galleys were strewn all over her bed as well as anything else that "offered lodgement." It was slow, meticulous work and, when she stopped to write her sister that she was once more in Canada and had found Charlie and Lizzie a little more frail, she added that she was truly sorry she had ever embarked on the book. Viewing it with a detached mind, Adelaide thought the papers were dull and repetitious: "It does offer a page of history inasmuch as it deals with the efforts of one earnest young woman to grope her way through conditions that existed at the time. I hope somebody will want to read it or Putnam's will wash their hands thoroughly of me and my doings."[44]

Adelaide's faculty apartment in Emerson Hall had been rented for the school year 1926–27, and she again took a small apartment on the eleventh floor of Butler Hall. It was close to Teachers College, many of her friends lived in the building, and there was an excellent, reasonably priced restaurant on the roof. A few weeks later Minnie and Gilbert, on their return from Newfoundland, would visit her there, but she could not prevail upon them to spend the winter in New York. Arthur Gosling was in the city at the same time, and Adelaide had an opportunity to see her favorite nephew again. She was confident that, if Arthur ever decided to give up his position with the publishing company, he could enter the field of English and become an excellent, perhaps distinguished, teacher and scholar.[45]

By November, 1926, "A Sound Economic Basis for Schools of Nursing" and Other Addresses was off the press. It was a relief to see the twenty-six papers and addresses culled from the large number

[43] Adelaide Nutting (Waterloo) to Isabel M. Stewart (New York), August 20, 1926, *ibid.*
[44] Adelaide Nutting (Waterloo) to Armine N. Gosling (St. John's), August 21, 1926, MAN Papers.
[45] Adelaide Nutting (New York) to Armine N. Gosling (Bermuda), November 6, 1926, *ibid.*

written between 1901 and 1923 in hard covers. Many expensive corrections had been made, and Adelaide wondered what the reviewers
would say and how the book would sell. After the expenses of publication were paid she planned to turn the 10 percent royalties over to
the NLNE. Among the first comments was a reassuring note from
Lavinia Dock. "Dearest Adelaide . . . Your articles sound more excellent than ever, and have a ring of truth and conviction which make
me wish everyone with money to give to colleges would read them. I
wish everyone could know that they are simply the expression of your
daily life thoughts."[46] Dr. Haven Emerson of the College of Physicians
and Surgeons wrote: "How like you is your book, so simple and pre-
cise. The pages reflect and glow with your enthusiasm and inspiration.
Long may the thoughts and hopes you express cheer and illumine you
and your friends."[47] Dr. Rufus Cole of the Hospital, Rockefeller Institute for Medical Research, wrote: "To read those moving addresses
brings vividly before me the realization of all you have tried to do for
the better education of the nurse. I am sure that your efforts which
have already produced such great results will continue to exert a profound effect for many years to come. This must be a great satisfaction
to you as it is to all your friends."[48] Putnam's was. pleased with the
volume and asked Miss Nutting to write another book, on any subject
she might choose.[49]

Soon after this, J. B. Lippincott asked Adelaide to prepare a textbook on nursing ethics. Adelaide felt committed to Macmillan and the
work on Florence Nightingale. Some time later she penciled notes for
a reply on the back of the Lippincott letter, regretting the delay and
her absence and saying that the subject was far too complex and that
she did not feel competent.[50]

The Nightingale book really interested Adelaide. Ever since her
Hopkins days, when she acquired her first copy of Florence Nightingale's *Notes on Nursing*, she had been an avid collector of books,
essays, and articles by and about Miss Nightingale. She had engaged
the services of Francis Edwards, a rare-books dealer in London, to
assist her in procuring personal letters, manuscripts, and special

[46] Lavinia Dock [Fayetteville, Pa.] to Adelaide Nutting (New York), [1926],
ibid.
[47] Haven Emerson (New York) to Adelaide Nutting (New York), November 8,
1926, *ibid.*
[48] Rufus Cole (New York) to Adelaide Nutting (New York), November 11,
1926, *ibid.*
[49] Adelaide Nutting (New York) to Armine N. Gosling (Bermuda), November
6, 1926, *ibid.*
[50] E. W. Bacon (Philadelphia) to Adelaide Nutting, [New York], December 3,
1926, *ibid.*

items. By the time of her retirement, Adelaide's collection was the second largest and most comprehensive collection of Nightingaliana in existence. A book on Florence Nightingale offered her a special way of putting her treasures to work and of sharing them with others. Having been instrumental in founding the Florence Nightingale memorial, Adelaide with characteristic generosity planned that royalties from the book would be her gift to the fund.[51] It might take several years to prepare the work she had in mind. Happily there were no deadlines, and she was free to take time out for other projects such as the Hopkins Endowment Fund or to travel. It was pleasant to lunch leisurely with friends at the Cosmopolitan Club and go to a matinee, or to have dinner downtown and spend an evening at the opera, without feeling the pressure of classes to meet and lectures to prepare.

Adelaide was serious and enthusiastic about the Nightingale studies, however, and immediately began an article on Miss Nightingale's use of statistics, which appeared in the May, 1927, issue of *The Public Health Nurse* under the title "Florence Nightingale as a Statistician." She hoped to write other articles soon.

As revealed in letters to her sister, Adelaide's social calendar explains some of her difficulties in settling down to work in the fortnight after Armine and Gilbert returned to Bermuda. On October 30 her nephew Arthur had dinner with her, and on November 1 she attended a dinner given for Sir Gilbert Murray by the League of Nations Association. On November 4 a tea was given in her honor by the Department of Nursing of Teachers College, and she spoke informally to a "great big room full of our students, several hundred they said, among them, sixteen Johns Hopkins nurses." The next evening she talked on Tunis to a small group of faculty women known as the Discussion Club. On November 7 she read aloud with Willystine Goodsell for two hours, and the next day she attended a luncheon welcoming Anna Maxwell home again. On November 11 there was a dinner for trustees and faculty to which Dean Russell had sent her a special invitation. On November 12 she went with a friend to hear Raquel Miller, a Spanish entertainer, impersonator, dancer, and singer. The next day she attended a luncheon of the Foreign Policy Association, where again "about 1,200 of quite the most interesting people in the city . . . gather to hear some other people talk about reshaping the League of Nations." At the end of the two-week period she concluded, "I doubt

---

[51] Isabel Maitland Stewart, "Notes relative to Miss Nutting's Projected *Mind of Florence Nightingale*," Florence Nightingale Packet, Department of Nursing Education Archives, Teachers College.

if ever this wild pace can be kept up, for already I am getting tired and sleep abominably, but there is no denying the interest of life in this particular spot on this distracting planet." To keep going at such a rate would necessitate new clothes. "If there is anything I grudge spending money for, it is clothes. Yet I like to look well-dressed."[52]

In her temporary quarters in Butler Hall, Adelaide often thought she should reach a decision relative to her declining years. Armine and Gilbert had discussed the matter with her on their recent visit. Would she not consider coming to Bermuda? The pace was slower there, the winters milder, the skies brighter, the air fresh and clean, and she would be surrounded by loved ones. Perhaps she would come for a long visit and then decide. An unexpected gift from alumnae and friends in early February, 1927, made the journey possible,[53] and on March 19 friends from the Nursing Department gathered at the dock to see her off.

After a long night of deep sleep aboard ship, "the very best in months," Adelaide began a letter to Isabel about some professional matters that had long concerned her—among them, a small conference for the nurses who were trying to direct university schools. Adelaide suggested "the next autumn at a convenient place and under the most favorable conditions." She was confident that Annie Goodrich would want to have the conference at Yale, but she personally favored Teachers College as the "Mother House" of all university schools. She already had "a fairly well-mapped-out program in mind." After retirement Adelaide was careful not to express unsolicited opinions on departmental affairs, but she made it clear she had not abandoned her interest in nursing affairs in general.

Of the visit to Bermuda, Adelaide wrote: "I am under no illusions. . . . just everything that I have no use whatever for, much less today than when younger, will surround me; but my sister and that small boy of Frances will bring happy moments if anything can in this Sahara of a life."[54]

In her next letter she described the Goslings' new home, "Step-A-Side," a very comfortable, quiet, and beautiful place in Paget, as well as their activities, "short walks, some drives, a tea, a luncheon, here and there among old friends—all in this smooth back water of life

[52] Adelaide Nutting (New York) to Armine N. Gosling (Bermuda), November 6, 1926, MAN Papers.
[53] Anna D. Wolf (Chicago) to Adelaide Nutting (New York), February 2, 1927, ibid.
[54] Adelaide Nutting (aboard the Holland-American Line's S.S. Verndam, en route to Bermuda) to Isabel M. Stewart (New York), March 20, 1927, ibid.

where nature is so kind and nothing matters much apparently." She
was quite concerned

> about what the awful tranquility might do for her [sister] because in
> Newfoundland, with her work for suffrage, for education, for protection
> of animals, for sundry other matters of importance, all depending a good
> deal on her constant effort and intellectual guidance, her life had some
> meaning. . . .
> It was a good idea to come down here at this time, for I have satisfied
> myself and also my sister, that this is not the place for me. For the first
> time she sees clearly and she says, "There is really nothing here that
> you want." So I go back to New York shortly . . . with this question at
> least settled and rightly. It will be easier to go ahead with other plans,
> with this old hope well out of the way.[55]

On May 1 Adelaide was back in New York. The S.S. *Avon* docked
early that morning, and the next day she was writing letters and telephoning her friends. Soon she began a rigorous schedule of luncheons
and dinners. On Thursday she went shopping downtown for her
sister. The next day her old friend Dr. Florence Sabin of the Rockefeller Institute came out for lunch, and in the evening Adelaide went
to Mrs. Jenkins' home for dinner. On May 10 there was a dinner at
the Faculty Women's Club, and on May 13 Arthur Gosling called and
Adelaide invited him to the Faculty Men's Club for dinner. Afterward
they played her favorite game, Russian Bank. The next week was even
busier: on Monday Adelaide went to the Cosmopolitan Club for dinner and to the theater with a friend; on Tuesday, at the Faculty
Women's Club, she heard two men speak on China; on Wednesday
she invited Arthur and a young woman he seemed interested in to
join her for lunch at the Cosmopolitan Club; the next night Arthur
took her to dinner at Galico's, and afterward they went to see Ethel
Barrymore in *The Constant Wife*; on Friday she again had tea with
Arthur at the club; and on Saturday an old friend, Kate deLong, came
out for dinner.[56]

It was good to be back in New York. For twenty years Morningside
Heights had been Adelaide Nutting's home. On a bright May morning
shortly after she returned from Bermuda, she wrote a description of
the view from Butler Hall.

> My home is on the Acropolis which lies between the lordly Hudson
> on the west and Morningside Drive on the east, narrowing down to a

[55] Adelaide Nutting (Paget, Bermuda) to Isabel M. Stewart (New York), April
10, 1927, MAN–IMS Correspondence.
[56] Adelaide Nutting (New York) to Armine N. Gosling (Paget), May 5, 15,
1927, MAN Papers.

space between the three domes of the University, the classic one pillars the Library; its intellectual heart and soul, its Book of Revelations; and Earl Hall, busy meeting place, center of life; and the beautiful dome of the sacred fount for spiritual thirst, St. Paul's chapel. Other domes, the exquisite little Roman chapel on Morningside, with the huge unfinished symphony of St. John the Divine looming up behind, and the roofs and domes of St. Luke's Hospital lying in between, and the charming little Morningside Park covering the hillside to the East.

From my wide window on a high floor of the newest and most pretentious apartment house my eyes sweep the Universe apparently . . . a lovely city of clouds and towers lies a far off to the Southeast, the Ritz, the new Savoy, the Metropolitan with its eternal light which glows far into the night. Sometimes I think I see a peep of the still most beautiful of all, the Woolworth. . . .

Other things stand out menacingly against the horizon—four tall huge chimneys pour forth an unending stream of smoke, at times belching. A menace either disregarded or against which helpless.

To fly back to my home, a northern sweep puts me near the tower of the beautiful Russell Hall of Teachers College, and the still more beautiful ones of Union Seminary. Far in the distance loom the stern towers of the new Medical Center of Columbia Presbyterian—great, grim defenses, appropriate enough, for is not their task one endless battle against disease. . . .

The city college, beautiful dream of [architecture]—steps up to the library, fields beyond. The architecture of the University, solid, substantial, conventional; on the whole they must be called unbeautiful but one most lovely and refreshing, the oasis in a desert of uninteresting apartment houses, the Casa Italiana, corner of Amsterdam and 117 St., beautiful in plan and proportions, in material and detail. It is a delight to the eye and I walk around that corner just to look at it and read its inscription.

Apartment houses, curiously sordid . . . food, many dining rooms, like Paris yet, not yet tables on the pavement but the garbage is . . . great cans uncollected at front doors and gates. Attractive little rooms, dining [out] steadily increasing, go from basement, first floor to roof, and one with a little courtyard, gay with red umbrellas, and the beginning of vines, doing a thriving business on 121 Street. . . .

On the whole this hill top expensive but what does man care how fares his body only if his spirit is fed, and the very stuff of life is obviously here.[57]

When she laid down the pen, Adelaide had made her decision. She might take holiday trips to Maine, Canada, Bermuda, or Europe, but she knew she would always return to Morningside Heights.

In the fall of 1927 she moved back to Emerson, to her apartment near the faculty dining room, where for years a special table had been reserved for her. Sometimes she ate alone, but more frequently she was invited to join Dr. and Mrs. Thomas Wood, Dr. and Mrs. Eugene Smith, or Willystine Goodsell, or they came to her table, and the conversation ran the gamut from physical education and mathematics to travel, politics, the newest books, and plays on Broadway. When Dr. and Mrs. Smith returned from abroad, they brought some rare seventeenth- and eighteenth-century documents from French hospitals and gave them to the Adelaide Nutting Historical Nursing Collection, which had been set up at Teachers College by the students and alumnae of the Nursing Education Department on its twentieth anniversary.[58] It was comforting to have friends nearby who enjoyed discussing philosophy, literature, and politics, and, when Adelaide did not have more pressing things to do, she gladly made a fourth at bridge.

Adelaide took pleasure in the social affairs she had never before been able to indulge in to any great extent, but her heart never strayed far from nursing and the projects and reforms she wanted to see initiated. The reorganization of the Hopkins School of Nursing and the establishment of the $1,000,000 endowment were still unattained goals. While Adelaide was abroad, the Training School Committee drafted a reorganization plan which it passed along for the consideration of the Medical Board of the Hospital and recommended to the trustees. The principal feature of this plan was the appointment of a director of the school whose duties were separate from those of the superintendent of nurses. Reluctant to see the school removed any distance from the hospital's nursing services, the Medical Board favored instead an educational director under the superintendent of nurses. The trustees were amenable to the committee's suggestion, but objections arose from the alumnae. At a breakfast for Johns Hopkins alumnae during the 1926 spring meeting of the three national nursing bodies, the ANA, the NLNE, and the NOPHN, Elizabeth Fox (class of 1910) had proposed that a group of alumnae of outstanding ability present a detailed plan for the future development of the training school to the trustees. A committee consisting of Miss Fox, Anna Jammé, Marion Vannier, Anna Wolf, and Effie Taylor was elected. Miss Taylor was chosen chairman and Miss Fox served as secretary.[59] After a twelve-month study of the Training School Committee's plan, the Alumnae Committee was granted the privilege of presenting its case directly to the Board of Trustees.

[58] *The Adelaide Nutting Historical Nursing Collection, Teachers College, Columbia University* (New York: Teachers College, 1929), pp. 3–6.
[59] Amy P. Miller, "A Short History of the Endowment Fund of The Johns Hopkins Nurses Alumnae Association," n.d., MAN Papers.

Adelaide had kept in close touch with Miss Taylor during much of the study, as she had with Miss Gray during her survey four years before. The week before the report was submitted to the trustees, Adelaide was busy with conferences. After the Philharmonic Concert on Sunday, January 15, Carolyn Gray came to Adelaide's apartment for a long talk, and on Monday Miss Nutting met with the consultant group. On Tuesday, Adelaide saw Carolyn Gray again, and on Wednesday she had dinner with Clara Noyes, an influential graduate of 1896 and a member of the original Endowment Committee. On Thursday Miss Nutting had a 9:30 A.M. appointment with Miss Gray, and on Friday the committee met again. At three o'clock on Sunday afternoon, January 22, Adelaide conferred with John M. Glenn, director of the Carnegie Foundation and a member of the Hopkins Board of Trustees. That same evening Anna Wolf came to Adelaide's apartment and was later joined by other members of the committee for their final meeting. Effie Taylor came by on Thursday and went on to Baltimore with Miss Nutting for the trustees' meeting on Friday, January 27.[60]

Succinctly and without reservation the committee reported that "the ambition and hope of the Alumnae" was to see their school become a part of The Johns Hopkins University. To that end the graduates had directed their efforts to secure "an endowment that would place the school on a sound financial basis and enable it to make that connection." Finally, the committee recommended that The Johns Hopkins University be asked again to consider the possibility of affiliating with The Johns Hopkins Hospital School of Nursing on the closest terms the policies of its organization would permit. It asked further "that a committee be appointed immediately to discuss with the University a means of establishing a connection between the School of Nursing and the University."[61]

The trustees listened with sympathy to the alumnae proposals, but the Medical Board of the hospital did not favor university recognition, and the hospital administration held doubts. It was disappointing, but Adelaide was not ready to write off university affiliation of The Johns Hopkins Training School for Nurses as a lost cause.

In the meantime, two other interests held promise of achievement. Adelaide's ambition for a new and distinct nursing periodical was partially fulfilled in January, 1928, by the appearance of the first issue of *The Nursing Education Bulletin*, a semiannual publication by the

[60] Adelaide Nutting, personal calendar, 1922, *ibid.*
[61] Johns and Pfefferkorn, *The Johns Hopkins Hospital School of Nursing*, p. 205.

alumnae, students, and staff of the Department of Nursing Education, Teachers College. Isabel M. Stewart was its editor, and Adelaide was a contributing editor.[62] The bulletin served the purpose of an alumnae organ by setting forth departmental developments, student organizations and activities, notes on graduates, appointments, and deaths, but it performed a larger professional function through its recording of experiments and studies in the field of nursing and its reviews of books and significant articles in other periodicals. In her first editorial, "In Salutation," Miss Nutting wrote hopefully, "The cherished hopes and plans of many years take form and substance in the pages of this *Bulletin*."[63] She predicted a warm welcome for the new publication inasmuch as it sought to bring together the teachers, supervisors, and executives guiding the activities and destinies of the student nurses who were acquiring their education largely in 2,000 hospital training schools. Although the 76,000 student nurses in these schools were the major concern of the magazine, the editors were alert to the "vast and strategic importance of developing and strengthening the equipment of graduate nurses for their several fields of work."[64] Through education, nursing's ultimate goals of improved care for the sick and the protection of health might be reached. The new journal would be "hospitable to new ideas, generous in its encouragement of all study and experiment which holds promise of enlarging our knowledge of our work [and] vigorous and fearless in criticism, particularly of ourselves."[65]

The long-planned-for Conference on Nursing Schools Connected with Colleges and Universities was held at Teachers College from January 21 through January 25, 1928. Miss Nutting presided at the opening session and traced the history of university-connected nursing schools from the beginnings at Teachers College in 1899–1900. The highlights of her talk were the 1903 association between the Chicago Presbyterian School of Nursing and Rush Medical, where science courses for nurses were taught; the opening of the University of Minnesota School of Nursing in 1909 under the direction of the medical school there and the establishment of special degrees for nurses;

---

[62] Miss Nutting's name appeared on the masthead of the first two volumes (four issues) of *The Nursing Education Bulletin*. The new series, begun in 1930, carried only the names of the editor, Isabel Stewart, the assistant editors and associates, the circulation manager, and the treasurer. Issues appeared when ready rather than on specified dates.

[63] M. Adelaide Nutting, "In Salutation," *The Nursing Education Bulletin*, January, 1928, pp. 1–3.

[64] *Ibid.*, p. 2.

[65] *Ibid.*, p. 3.

the opening of other university schools, such as Cincinnati, Indiana, Michigan, Nebraska, Leland Stanford, Northwestern, and Washington, where five-year courses led to a diploma or a degree; Simmons in Boston, which specialized in public health nursing; and the endowed schools, such as Yale and Western Reserve. For years Teachers College had been the solitary outpost for graduate-nurse training courses for advanced work, but by 1928 forty-five courses were offered by schools throughout the country.

The purpose of the conference, Miss Stewart said, was to study the progress of the university school movement, to evaluate the assets and liabilities in this new kind of educational partnership between nursing schools and universities, and to gather advice from all sources, especially from those who had had experience in other forms of professional education. For three rewarding days the conferees discussed the variety of relationships between university schools and colleges, the better training of women for the nursing profession, and the development of leadership within nursing.

In the second issue of *The Nursing Education Bulletin*, Adelaide's editorial touched on the recent conference by pointing out that thirty years earlier Isabel Hampton Robb had urged that special educational qualifications be required of those who would assume the responsible positions of superintendent and teacher in the nursing profession. Mrs. Robb had suggested that training such as that recently established through affiliation with Columbia University could provide some of the needed preparation. Adelaide regarded this first small conference on universities and schools of nursing as a historic one and in her editorial recommended that its *Proceedings* be attentively read as a historical document and placed in the libraries of all nursing schools, associations, and clubhouses.[66]

Another of Adelaide's dreams for nursing was an annual yearbook which would provide statistical information about the profession, its branches, main divisions, and activities, as well as the approximate number of persons engaged in each. Each topic would be accompanied by a brief presentation not only of the present situation and certain current problems but also of changing conditions and progress made. Matters of a controversial nature would be excluded. Roughly, the topics would cover state, national, and international nursing organizations, the Red Cross, the army and navy, periodicals, clubs, registries, private nursing, student hours of duty in various states, legislation, scholarships, pensions, and annuities. In the summer of 1927 Adelaide

[66] M. Adelaide Nutting, "Reflections on the Conference on University Schools," *ibid.*, August, 1928, pp. 1–6.

had discussed the idea of a yearbook with Carrie Hall, president of the NLNE. Miss Hall had expressed an interest and had agreed to take up the matter at the directors' meeting in January.[67]

The Board of Directors of the NLNE approved the idea and authorized the formation of a subcommittee of the Publications Committee to prepare a yearbook. The board requested that Miss Nutting serve as chairman and name her own committee members. The headquarters of the NLNE would provide clerical help. Adelaide began work at once and drafted a tentative table of contents, cited the necessary historical information, census reports, the professional fields, special organizations, registries, and state laws to be included.[68] Despite the enthusiasm with which the directors and the Publications Committee greeted the proposal, however, the necessary funds to carry out the project were not appropriated and the matter was tabled.

Among the projects being partially underwritten by the NLNE was the Committee on the Grading of Nursing Schools, which had been approved by the three national nursing organizations in 1925. A year later the autonomous committee had expanded to include representatives of other organizations "assumed to be interested in the quality and availability of nursing service." When the twenty-one-member committee was deemed ready for organization in 1926, it represented fourteen national organizations, including the three nursing organizations, the American Medical Association, the American College of Surgeons, and the American Public Health Association; of its seven members at large, four were educators. Adelaide was especially interested because the NLNE had been trying ever since her report on nursing education in 1911 to secure the Rockefeller Foundation's interest in a comprehensive study of nursing education. Following World War I the NLNE had doubled its efforts to find ways and means of sorting out good schools from the mediocre and poor among the 2,000 training schools. Far-sighted young women who desired the best training for careers in nursing wanted more data than the mere fact that a school had been approved by state examiners or that its graduates were eligible for Red Cross enrollment.[69]

Representing the American Medical Association, Dr. William Darrach of the College of Physicians and Surgeons was elected chairman of the Committee on Grading, and Mrs. May Ayres Burgess, a

[67] Adelaide Nutting (New York) to Carrie E. Hall (New York), January 14, 1928, MAN Papers.

[68] Blanche Pfefferkorn (New York) to Adelaide Nutting (New York), July 13, 1928, ibid.

[69] Mary M. Roberts, American Nursing: History and Interpretation (New York: Macmillan, 1954), pp. 183–84.

statistician who had assisted in a survey of private-duty nursing in New York State, was asked to direct the study. The five-year program, which ultimately extended over eight years, was more ambitious than any previous plan for classifying nursing schools, for it embraced three projects: a study of supply and demand for nursing services, an analysis of jobs, and the grading of schools.

First of all, it was imperative to know if there was a shortage of nurses and whether the kind of nurse the hospitals wanted was the kind of nurse that the public wanted. Questionnaires were sent to doctors, hospitals, registries, patients, and nurses from the public health field, institutions, and private duty. The first study, *Nurses, Patients, and Pocketbooks*, revealed that there were far more inadequately prepared nurses than could be employed under existing conditions, but that there were too few well-prepared nurses of all types to meet the country's special needs. It also pointed out the faulty distribution of nurses throughout the country and the nurses' need for reasonable hours, adequate income, opportunity for growth, and constructive leadership.[70]

All of the 2,000 nursing schools were invited to participate in the grading studies; 1,458 schools, 74 percent of the schools accredited by state boards, participated in the first grading, and 81 percent took part in the second. Because of the expense, surveying the schools through visitation was rejected in favor of the statistical method, and the items selected were weighted in importance.[71] Each participating school was graded on each item of the questionnaire in relation to all other schools and was sent two copies of the report indicating its comparative standing. The schools were not classified as A, B, C, or first, second, third, and fourth rate, and no list, so greatly desired by vocational and other advisors, was ever published. At first Miss Nutting and Miss Stewart were disappointed that the committee had not set up more arbitrary standards, but the summaries presented later showed how difficult, unfair, and damaging any other system of rating would have been.[72] The rating of most schools improved on the second grading, but, without a classified list, no weight of public opinion could be brought to bear on the schools needing change and reform.

70 May Ayres Burgess, *Nurses, Patients, and Pocketbooks* (New York: Committee on Grading of Nursing Schools, 1928); Roberts, *American Nursing*, pp. 234–35.

71 Roberts, *American Nursing*, p. 186; *ANA Bulletin*, 1932, MAN Papers.

72 May Ayres Burgess (New York) to Adelaide Nutting (New York), November 13, 1926; and May Ayres Burgess [New York] to Elizabeth Burgess (New York), January 3, 1929; MAN Papers.

Some of the committee's critics believed "the continuous release of vivid, well illustrated and informative material through professional and other media, month after month, through the life of the Committee," contributed more to raising the level of nursing education than the carefully detailed reports to the schools.[73] The ANA was spurred to make a study of professionally sponsored registries in search of a clue to ineffective methods of distributing nursing services. Adelaide never believed that the committee brought about all the vast improvement claimed for it, and she thought its philosophy was couched in old platitudes.[74] The committee's basic conclusion that there were too many poorly trained nurses and too few well-educated nurses was not new or startling to her, and, while it may have underscored the need for university schools and better-qualified candidates, it provided no blueprint for implementation. This was particularly discouraging because the profession had provided half of the $300,000 the survey had cost.[75]

Through committee work and an enriched social life, Adelaide had adjusted to retirement. At conventions and in visits from colleagues, nursing friends, and former students, she was made to feel that she was still part of the nursing profession. It pleased her when Florence Johnson wrote that it was the unanimous wish of the Nurses Committee for the annual Nightingale service that she be asked again to lead the procession to the Cathedral Church of St. John the Divine, although she no longer felt strong enough for parades and marching.[76]

Adelaide did not like the thought of growing old and infirm when there was so much still to do. The deaths of her friends Mrs. David Eugene Smith and the Baroness Sophie Mannerheim in January, 1928, of Lady Grace Osler the following August, and of Anna Maxwell in December drove home the fact that time was fleeting. From Bermuda word came that Gilbert's health had failed and that Armine was greatly worried. Lizzie had a stroke in October, and Adelaide went to

[73] Roberts, *American Nursing*, p. 187.

[74] M. Adelaide Nutting, pencil notes on margin of May Ayres Burgess' address, "Quality Nursing," before the American Hospital Association, Detroit, September 15, 1932, MAN Papers.

[75] The four large publications of the Committee were: May Ayres Burgess, *A Five Year Program for the Committee on the Grading of Schools* (New York: Committee on the Grading of Nursing Schools, 1926); May Ayres Burgess, *Nurses, Patients, and Pocketbooks* (1928); Ethel Johns and Blanche Pfefferkorn, *An Activity Analysis of Nursing* (1934); and the final report, *Nursing Schools Today and Tomorrow* (1934).

[76] Florence Johnson (New York) to M. Adelaide Nutting (New York), April 30, 1928, MAN Papers.

Waterloo to comfort Charlie, who seemed a shadow of his former self. His steps faltered, his memory had failed, and Adelaide wondered whether he or Lizzie would be first to go.[77]

Not feeling well herself, Adelaide did not attend the meeting of the International Council of Nurses in Montreal in July, 1929. She had been invited to address the general evening session on July 9 and had met the February 1 deadline, which would allow time for the translation of the papers into the official languages of the congress, English, French, and German, and for the printing of the papers well in advance of the meeting. In inviting her, Lillian Clayton had said, "Negotiations are still under way to determine which organization will have the pleasure of paying your expenses."[78]

As usual, Adelaide was not satisfied with her paper, but she had looked forward to talking with leaders from different parts of the world and to greeting her former students. She was especially happy that Mrs. Fenwick and Margaret Breay would be there because she wanted to discuss with them the Florence Nightingale memorial, which they had helped her launch at the Cologne meeting in 1912. At that time the plan most favored had been a Chair in Nursing Education at the University of London, but the legal obstacles in the university's charter had interfered, and nothing had been done before World War I. Then, because of the war, the council's activities had been almost entirely suspended for ten years.[79] In the meantime, the League of Red Cross Societies had started the International Public Health Nursing Course at Kings College in 1920. Later it had transferred the course to Bedford College for Women, another part of the University of London, where it became a unit separate from the regular college program, but it was doubtful that the League of Red Cross Societies would be able to continue the program indefinitely.[80]

It was very warm in New York the summer of 1929, and Adelaide went to Ogunquit a week early in the hope that she could gain enough strength to go to Montreal for the convention. On July 6, however, she wrote Isabel Stewart that she would not be able to make the trip.[81]

[77] Adelaide Nutting (Waterloo) to Isabel M. Stewart (New York), October 17, 1928, MAN–IMS Correspondence.
[78] Lillian Clayton (New York) to Adelaide Nutting (New York), October 5, 1928, MAN Papers.
[79] Isabel M. Stewart and Anne L. Austin, *A History of Nursing from Ancient to Modern Times: A World View* (New York: G. P. Putnam's Sons, 1926), pp. 472–74.
[80] *Ibid.*
[81] Adelaide Nutting (Ogunquit, Maine) to Isabel Stewart (New York), July 6, 1929, MAN–IMS Correspondence.

She asked that Elizabeth Burgess read the paper, and she also sent
some notes to Nina Gage about the Florence Nightingale memorial,
which was to come up for review. Adelaide believed that the memorial
should involve more than the courses offered under the auspices of
the League of Red Cross Societies at Bedford College. She proposed
instead a Florence Nightingale foundation of such scope as to form an
international center for study and research in nursing and the kindred
problems of hospitals and public health, upon which Miss Nightingale's mind had played with such amazing power and originality. One
of the first acts of such a foundation, she said, would be to secure
quarters in which to house its staff, carry on its work, and assemble
all Miss Nightingale's books, letters, manuscripts, portraits, personal
belongings, and other things intimately associated with her life and
work. Such a center would be "open to be visited by nurses from all
over the world and the thousands of other persons who could thus
catch a glimpse of the nature of her surroundings and envisage in
some measure the vast range of her thought and labor." Although
Adelaide hoped Miss Nightingale's home might be available, she did
not conceive of it so much as a shrine as a living, working memorial.
There was much yet to be written about Miss Nightingale's own
work, and Adelaide hoped that in establishing such a foundation the
International Council of Nurses would provide fellowships for students of unusual promise and for the writing and publication of
studies, reports, and monographs. Adelaide envisaged a permanently
endowed trust fund under the direction of trustees representing men
and women of great eminence from different countries and including,
if possible, a member of Miss Nightingale's family.[82]

Isabel Stewart sent Adelaide daily letters about the convention that
7,000 people were attending. She reported who had asked about her
and how her paper and the Education Committee report had been received. She described the Teachers College Alumnae dinner and the
joint luncheon of the History of Nursing societies of McGill University and Teachers College. The societies had voted to offer $100 for
the best contribution to nursing history written between 1929 and the
interim meeting of the International Council of Nurses in 1931; it was
to be known as the Adelaide Nutting–Lavinia Dock prize. The Nightingale memorial had been discussed, but no positive action had been

[82] Adelaide Nutting (Ogunquit) to Nina C. Gage (Montreal), July 3, 1929,
quoted in H. R. Hamley and Muriel Uprichard, *A Study of the Florence Nightingale International Foundation* (London: Grand Council of the International
Council of Nurses, 1948), p. 31.

taken except to invite further consideration.[83] At Ogunquit, Adelaide regretted her absence. She wrote Isabel Stewart: "It is simply awful to have petered out so completely mentally and physically. I shall never cease to hang my head over that paper."[84] A letter from Annie Goodrich describing the paper as "splendid" cheered Adelaide, and even she began to think better of it.[85]

The early months of 1930 found Miss Nutting in better health and spirits than she had been for some time. She decided to go to England to take up the matter of the Florence Nightingale memorial with nursing leaders there and to investigate the Bedford course and help decide if it should be taken over by the Florence Nightingale International Foundation. She wrote Isabel Stewart, who was then on a world tour and currently in India sightseeing and visiting former Teachers College nursing students, that she planned to go abroad the first moment it seemed feasible. Between visits to the doctor, she explained,

> the months have been crowded—and so they have, packed first with music more than I have heard for many years—a feast—a banquet, indeed, with the Philharmonic, the Boston Symphony and now recently and unexpectedly—the Philadelphia Orchestra—Florence Sabin who is really a musician (as was Miss Dock and still is) a devotee of the latter. Then we have had some good Foreign Policy luncheons. . . .
>
> And besides these great events there have been some lesser ones—a pleasant luncheon at the [Cosmopolitan] Club downtown to meet Grace Abbott. . . .
>
> At another luncheon, a larger one, I met Frances Perkins, the State Commissioner of Industry. She spoke extremely well, and has grown steadily since I used to see her years ago. She says she will come up here to speak at our Women's Faculty Club later on if we want her, and I am going to try to stir them up to arranging a dinner for her.

Adelaide had also been to a play and to dinner with Katharine Fisher, who had left Teachers College to become an editor on the staff of *Good Housekeeping*.[86]

Preparatory to going abroad, Adelaide began to resign from com-

[83] Isabel M. Stewart (Montreal) to Adelaide Nutting (Ogunquit), July 5, 11, 1929; Isabel M. Stewart (New York) to Adelaide Nutting (Ogunquit), July 14, 1929; Isabel M. Stewart (West Cornwall, Conn.) to Adelaide Nutting (Ogunquit), [August 3, 1929]; and Isabel M. Stewart (Ossining, N.Y.) to Adelaide Nutting (Waterloo), August 25, 1929; MAN–IMS Correspondence.

[84] Adelaide Nutting (Ogunquit) to Isabel Stewart (New York), July 17, 1929, *ibid.*

[85] Adelaide Nutting (Ogunquit) to Isabel Stewart, [Ossining], August 9, 1929, *ibid.*

[86] Adelaide Nutting (New York) to Isabel Stewart, [in the Far East], February 2, 1930, *ibid.*

mittees and organizations. She sent Major Julia Stimson, superintendent of the Army Nurse Corps, her resignation from the Committee on
the Use of Library Facilities, and she resigned her membership in the
American Social Science Association, which had conferred a liberty
medal on her in 1918. Henceforth she would devote her energies to
nursing projects and the book on Florence Nightingale. She then
booked passage to England on the S.S. *Minnewaska*, which would
sail from New York on June 7.

April 8 was Dr. William Welch's eightieth birthday, and he was
being feted as he had been on his sixtieth and seventieth birthdays.
Physicians, former students, and friends in various cities were gather-
ing to pay him tribute. Adelaide went to Washington to join Georgia
Nevins at a dinner where 1,600 persons were honoring Dr. Welch.
The principal speaker for the occasion was President Herbert
Hoover.[87] Clara Noyes, one of Adelaide's former students and now
director of the American Red Cross Nursing Service, met her at the
train. She drove her out to see the cherry blossoms and then on to
Georgia's apartment, which was quite near the Daughters of the
American Revolution Building, where the dinner was to be held.[88]
Dr. Welch had retained that zest for life which had always endeared
him to colleagues, students, patients, and friends. For Adelaide it was
a nostalgic occasion. Her thoughts raced back to the days when the
Big Four—Welch, Kelley, Halsted, and Osler—were just starting their
careers at Hopkins and Isabel Hampton was superintendent of nurses.
Dr. Welch had always prided himself on his loyalty to the nursing
profession. As a pathologist and a believer in preventive medicine, he
appreciated the teaching role of the nurse in public health and he
agreed with Miss Nutting that the preparation of all nurses should be
strengthened. He never specified just how this should be done, but he
called nursing "a great profession" and in his inimitable way inspired
nurses to want to make it worthy of that accolade.[89]

On Adelaide's return to New York, word came that Charlie was
not well. On April 30 she canceled her passage to Europe and went to
Waterloo. By May 22, Charlie seemed better and Adelaide returned to
New York, but an hour or two after she arrived a telegram came say-

[87] "Souvenir Program, Dinner Honoring William Henry Welch on his Eightieth Birthday, Centennial Hall, Washington, D.C."; and clipping from the *Baltimore Sun*, May 1, 1934; MAN Papers.

[88] Clara Noyes (Washington, D.C.) to Adelaide Nutting (New York), April 1,
1930, *ibid.*

[89] Adelaide Nutting, "Pencilled Notes on H. W. Welch, Perhaps for a Tribute
in *The Johns Hopkins Nurses Alumnae Magazine*," n.d., *ibid.*

ing Charlie had died during the night. Prostrated with shock and grief, she was too weak to return to Waterloo for the funeral.[90]

In Bermuda, Gilbert Gosling's condition was steadily worsening. Adelaide wanted to be with her sister, but wrote: "I am too low in spirits, too insecure in the control of my emotions, too tearful over things, and altogether worthless to be a good companion. . . . I would but add to your burdens."[91]

Charlie's death was a hard blow. He was the oldest brother. When in need of funds for travel and study, Adelaide had always been able to borrow from him. In recent years he seemed to have grown strangely fond of her and turned to her in moments of trouble. "His last letters . . . had a kind of pathos about them that often brought tears."[92] Charles Nutting had been an upright citizen and he had sustained his family in time of need. Surely he deserved a memorial that would perpetuate his generous and kindly deeds. With only her pension and a small income from royalties and a few securities, Adelaide did not have a large sum at her command. She wrote to the dean of the Law School, McGill University, inquiring about the possibility of setting up a $1,000 scholarship fund in honor of her deceased brother, a law graduate of the class of 1872. After some correspondence it was decided that a prize of $50 or $60 would be offered annually to the law student writing the best essay on some phase of Canadian history or jurisprudence.[93] Adelaide then wrote Lizzie, "I have seldom done anything in my life which has given me so much pleasure as this gift in honor of my beloved brother."[94]

In October, Gilbert Gosling suffered another heart attack, and Arthur was called home. In November, just after Adelaide had gotten new tenants settled in her sleeping rooms and was preparing to go to Minnie's, a telegram arrived with the news that Gilbert had died on November 5. In less than a week Adelaide was on her way to Bermuda. She hoped that she would be of some comfort to Minnie and could persuade her to return to New York for Christmas and the rest

[90] Adelaide Nutting (New York) to Armine N. Gosling (Bermuda), June 5, 1930, ibid.

[91] Ibid.

[92] Adelaide Nutting (East Gloucester) to Armine N. Gosling (Bermuda), July 29, 1930, ibid.

[93] Adelaide Nutting (East Gloucester) to Prof. P. E. Corbett (Montreal), July 31, 1930; P. E. Corbett (Montreal) to Adelaide Nutting (New York), October 14, 1930; and to Adelaide Nutting (New York), receipt, McGill University, acknowledging check for $1,000 from Miss Nutting for prize in the Faculty of Law, October 20, 1930; ibid.

[94] Adelaide Nutting (New York) to Lizzie N. Nutting (Waterloo), October 25, 1930, ibid.

of the winter. Perhaps later on they might take a Mediterranean cruise and fulfill their dream of visiting Greece.[95]

Minnie was deeply broken up over Gilbert's death. They had been married nearly forty-three years, and in retrospect every hour together had been happy. Before the children and friends, she held up extraordinarily well, appearing strong and calm, but the minute she and Adelaide were alone she burst into tears. Many, many letters and messages of sympathy arrived from Newfoundland, Canada, and England. Gradually Adelaide was able to get her sister's thoughts off her grief a little at a time.[96] Armine seemed grateful to have her sister there; Adelaide's reassuring presence had always been a part of her life.

Armine returned to New York with Adelaide, but she stayed only a short time. She was worried about leaving Arthur alone, and financial matters had to be looked into. Gilbert's long illness had cost dearly, and their savings and investments had suffered heavy losses. Minnie felt she should go back to Bermuda and salvage something for her declining years.[97]

Before a year had passed, death came again to the Nutting family. On September 25, Charlie's widow died. Lizzie had long been deaf, and much of her life she had not been well, but she had managed to look after Charlie in his last illness and had tried to put his troubled mind at ease. After her funeral, Joseph Gingras, Charlie's law partner, wrote Adelaide that she and Armine were the principal beneficiaries of the will.[98] Adelaide had protested when Lizzie told her that she was remembering her in her will, asking instead that the money be given to more needy members of the family.[99] Lizzie had not made the change, and Adelaide now decided that her sister should have the money.[100]

Although Adelaide had been retired for almost seven years, she was not forgotten by the alumnae who had sat in her classes. To them she was still a great inspiration. In New York they made it a point to

[95] Adelaide Nutting (Paget, Bermuda) to Isabel Stewart (New York), November 14, 1930, MAN–IMS Correspondence.

[96] Adelaide Nutting (Paget) to Isabel Stewart (New York), November 21, 1930, ibid.

[97] Armine N. Gosling (Paget) to Adelaide Nutting (New York), [January 11, 1931], MAN Papers.

[98] Adelaide Nutting (New York) to Joseph Gingras (Waterloo), January 12, 1932, ibid.

[99] Adelaide Nutting (New York) to Lizzie Haskell Nutting, [Waterloo], October 25, 1930, ibid.

[100] Joseph Gingras (Waterloo) to Adelaide Nutting (New York), September 10, 1933, ibid.

see her, and, upon returning home, wrote her how much they had received from talking things over. She spurred them to go forward, not to give up, and always to keep in mind the sacredness of their calling. At Christmas, Easter, and on her birthday there were cards, letters, and presents. In her apartment were many gifts from former students—a large brass tray from Etha Klosz in India, and baskets, vases, and books from others. "Our daughters, never forget," she often said to Isabel.

When Adelaide retired, the alumnae had honored her with a gift of money, but her associates had long wanted to show in some special way their recognition of her contribution to Teachers College. When a portrait was suggested, Miss Nutting's friend Dr. David Eugene Smith voiced "vehement opposition," declaring that portrait painting was a lost art; he proposed a library fund and a good photograph. About this time Adelaide spent a weekend with friends in West Cornwall, Connecticut.[101] Stanislav Rembski, a Polish artist, and his wife also were guests, and it proved to be a delightful holiday for everyone. The artist was greatly impressed by Miss Nutting's knowledge of European art and culture, her depth of feeling, human understanding, vision, poise, and serenity. As they talked he had the desire to paint this seventy-four-year-old woman in a mood of contemplation, of evaluating her life's work. He wanted to capture on canvas "that quality most characteristic and expressive of her—an empathy with all humanity which moved her so profoundly."[102] When reproductions of some of Mr. Rembski's portraits were shown to Dr. Smith, he reversed his position and assumed chairmanship of the portrait committee, insisting that Rembski be given the commission.

The portrait was painted in Miss Nutting's apartment. On the wall was a reproduction of a portrait by Andrea del Sarto, a favorite of Miss Nutting and Mr. Rembski, and he immediately decided to introduce it in the background in token of her love for classical art. At first Adelaide wanted to be painted in a simple dark dress rather than in academic robes. "I do not do my work in an academic gown," she smiled, saying further that her degree was honorary. Before starting the second sitting, however, she told Mr. Rembski that the committee was adamant about the academic costume and that she would support the artist in his decision. He assured her that he would not let the

[101] Abby Porter Leland, principal of P.S. 157, Manhattan, and Elizabeth Burgess, Department of Nursing Education, Teachers College, friends of Stanislav Rembski, introduced him to Miss Nutting.
[102] Stanislav Rembski (Baltimore) to Helen E. Marshall (Normal, Ill.), February 25, 1966, Marshall Papers.

gown overshadow or distort her character, and she agreed to put on the gown and hood. He refused to put the stiff mortarboard on her head, as was customary in women's academic portraits, and suggested a pearl necklace as a feminine touch, underscoring the fact that only a woman could have accomplished the mission that Miss Nutting had set for herself.[103]

The portrait, the first of a woman to hang on the walls of Teachers College, was presented on February 10, 1932.[104] The brief ceremony was attended by the trustees, friends, and colleagues. Adelaide, ill with a cold, was confined to her apartment. Dr. David Eugene Smith, his faith in the art of portrait painting restored, remarked:

> Adelaide Nutting arrived at the doors of the University with her four talents of the spirit, a great idea, high and inspiring ideals, successful experience, personality and culture—broad culture such as her colleague, Sir William Osler, possessed, the love of books and the appreciation of the value of history and poetry and modern science.[105]

She "transmuted the apprentice into a student and paved the way for the broader training of the nurse." Dean Russell spoke of Adelaide's personality, forceful professional acumen, and the inspiration of her example as a path-breaker and pioneer in the new field of education. President Butler said that it had been Miss Nutting's function to make a new integration of materials lying about in scattered units—medicine, natural science, social service—and to bind them together with that real human insight which characterized her and gave her a unique prestige on Morningside Heights.[106] In accepting the portrait for the trustees, Cleveland Dodge commented, "When we think of her influence passing from her to her students and of those students influencing and training others, it is impossible for us to measure the worth of the fruit of this woman's life."[107]

As soon as the presentation was over, Isabel Stewart hurried to Adelaide's apartment to tell her how beautifully it had been done; when the remarks were typed, she would bring a transcript. Among Miss Nutting's papers were found penciled notes she had jotted down to use in letters to those who had spoken. To David Eugene Smith she wrote:

[103] *Ibid.*
[104] Clippings from *New York Times*, January 3 and February 17, 1932, MAN Papers.
[105] Isabel M. Stewart, "Teachers College Receives Portrait of Adelaide Nutting," *Teachers College Record*, March, 1932, pp. 481–82.
[106] *Ibid.*
[107] Isabel M. Stewart, "Memorandum on Presentation of Portrait of A. Nutting to Trustees, Teachers College, February 10, 1932," MAN Papers.

How to find words to tell you how great is my gratitude for your friendship which has been such a sustaining thing during the past few years, for the all too generous words you found yourself able to say for the work I tried to do.

If I could write an Ode to Friendship like Christopher Smart's glorious ode before me, it might partly speak my appreciation. But friendship and gratitude are timeless things. They do not fade, they grow and strengthen.[108]

To President Butler she expressed "immeasurable gratitude for the distinction of his dignity, presence and his words to the occasion."

In a sense that portrait does not seem to me to portray a person except for a brief moment she was given a chance to represent a work—the door was opened in the University. . . . Your presence and your recognition of nursing as a part of medicine and hygiene is an encouragement to the body of women I represent.[109]

[108] Adelaide Nutting, "Notes for Letter to Eugene Smith Following His Presentation of the Portrait," [February, 1932], *ibid.*

[109] Adelaide Nutting, "Notes for Letter to Nicholas Murray Butler, President, Columbia University," [February, 1932], *ibid.*

XXII

Nursing's Elder Stateswoman, 1932–1948

By 1932, economic depression had settled over America like a heavy pall. Evidence of the blight could be seen everywhere. Thousands of small shops and factories had been forced to close; sixteen million of the forty-eight million employables in the United States were idle; and bread lines leading to soup kitchens formed along the sidewalks, often blocking entrance to the small stores that managed to stay open for business. On the haggard faces of men, women, and children were the marks of hunger, disillusionment, and despair; on their bodies were disease and the worn and soiled garments of poverty. On winter days, rags and papers were often bound about their feet. New York City was especially hard hit. Thousands were homeless. Rents went unpaid, and either the tenants were evicted or the heat was shut off. Unsuccessful at begging, many turned to larceny.

All her life Miss Nutting had tried to alleviate the suffering of others, but now her strength, as well as her means, was limited. When she learned that homeless, jobless men were shivering in makeshift packing-box shacks on the hillside between Riverside Drive and the New York Central tracks along the Hudson below, almost in the shadow of the great Riverside Church, however, she took action. She called Clyde Miller and asked him if he would do a favor for her and take some blankets to the men in "Hooverville," as the shantytown was called. He agreed. Adelaide had collected enough blankets to fill a taxi. She was unable to assist in the distribution, but she insisted on paying the taxi fare. Years later Mr. Miller commented:

> It gave her personal satisfaction to relieve suffering. She said she could sleep better if she knew these blankets were keeping others warm. The act of simple charity and kindness . . . was not in her case a gesture to get the victims of the Great Depression out of her thoughts and off

her conscience. She knew that changes must come in economics, and politics, and public education to prevent the vast suffering which accompanied needless and recurring depression.[1]

Thousands who were ill could not afford hospitalization. Reports from Adelaide's former students revealed that many hospitals with training schools had lost so much income that they had been forced to close. Nurses who had depended on private duty prior to World War I received few calls; registries bulged with the names of unemployed nurses. Dr. May Ayres Burgess told a reporter for the *New York Sun* that since November, 1931, 500 nurses had applied to the Emergency Work Bureau. Sixty-eight percent were in absolute need, while 19 percent had enough money to last one or two weeks. Dr. Burgess attributed the large number of unemployed nurses to an overproduction of graduate nurses, citing that in the 1920s the total population of the United States had increased only 7 percent while the increase in graduate nurses had been 78 percent.[2] Fifteen hospitals in New York were compelled to close because of lack of funds.[3]

What did this mean for nursing as a profession, Miss Nutting asked. She had been deeply concerned about unemployment in other fields. Her files contained notes on labor surveys and clippings and penciled notes on unemployment. "What values could be salvaged out of this economic chaos?" On August 31, 1931, she wrote to Janet M. Geister, director at the headquarters of the ANA. Relating the gravity of the problem of overproduction and unemployment, she implored that something be done quickly to restrict the number of student nurses and to bolster the employment of graduate nurses. "If I interpret aright the function of our national nursing association it lies in just such efforts to protect and safeguard the well-being of our members. That would appear to be among their most important, essential and indeed inescapable duties."[4]

At the ANA's Board of Directors meeting in September, headquarters was instructed to outline suggestions to be made to registries, with special emphasis on the study of vocational trends and methods, in an attempt to help ease the anticipated unemployment situation

[1] Clyde R. Miller (New York) to Isabel M. Stewart (New York), May 8, 1958, IMS Papers.

[2] Clipping from the *New York Sun*, February 4, 1932, MAN Papers.

[3] Marie Rose (New York) to Adelaide Nutting (New York), February 9, 1932, *ibid.*

[4] Adelaide Nutting (New York) to Janet Geister (New York), August 31, 1931, *ibid.*

during the coming winter.[5] At the convention of the three nursing organizations held in New York in October, Miss Nutting spoke of the imperative need to decrease the number of nursing students and cited the weaknesses of the present system. Currently hospitals were employing graduate nurses for administrative positions, not for the bedside care for which they had been prepared.

In January, 1932, Elizabeth Burgess, president of the NLNE, pointed out to the joint boards of the ANA, the NLNE, and the NOPHN that, psychologically, this was the time to make public the range and extent of unemployment. She stressed the fact that it was an educational problem as well as an economic problem, and that a letter should be sent to hospital boards, superintendents of hospitals, and directors of nursing schools. A committee from the three organizations then drew up a form letter, which they sent to the 6,116 hospital directors listed by the American Medical Association, and a news release, which was sent simultaneously to 1,000 newspapers. The letter appealed for effective action: thousands of nurses were unemployed; there were too many nursing schools and too many nurses. The Duke Foundation had reported in 1931 that small hospitals could operate more economically without a nursing school. The program outlined by the ANA recommended that hospitals select nursing school candidates more carefully because the practice of carrying large numbers of probationary students and dropping 25–50 percent of them was costly; that non-training duties presently performed by student nurses be performed by hired orderlies; that tuition be required of all student nurses and that their allowances be abolished; and finally that the hiring of graduate nurses would lend stability to hospitals.

The letters to hospital directors and the news releases (which contained a bibliography for those wishing to study the situation) were sent out on July 2.[6] By September 2, responses had been sent in by 115 hospital directors in 32 states, 80 of which were from accredited institutions. These replies, Miss Nutting noted, amounted to less than 5 percent of the number of letters sent.

The ANA Bulletin, a monthly publication which had been sent out in cooperation with the Grading Committee since 1930, observed on April 1, 1933, that the picture of the nursing school situation appeared "happier" than it had been at the time of the committee's report in 1928, but this statement was open to question. The number of ac-

---

[5] Rough draft, "ANA Special Letter to Presidents of Hospital Boards, Superintendents of Hospitals, and Directors of Nursing Schools," ibid.
[6] Ibid.

credited nursing schools had decreased by 104, but the number of students had increased by 5,519.[7]

The Federal Emergency Relief Administration (FERA) provided some unemployment benefits for nurses,[8] but the National Recovery Act took no cognizance of their needs. The ANA seized the opportunity afforded under the FERA to launch an all-out campaign for the eight-hour day for nurses employed on a daily basis and a forty-hour week for those working on a weekly or monthly schedule. The New Deal's provision for leisure was meaningless for nurses on twelve-hour duty.

Although Miss Nutting was not well enough to take an active part in the programs undertaken by the national organizations to safeguard nurses and nursing in the dark days of the depression, she tried to keep up with what was taking place through Isabel Stewart and Effie Taylor, who had been elected president of the NLNE in 1932 and was deeply concerned about the overstocked profession and the exploitation of students committed in the name of education.[9] Adelaide also talked frequently with Lillian Wald by telephone. Three hundred thousand families were on relief in New York City in October, 1934. The Henry Street Settlement had expanded into twenty-one nursing centers, twelve of which were located in Manhattan, seven in The Bronx, and two in Queens. Trained nurses on the staff numbered 265. They answered 550,000 calls, 300,000 of which could not be paid for. Mayor Fiorello La Guardia headed an appeal for $550,000 to help the settlement care for 100,000 patients during the winter of 1934.[10] It distressed Adelaide that she had to content herself with contributing "a mite" here and there and with trying to keep up the morale of her young friends, but a former Teachers College student wrote: "My dear Miss Nutting, Seeing you Wednesday was a delightful interim in the trend of daily life. Having recharged my batteries I now feel ready to meet all problems of the next four months."[11]

Despite her unusual ability to inspire others to greater deeds, there were times when Adelaide felt insecure and unworthy. She believed she had been overrated by her friends in the profession, and she grieved that she had not accomplished more. Among her papers were

[7] Copy of the ANA Bulletin, April 1, 1933, ibid.
[8] Mary M. Roberts, American Nursing: History and Interpretation (New York: Macmillan, 1954), p. 228.
[9] Effie J. Taylor (Dean, Yale School of Nursing, New Haven, Conn.), Circular letter to Deans of University Schools of Nursing; and Effie Taylor (New Haven) to Adelaide Nutting (New York), March 5, 1935; MAN Papers.
[10] Clipping from the New York Times, October 10, 1934, ibid.
[11] May Esenwein (Meriden, Conn.) to Adelaide Nutting (New York), ibid.

numerous memoranda relating to "Lost Causes prior to 1925," the year of her retirement, and "Lost Causes since 1925." They were, she wrote, "a rough summary of a number of attempts to do certain things which were either initiated by me or undertaken supposedly with my approval." She listed the failure to secure an endowment for The Johns Hopkins Hospital School of Nursing in 1914, a permanent connection between Teachers College and the Presbyterian Hospital School of Nursing in 1916–17, or a school of nursing under the auspices of Columbia University and Presbyterian Hospital. Adelaide opposed the Committee on the Grading of Schools of Nursing as she had from its beginning in 1926, insisting that "the results of the study are of little consequence, the cost of the seven years labor has been enormous, and the expense of the meetings has been little short of a disgrace, to those in charge of a responsible piece of professional investigation and reform."

Another lost cause was Miss Nutting's proposal in 1927 to use the money given to her by students and friends upon her retirement to publish a small quarterly or semiannual nursing education magazine wholly devoted to educational advances. Nursing leaders had agreed that such a publication was undoubtedly needed, but argued that it would be a very difficult venture. "It was clear no cooperation could be looked for," and the idea was reluctantly abandoned.

In 1928 Adelaide had proposed that the NLNE issue a yearbook. The idea was approved by some, and Nina Gage, executive secretary of the NLNE, gathered together a vast amount of material. The project was overshadowed by the Grading Committee, however, and was postponed for two years; by then it was too late for Miss Nutting to go ahead with the work. She had envisaged it as a mirror held before the world at large as well as before nurses, a device for quickly disseminating new information, for alerting the profession to its goals and purposes and pointing the way to their attainment, and for keeping before nurses their divine commission to heal the sick.[12]

At about the same time, Adelaide had proposed that the Isabel Hampton Robb Memorial Fund be used to provide one or two large loans to students, but she was outvoted; instead, scholarships of $50 to $100 were made available. She was also unsuccessful in getting the American Nursing Association to support a new kind of registry and a group insurance plan.

[12] *Facts About Nursing* has been published annually since 1935 by the ANA; by mid-century it had become an answer to Miss Nutting's appeal for a nursing yearbook.

Under the dateline "1932" Miss Nutting listed two lost causes: one, her unsuccessful efforts to sustain a nursing colleague who had been asked to resign her position as head of a collegiate nursing school because her forthright stand on hours and curriculum had antagonized some of the trustees; and the other, her inability to convince the NLNE of the value of the yearly publication of a calendar featuring photographs, brief biographies of twelve prominent nursing leaders, and appropriate inspirational quotations on nursing.[13]

Biography had always been a source of inspiration to Adelaide, and another of her "lost causes" was a biography of Isabel Hampton Robb. Ever since Isabel's death in 1910 Adelaide had wanted to write Isabel's life story so that future generations of nurses might know of her work for the profession. Through the years she had collected materials on Isabel. She first suggested the biography to The Johns Hopkins Nurses Alumnae in 1928. She had even drafted a rough outline for the book, but the proposal did not meet with the enthusiastic response she desired. Lavinia Dock, who had loved and worked with Isabel, questioned the feasibility of the project, and, when Adelaide revived the idea in 1933, Miss Lawler agreed with Lavinia, who tried gently to dissuade Adelaide.[14] Later, Lavinia would bring up the argument of expense and eventually take a firm stand against having a part in the preparation of the book.[15] Years before, when a similar difference of opinion had arisen, Adelaide had laid down the rules of their friendship, and now nothing that Lavinia said could alter Adelaide's belief that the biography should be written. In 1939, The Johns Hopkins Hospital would celebrate its fiftieth anniversary, a propitious time, Adelaide thought, to bring out a biography of the school's first principal. She wrote a letter to Miss Lawler, asking that it be read at the annual meeting and saying it was highly desirable that the biography of Mrs. Robb be written, and that it was no longer wise to wait, hoping that someone from the alumnae would "arise to assume the task of writing her history. You know how gladly I would have undertaken it had it not been clearly beyond my powers." Adelaide thought it should be written by a trained historian and financed by The Johns Hopkins Nurses Alumnae Association; she

---

[13] Adelaide Nutting, "Lost Causes" (a folder of clippings, letters, and notes in Miss Nutting's handwriting), MAN Papers.

[14] Lavinia Dock (Fayetteville, Pa.) to Adelaide Nutting (New York), December 27, [1933 or 1934], ibid.

[15] Lavinia Dock (Fayetteville) to Adelaide Nutting (New York), June 19, 1938, ibid.

had in mind a woman who had been working for the Carnegie Endowment for International Peace.[16]

The alumnae present at the annual meeting received Miss Nutting's suggestion with enthusiasm and appointed a committee to explore and consider the possibilities of financing the project. Mary Cloud Bean, class of 1895, was chairman. On February 26, 1938, she wired Miss Nutting that the Alumnae Association had endorsed the Robb biography and had authorized the committee to proceed.[17] Dr. Edith Ware, a competent and capable historian, was employed and set to work at once in the hope that the book might be finished in time for the fiftieth anniversary. Meanwhile, the search for funds to underwrite Miss Ware's research and publication continued. In her enthusiasm, Adelaide suggested that, as soon as the Historical Committee finished the biography of Isabel Robb, the biography of Lavinia Dock should be written. "No one in nursing," she wrote, "has given more in certain ways than she. Her influence . . . has been very strong and good. In her judgment about people, [however] she goes astray."[18]

Later, Adelaide cautioned the Historical Committee to overlook Miss Lawler's indifference and Miss Dock's opposition.[19] On July 31, 1939, she wrote Isabel Stewart that Miss Ware was at Briarcliff Manor working on the biography of Mrs. Robb. "I know I am disappointing her but that cannot be helped I fear. There are just two words that keep ringing in my ears. 'Too late, too late.' "[20]

The preparation of Mrs. Robb's biography involved more time, labor, and expense than the Hopkins alumnae committee anticipated. Certainly it would not be completed in time for the fiftieth anniversary of the opening of the hospital and school, but for a few months Miss Nutting, Miss Bean, and the committee were hopeful that funds would be forthcoming and that the book would be completed by the fiftieth anniversary of the first graduating class. When it became clear that funds were not forthcoming to complete the task, Miss Ware turned over her notes, so painstakingly gathered, to The Johns Hopkins Nurses Library, in the hope that some future historian might use

[16] Adelaide Nutting (New York) to Elsie Lawler (Baltimore), May 28, 1937, ibid.

[17] Mary Cloud Bean (Baltimore) to Adelaide Nutting (New York), February 26, 1938, ibid.

[18] Adelaide Nutting (New York) to Mary Cloud Bean (Baltimore), January 9, 1938, ibid.

[19] Adelaide Nutting (New York) to Mary Cloud Bean (Baltimore), June 15, 1939, ibid.

[20] Adelaide Nutting (New York) to Isabel Stewart (New York), July 31, 1939, ibid.

them and accord to Isabel Hampton Robb the place she deserved in the history of nursing education.[21]

It annoyed Adelaide that age and its infirmities deprived her of seeing friends. By the spring of 1934 Miss Nutting was no longer able to attend conventions or banquets, but she enjoyed sending greetings. Often they were historical and inspirational, and they never failed to take into account the contributions of colleagues and other leaders in nursing such as Isabel Robb, Lillian Wald, and Annie Goodrich. On the fortieth anniversary of nursing education at Teachers College, she noted that not one of them had started out with the intention of becoming a leader. "There was before each of them a new, difficult and profoundly important task, calling for their highest energies and these they gave in full measure. I doubt if there is anyone whom we should fear more than that person, man or woman, who is determined to be a leader."[22] With genuine regret Adelaide wrote the secretary of the Cosmopolitan Club on March 13, 1934, that the time had come when her withdrawal from membership could no longer be deferred.[23] The secretary asked her to change her mind before the request was passed on to the Board of Governors, Adelaide's answer was final.[24]

The professional organizations with which Miss Nutting had been associated were reluctant to remove her name from their rolls. Aware that her poor health and retirement meant reduced income, a number of them conferred honorary membership upon her. The Faculty Women's Club, which she had worked so hard to organize in her early years at Teachers College, made it known that she would pay no more dues and that she was welcome to use its facilities as long as she lived. In 1934 the NLNE conferred honorary membership upon her. Effie Taylor, president of the league and an old Hopkins student, wrote:

> Nothing which the League of Nursing Education has in its power to confer, can in even the smallest measure express to you the esteem and the deep affection in which you are held by the nurses who have had

[21] Subsequently Edith Ware's notes proved invaluable to Ethel Johns and Blanche Pfefferkorn in writing *The Johns Hopkins Hospital School of Nursing*, sponsored by The Johns Hopkins Nurses Alumnae Association, Inc., and published by The Johns Hopkins Press in 1954.

[22] Adelaide Nutting, "A Message for Teachers College Nurses Alumnae Dinner," October 13, 1939, MAN Papers.

[23] Adelaide Nutting (New York) to Mildred Adkins (New York), March 13, 1934, *ibid.*

[24] Mildred Adkins (New York) to Adelaide Nutting (New York), March 20 and April 17, 1934; Adelaide Nutting (New York) to Mildred Adkins (New York), April 26, 1934; and Mildred Adkins (New York) to Adelaide Nutting (New York), May 10, 1934; *ibid.*

the honor to be associated with you in the building up of our beloved profession.

You have been the torch which has shown the way and we are eager to follow on.[25]

In 1935 Miss Taylor was saddened to learn that Miss Nutting would not be present at the meeting to read her paper.[26] At the fourth annual meeting of Collegiate Schools of Nursing at Catholic University, Washington, D.C., on January 21 and 22, 1934, Miss Taylor as secretary presented a recommendation that Adelaide Nutting and Annie Warburton Goodrich, dean emeritus, Yale University School of Nursing, be made honorary members.[27]

Miss Nutting's awareness that she would not accomplish all her goals and that the time was coming when she would not be able to look after herself was frustrating. In June, 1937, Teachers College closed the dining rooms on the eighth floors of Whittier and Lowell, where for twenty-one years she had taken most of her meals. Food service would be confined to the Dodge Hall cafeteria. Adelaide wrote her sister, "This frail old body is now wondering how it will stand a distant dining room."[28]

Miss Nutting had always rented her apartment during the summer school session, and in 1937 she stayed at Briarcliff Manor until it was nearly time for school to open in the fall. For years she had rented two rooms to students during the school year. Miss Stewart was careful to send her tenants from the Nursing Department who would bring in food and serve it to her if she did not feel up to going to the dining room.

Adelaide weathered the stifling heat of the summer of 1938 until the close of summer school, when Isabel took her to Old Greenwich, Connecticut, where there were cool sea breezes, and stayed with her for ten days. There was no elevator, the place was expensive, and she was so lonely after Isabel left that Katharine Fisher drove out, brought her back to New York, and found someone to cook her meals.[29] The

[25] Effie J. Taylor (New York) to Adelaide Nutting (New York), May 26, 1934, ibid.

[26] Effie J. Taylor (New Haven, Conn.) to Adelaide Nutting (New York), May 23, 1935, ibid.

[27] Report of The Fourth Annual Convention of the Association of Collegiate Schools of Nursing, Catholic University, Washington, D.C., January 21–22, 1934, p. 4.

[28] Adelaide Nutting (New York) to Armine N. Gosling (Bermuda), May 28, 1937, MAN Papers.

[29] Adelaide Nutting (New York) to Armine N. Gosling (Bermuda), September 7, 1938, ibid.

hour-and-a-half drive from Connecticut was so exhausting that Adelaide wondered if she should not find another place to live, and she began making inquiries about homes for the aged.[30]

Again Armine invited her to move to Bermuda and "to lay aside her prejudices against this little island." She told her to bring her books, whatever furniture she wished, a desk for her room, rugs and household linen, to let her friends arrange for the sale of her things, and to come to "Step-A-Side" as soon as possible.[31] Adelaide replied at once, thanking her sister, but saying she had decided not to go to Bermuda.[32] Lavinia Dock wrote from the family farm in Pennsylvania, where she had long since retired with her four sisters, suggesting as alternatives a nursing home or an old ladies' home. She told Adelaide about a friend who was very happy in a lovely Episcopal home in Philadelphia, but warned her that she herself "would not be able to stand the old tabbies and pussycats."[33]

Adelaide decided to continue living in the apartment that had been her home for so many years. She enjoyed the companionship of the young nurses Isabel Stewart selected to share the apartment with her: Jessie Black, a bright Scottish girl who had come to America to take her training at Johns Hopkins; Helen Bunge and Peggy Hart from Canada; and Florence Hixon; all of whom eventually became nursing leaders in their own right.

In 1944, on the occasion of its fiftieth anniversary, the NLNE created the Mary Adelaide Nutting Award, which from time to time would be conferred upon leaders and organizations for their outstanding contributions to nursing education. The award was intended not only to honor Miss Nutting but to recognize and encourage leadership in nursing education and to stimulate scholarly investigation and research in the field. The silver medal, honoring individuals, and the bronze plaque, for organizations, were designed by Malvina Hoffman, a renowned sculptor. One side bore a profile likeness of Miss Nutting and the other the lamp of knowledge. It was a stirring moment when the Award Committee presented the medal and plaque to the league and announced that Adelaide Nutting herself would be the first recipient. On April 27, in a simple ceremony attended by a few close

[30] Alice Snyder (New York) to Adelaide Nutting (New York), December 9, 1938, ibid.

[31] Armine N. Gosling (Bermuda) to Adelaide Nutting (New York), September 2, 1938, ibid.

[32] Adelaide Nutting (New York) to Armine N. Gosling (Bermuda), September 12, 1938, ibid.

[33] Lavinia Dock (Fayetteville) to Adelaide Nutting (New York), October 22, [1939], ibid.

friends, Stella Goostray, president of the league, presented the award to Miss Nutting in her apartment. No other awards were made until after World War II.[34] The award brought numerous letters of congratulation. Seeing the notice in the morning *Tribune*, Dean Russell wrote: "I rejoice not only in your great accomplishment but in the fact that you beat out a new path and had pleasure in doing it. Surely the world has followed that path to your door."[35] J. Norris Myers, manager and editor in chief of Macmillan Company, wrote:

> I received a thrill from reading in the New York *Times* last week the account of the presentation to you of the newly established medal which is so well deserved by you. My mind could not help running back over those years to those days when you were building nursing education so splendidly in Baltimore and New York and particularly to the broad sympathy and advice through which you helped a struggling young publisher to establish a nursing textbook literature of which I hope you too can be proud.[36]

In July and early August, 1944, Miss Nutting was ill in St. Luke's Hospital, but after a few days at home she rallied and was up and about again, visiting with her housekeeper, Rachel Brooks, reading professional journals, catching up on her correspondence, and planning for the future. She had not given up hope for the Johns Hopkins Endowment, the Isabel Hampton Robb Memorial Fund, the biography of Mrs. Robb, or the Florence Nightingale book. In 1941 she had found time and strength to write an introduction to the new, one-volume edition of Sir Edward Cook's *Life of Florence Nightingale*. Of this, J. Norris Meyers had written:

> It is beautifully done with that masterly English which I have long known to flow from your pen. . . . There is also . . . deep significance in the junction in the one volume of the names of Florence Nightingale in Europe and of Adelaide Nutting in the America she has served so well.[37]

[34] *New York Times*, May 5, 1944, p. 4. Subsequent awards of medals have been made to Isabel Stewart (1946), Annie Goodrich (1949), Mary M. Roberts (1949), Hon. Frances Payne Bolton (1951), Stella Goostray (1955); plaques have been awarded to the International Council of Nurses (1947) and The Maternity Center Association (1951).

[35] James E. Russell (Trenton, N.J.) to Adelaide Nutting (New York), [May, 1944], MAN Papers.

[36] J. Norris Myers (New York) to Adelaide Nutting (New York), May 8, 1944, *ibid.*

[37] J. Norris Myers (New York) to Adelaide Nutting (New York), April 30, 1942, *ibid.*; Adelaide Nutting, Introduction to *Life of Florence Nightingale*, by Sir Edward Cook (New York: Macmillan, 1941).

Encouraging words from Dr. Meyers had always inspired Adelaide. She hoped her book on *The Mind of Florence Nightingale* would partake of Miss Nightingale's greatness, her courage, dedication, and determination; the verve and incisiveness of her reports, such as "Our Soldiers Enlist to Death in the Barracks" (1855), "How People May Live and Not Die in India" (1863), and "How Some People Have Lived and Not Died in India" (1873); and her dramatic use of charts and statistics. "The great ideal [Florence Nightingale] set before nurses," Miss Nutting wrote, "was first and foremost courage reaching heroic heights physical and spiritual, in lifting one's self to truly super-human effort in actual labor over the sick, moral courage in moving above paralyzing official military routine in order to protect her sick men."[38]

The longer Miss Nutting thought of the project, the more majestic its proportions became. She was humbled by her design and felt she had neither the ability nor the strength to carry out the plan. Thus she modified her original plan so that it embraced a series of essays by leading scholars and writers of the day on some phase of Miss Nightingale's life and character. She wanted the volume to be one of fact and inspiration. In his poem on the one hundredth anniversary of the birth of Florence Nightingale,[39] John Finley, editor of the *New York Times*, had caught the vision Adelaide wanted to bring to nurses. He now agreed to become co-editor of the book, and Macmillan accepted the arrangement whereby royalties would be paid to the Florence Nightingale International Foundation. Mr. Finley's health soon failed, however, and Adelaide was left to do the work alone. She especially wanted Dr. Harry Emerson Fosdick to write the article on Miss Nightingale as a religious thinker. After visiting with Miss Nutting several times, however, Dr. Emerson said he could not write the essay and suggested instead Dr. D. E. Bowie of the Union Theological Seminary. Dr. Bowie was interested, but he was in the midst of a translation of the Bible and died before he got around to the essay. Then World War II came, and a paper shortage led Macmillan to withdraw its offer of publication. After the war Adelaide turned her materials over to Isabel Stewart, telling her to do with them as she saw fit.[40]

Ever since her student days at Hopkins, Adelaide had been acquiring books—professional books, history books, fiction, and poetry. She had given the rare books on hospitals, nursing, and Florence

[38] Nutting, Introduction to *Life of Florence Nightingale*.
[39] John H. Finley, "Florence Nightingale," 1920, MAN Papers.
[40] Isabel Stewart, "Notes on *The Mind of Florence Nightingale*," *ibid.*

Nightingale to Teachers College some years before, to the Adelaide Nutting Historical Nursing Collection. As she grew older she realized it behooved her to dispose of her books while she could, lest the time should come when she would not be able to give them to those who would truly appreciate them. On December 16, 1938, she sent 175 books to the Hopkins Nurses Library in Baltimore, and the following January she sent 47 more. She had a set of Shakespeare rebound before sending it in 1940. With this consignment of books she also sent her copy of the picture *The Book Hunter* for the Nurses Library.[41]

In April, 1940, Adelaide sent the Nurses Library of St. Luke's Hospital, New York, a parcel of books which included five volumes by Lytton Strachey, Nijensky's *Nijensky*, T. R. Lawrence's *Seven Pillars of Wisdom* and *Revolt in the Desert*, and books on interior decoration, furniture, sculpture, and travel.[42] In January, 1941, John French, librarian at The Johns Hopkins University, acknowledged the receipt of "40 miscellaneous volumes on Byron, Shelley, etc.," and the following month her "generous gift" of 95 steel engravings from Finden's *Life and Works of Lord Byron*.[43] Adelaide also had a large collection of little books (reprints in small type) that could easily be tucked into a coat pocket or handbag and read while waiting in an office or station, a train or bus. Some of these she gave to former students or friends. The two she especially prized had been given to her by Dr. Osler, and she sent them to Elsie Lawler, along with the large brass tray Etha Klosz had brought her some years before from India. "It has long hung high on the walls of this living room. During her [Mrs. Klosz] recent visit here I told her I would like to send it to you for any use you might like to make of it but coming as a gift from her to you."[44]

From year to year the circle of Adelaide Nutting's friends grew smaller. Rachel Bonner, first matron of Johns Hopkins Hospital, died

---

[41] "Gifts of books," *ibid*. Miss Nutting kept a record of the books she sent to institutions and a folder of acknowledgments. Usually she inquired if a library needed certain books before dispatching a parcel. Entries as early as 1929 record the gifts of rare editions to the library of Columbia University, and the folder of acknowledgments contains a number of the elaborate certificates then sent to donors.

[42] Helen Olandt (New York) to Adelaide Nutting (New York), May 3, 1940; and C. W. Munger (New York) to Adelaide Nutting (New York), May 3, 1940; *ibid*.

[43] John French (Baltimore) to Adelaide Nutting (New York), January 27 and February 27, 1941, *ibid*.

[44] Adelaide Nutting (New York) to Elsie Lawler (Baltimore), June 20, 1939, *ibid*.

in January, 1934, and Dr. Welch passed away in April of that year.[45] Mrs. Jenkins and Jane Addams died in 1935, Clara Noyes in June, 1936, Carolyn Gray in December, 1938, and Adelaide's sister-in-law Claire, the widow of her brother Jim, in November, 1938. Adelaide worried a great deal about Lillian Wald, who was not well. She had given up her place as head worker at the Henry Street Settlement in 1933 and four years later had resigned from its Board of Directors and retired to her country home, "House-on-the-Pond," at Saugatuck, near Westport, Connecticut. Miss Wald was greatly disturbed over the situation of the Jews in Germany, and in 1936 Lavinia Dock wrote Adelaide that she often wished Lillian could go before the situation got worse, as she feared it would.[46]

The loss of so many friends brought solemn thoughts to Adelaide and her family. She wrote her nephew Harold Nutting what she would like to have done in the event of her death. Bruce's wife, Lu, had written to ask if she wanted a burial plot in Waterloo. Adelaide replied: "First, there will be nothing to bring any member of my family here after my death since there will be nothing to be done. I have arranged to be cremated and if there is any service it will be brief." In her will she was leaving a small amount to each of her nephews and nieces and the remainder to her sister. She feared that, if she were sick for a long period, there might not be anything for anyone. She assured her nephew that Isabel Stewart and Dr. Benjamin Andrews of the College faculty would look after everything.[47]

Reading had always been one of Adelaide's greatest pleasures. She might economize on clothes, travel, and other entertainment, but books and magazines were as essential to her mind as food was to her

---

[45] William Henry Welch was born in Norfolk, Conn., on April 8, 1850; he died in Baltimore, Md., on April 30, 1934. After receiving the M.D. degree from Columbia University in 1875, he interned at Bellevue Hospital in 1875 and 1876. He studied abroad with Pasteur, Koch, Lister, and others from 1876 to 1878, and in 1879 returned to Bellevue to practice and teach. In 1884 he was invited to join the first faculty of The Johns Hopkins University School of Medicine, but returned to Europe to study before going to Baltimore. Dr. Welch served as dean of the Hopkins medical faculty from 1893 to 1908; he then taught pathology until 1916, when he was appointed the first director of the Hopkins School of Hygiene. He was elected president of the American Medical Association in 1911. In 1926 he became professor of the history of medicine and director of The Johns Hopkins Institute of Medicine. On his eightieth birthday Dr. Welch was honored by simultaneous dinners across the nation. He never married. For further details, see Simon and J. T. Flexner, *William Henry Welch and the Heroic Age of Medicine* (New York: Macmillan, 1941); *Baltimore Sun*, May 1, 1934.

[46] Lavinia Dock (Fayetteville, Pa.) to Adelaide Nutting (New York), March 29, 1936, MAN Papers.

[47] Adelaide Nutting (New York) to Harold Nutting (Ottawa), February 20, 1939, *ibid.*

body. Long after her retirement she continued to subscribe not only to nursing periodicals but to *The New Republic*, *Atlantic Monthly*, *Harper's Monthly*, the *Manchester Guardian Weekly* (England), and the *Saturday Review of Literature*. She remained an inveterate clipper. She constantly exchanged papers, books, and opinions with her sister. "The papers are full of the Ethiopian trouble," she wrote in July, 1935, in reference to some marked copies she was sending Armine. "Somewhere I feel in my bones that Mussolini is rushing to his doom, which I would not mind if it did not mean also an awful time for our beloved Italy." About Germany and England, she was uncertain, but she sent Armine all her copies of the *Manchester Guardian*, which to her made the British position "quite clear."[48]

Adelaide tried to keep abreast of the times and alert to events on the local, state, national, and international scene. She never took out American naturalization papers, however, for, to her, patriotism transcended the lines of nationality. She once wrote:

> This whole world is God's beautiful world and we are first of all his children and only in a secondary sense, Americans or Canadians, or British, or any other race. . . . some day the mad ambition to dominate which is a form of insanity, wherever it is found, will be curbed.[49]

She followed the war in Europe in the papers and on the radio. "Over everything hangs the sombre cloud of war," she wrote Jessie Black,

> and no one can wholly escape its shadow, yet it must be a constant comfort to you, as it is to some of us here, to see how superbly the British are facing every aspect of the situation. And what a sad picture is our last view of Chamberlain, leaving behind him only memories of the most tragic failure in the history of British Statesmen.[50]

Adelaide was appalled by the Nazis' treatment of Jews in Germany, and when word came of Lillian Wald's death on September 1, 1940, she rejoiced with Lavinia Dock that Lillian had been spared the sadness and horror of the atrocities committed.

Of all Adelaide Nutting's many interests, The Johns Hopkins Hospital School of Nursing was her abiding concern. It was her alma mater, and to it she professed an undying loyalty. She had long desired to see it become a collegiate school, an integral part of The Johns Hopkins University. When Elsie Lawler retired in 1940, and

[48] Adelaide Nutting (Ogunquit, Maine) to Armine N. Gosling (Bermuda), July 19, 1935, *ibid.*
[49] "Miscellaneous Notes," *ibid.*
[50] Adelaide Nutting (New York) to Jessie Black, [Baltimore], September 3, 1940, *ibid.*

Anna Dryden Wolf was chosen to succeed her, Adelaide's hopes rose again for the future of Hopkins. Having received the bachelor's degree from Goucher College before training at Hopkins, and later having earned the master's degree from Teachers College, Anna Wolf brought to her new job experience that included teaching at the Vassar Training Camp and administrative positions in Peking, China, the University of Chicago, the New York Hospital, and the New York Hospital School of Nursing.[51] She took over her administrative duties with high hopes and true vision, and Adelaide Nutting observed approvingly from afar. Within six months the staff had been reorganized, and a clear-cut statement of faculty status, responsibilities, and prerogatives similar to those of faculties in institutions of higher education had been mutually agreed upon. Students were given the opportunity to form a student association and thus to create the channels for a cooperative working relationship between students and faculty. The students adopted an honor code and published a handbook, The Dome, which was designed to inform the students of what they should expect from the school and what the school might expect from them.[52]

Vigorous and widespread recruitment programs were launched by The Johns Hopkins Hospital School of Nursing and other nursing schools during the latter part of 1941 as a part of the national defense effort. Then came the bombing of Pearl Harbor, and the nation was again at war.

From her apartment in Emerson Hall, Adelaide kept informed of developments on the nursing front. Directives from the Procurement and Assignment Service of the War Manpower Commission defined the professional services that would be allocated to patients in hospitals. Surgeon General Thomas Parran declared nursing a strategic defense skill of which there was a serious shortage. At his request, two hospital units were organized at Johns Hopkins in 1942, and, of the sixty nurses who went overseas with General Hospital No. 18 and General Hospital No. 118, twenty-three were in teaching positions. By June, 1941, an additional seventy-one had joined the Army and Navy Nurse corps. Fortunately, the recruitment program was a success; 195 students were admitted in 1942 as compared to 101 in 1941 and 82 in 1940. To Adelaide's great satisfaction, 40 percent of the 195 students entering Johns Hopkins in 1942 held degrees, a slightly higher percentage than that for the preceding decade.

[51] Johns and Pfefferkorn, The Johns Hopkins Hospital School of Nursing, p. 245.
[52] Ibid., p. 247.

Adelaide believed the nursing profession was better prepared this time. The experience of World War I would serve as a guide, and there were still a few leaders from that time, such as Mary Beard, former president of the NOPHN and chairman of the Subcommittee on Public Health Nursing of the General Medical Board Committee on Nursing, who now gave of her wisdom and talents as director of the American Red Cross Nursing Service, and Isabel Stewart, who had done the arduous spade work for Miss Nutting's committee.

The retreat from Dunkirk and the Battle of Britain were only days away when the ANA, NLNE, and NOPHN met in Philadelphia on May 12, 1940. Telegrams were sent to President Franklin D. Roosevelt, offering the organizations' services to the country in the event they should be needed. Urged on by Isabel Stewart, in late July Julia C. Stimson, president of the ANA, called together representatives of five national nursing organizations, the American Red Cross Nursing Service, and federal agencies immediately concerned with nursing services.[53] Mary Beard's terse statement, "I have no words to tell you how serious I think this thing is going to be," stirred the group to action, and before the day ended the Nursing Council of National Defense had been organized and its functions in determining the role of nurses and nursing in national defense and in unifying the nursing activities related to it had been broadly outlined.[54]

The meeting reminded Isabel Stewart of that Sunday in 1917 when Miss Nutting had called together nursing's leaders in New York City, where plans for the National Emergency Council on Nursing were launched. Again a survey of nursing resources was conducted, this time through the U.S. Public Health Service and the American Red Cross, and 75 percent of the nurses responded enthusiastically. Of the 300,000 active nurses, 100,000 unmarried nurses under the age of forty would become eligible for military service if they passed the physical examination; of the inactive nurses, 25,000 were available for full-time service.[55]

The American Red Cross and the National Council on Nursing

[53] Originally represented on the council were the nursing member agencies: the ANA, NLNE, and NOPHN, the Association of Collegiate Schools of Nursing, the National Association of Colored Graduate Nurses, and the nursing service agencies, which included the Nursing Service of the American Red Cross, the Federal Children's Bureau, the U.S. Army Nurse Corps, the U.S. Navy Nurse Corps, the Division of State Relations and the Division of Hospitals of the U.S. Public Health Service, the Nursing Service of the U.S. Veterans' Administration, and the Nursing Service of the Department of Indian Affairs. See Roberts, *American Nursing*, pp. 303–4.

[54] *Ibid.*, p. 305.
[55] *Ibid.*, p. 306.

were progressing with their mutually agreed-upon programs for national defense nursing when, almost a year after Pearl Harbor, the Council of National Defense created a third agency, the Government's Subcommittee on Nursing.[56] Its functions, like those of the Nursing Council of National Defense, were to analyze the nation's military and civilian need for professional nursing services, to make plans for meeting the need, and, when necessary, to cooperate with the nursing services of the Allied nations.

The training of nurse's aides by the Red Cross, which had caused such concern in World War I, came up again. This time the aides were to prove an important national resource. After a year's study, the Red Cross outlined a new course and set up training programs for the aides. When the Office of Civil Defense was created, plans were included for the training of aides, but the American Red Cross volunteered to speed up its program and to prepare the 100,000 aides the Office of Civil Defense regarded as necessary, on condition that only those aides who were approved upon completion of the eighty-hour Red Cross course be assigned to duty.[57] In two years this seemingly impossible goal was attained under the leadership of Mrs. Walter Lippmann. The Red Cross also offered courses in home nursing which nearly half a million persons completed by the end of 1942. Many of the aides worked as volunteers. Somewhat reluctantly the nursing profession conceded that professional nurses could not perform all the services required by a nation at war. The Government's Subcommittee on Nursing set up quotas for nursing students: 50,000 in 1941 and 55,000 in 1942.[58]

During World War II there was no army school for training nurses, but the Bolton Cadet Nurse Corps Act, passed on July 1, 1943, provided a strong incentive for high-school graduates to enter nursing schools and "join the proud profession." The new legislation offered student nurses a free education, indoor and outdoor uniforms, and a monthly stipend for thirty months, while participating institutions were provided maintenance for students for the first nine months, tuition fees throughout the program, and financial assistance in expanding residential and educational facilities. Between July, 1943, and October 15, 1945, almost 170,000 cadets entered the 1,125 nursing schools participating in the program, and 124,000 had graduated

[56] The official title was The Subcommittee on Nursing of the Health and Medical Committee of the Office of Defense Health and Medical Service. There were five other subcommittees. *Ibid.*

[57] *Ibid.*, p. 308.

[58] *Ibid.*, p. 359.

by the time the program was terminated in 1948; in addition, 10,309 graduate nurses took concentrated postgraduate courses at fifty-seven universities.[59]

The valiant services rendered the nation by nurses during the war cheered Miss Nutting. Isabel Stewart, soon to retire, pointed out to her the long list of Teachers College nursing alumnae doing important work for the War Council, the United States Public Health Service, the Red Cross, in veterans' hospitals, the Army Nurse Corps, the Navy Nurse Corps, the Cadet Nurse Corps, preclinical summer programs modeled after the Vassar Camp, in heading the nursing services of hospitals and public health agencies all over the country, and in holding office in professional organizations. Daring to raise educational standards in the face of wartime emergencies, Anna Wolf announced in 1944 that in 1946 only students with baccalaureate degrees would be admitted to the Hopkins Training School.[60]

The war years were difficult for Miss Nutting. For some time she had been concerned about Arthur Gosling, once her favorite nephew. He was well educated and brilliant, but had succumbed to the weakness for drinking which had been the undoing of his grandfather Vespasion Nutting and his uncle Arthur Nutting. Medical science had been unable to help him, and he had returned to his mother's home in Bermuda. Anxiety over his condition, the events in Europe, and the well-being of her nephews on the front lines weighed heavily upon Adelaide. Then, on December 15, 1942, a cablegram from Bermuda brought news of the death of her sister, the last remaining member of her immediate family.[61]

Armine Gosling had not been well for some time, but Adelaide's own health and the war had prevented her from going to Bermuda. Until the war interfered with communications, they had corresponded weekly. Adelaide pondered a memorial to her sister. When Armine's husband, Gilbert Gosling, had died in 1931, Adelaide had encouraged her sister to write the story of their life together, and of his work as a civic leader and mayor of St. John's. Armine, too, had given of herself to Newfoundland, first as a teacher, then as a leader in the church and community, in the prevention of cruelty to animals, and in the movement for woman suffrage. Later, she and her son, Ambrose, had

[59] Ibid., pp. 383–92.
[60] Johns and Pfefferkorn, The Johns Hopkins School of Nursing, p. 382. During 1946 and 1947 all entrants to The Johns Hopkins School of Nursing had earned bachelor's degrees, but in 1948 the school reverted to the minimum requirement of a high-school diploma.
[61] Armine G. Campbell (Bermuda) to Adelaide Nutting (New York), December 15, 1942, MAN Papers.

helped to establish the Gosling Public Library in St. John's in memory of Gilbert Gosling. Adelaide thought perhaps a companion volume to the one Armine had written about Gilbert would be appropriate. She could not do it herself, but she planned to mention the matter to Armine's daughter, Armine Campbell, who wrote very well.

After Armine's death, Adelaide felt she had no one; her nieces and nephews were far away living their own lives. She turned to Isabel Stewart, as she had been doing unconsciously for years. Isabel had been her student, then her successor at Teachers College, and for years she had helped her in small ways, selecting students to live in her rooms, bring her meals up from the cafeteria, and make her a cup of tea, and seeing that she got to the doctor, the dentist, or the dressmaker. When it became burdensome for her to fill out the income tax forms, pay the rent, the housekeeper, and the other bills that came in, Adelaide turned over her dwindling bank account to Isabel and gave her the power of attorney.[62]

In April, 1944, Miss Nutting finally got around to rewriting her will. She had little money to bequeath. She had always given liberally to charity, professional organizations, and needy relatives, the amount depending on the cause and the state of her bank account. After sending a "substantial" check to her nephew Harold Nutting on the occasion of his wedding, her sister-in-law Claire had written, "I am afraid you are going to land yourself in the poor house, you are so generous."[63] Adelaide had lived frugally so that she might have the joy of giving. A bequest from Mrs. Jenkins years before had been carefully invested, against an illness or other mishap, and she now proposed to distribute any that remained of it among her five nephews and two nieces, her housekeeper, Rachel Brooks, Isabel Stewart, and Benjamin Andrews. She bequeathed her royalties to Isabel and her books to the Historical Collection at Teachers College. The residue of her property, if any, was to be divided, with one-third going to the Teachers College Division of Nursing Education for the Adelaide Nutting Historical Collection, one-third to The Johns Hopkins Hospital School of Nursing for the completion of the *Life of Isabel Hampton Robb* or, if it had been completed, to purchase books for the School of Nursing Historical Collection, and one-third to the International Council of Nurses as a memorial to Lavinia Dock. Her jewelry was to be divided

[62] Isabel Stewart, "Confidential Information on M. A. Nutting, August, 1945," compiled for Miss Nutting's relatives in the event of death while Miss Stewart was in London. *Ibid.*

[63] Claire Nutting (Ottawa) to Adelaide Nutting (New York), December 19, 1919, *ibid.*

among friends. She requested that her body be cremated and that her ashes be taken to Canada and buried beside her mother. Isabel Stewart, Katharine Fisher, and Benjamin Andrews were named as executors.[64]

Adelaide was now eighty-six years old and growing more frail each year. She no longer had the strength to leave the apartment in the heat of summer, and it seemed a long time since she had been able to go with a friend for a quiet walk through Morningside Park. Even on days when she felt especially strong she did not dare to venture out alone: it was difficult to find the way home. Visits from friends both roused and tired her. Birthdays and holidays still brought messages of love and gratitude and gifts of fruit, candy, red roses, and her favorite, white violets.

In the fall of 1947, Adelaide could no longer receive the care she required in her apartment, and friends arranged for her to be taken to the country branch of the New York Hospital. With an almost child-like trust she accepted their dictum. For over a year she lived on, slowly declining, but to the end of consciousness she maintained the dignity and gracious manner so characteristic of her.

Within a month of her ninetieth birthday Adelaide Nutting passed away in her sleep on Sunday evening, October 3, 1948. On Tuesday her funeral was held in St. Paul's Chapel, Columbia University. She had always said she did not want flowers at her funeral, but they were sent by the Nutting nieces and nephews, the Teachers College Division of Nursing Education, The Johns Hopkins Hospital Alumnae Association, the Florence Nightingale International Foundation, the National League of Nursing Education, and the American Red Cross. Chaplain Knox, an old friend of Miss Nutting, came out of retirement to conduct the impressive Anglican service. The Columbia choir sang her favorite hymns, and her casket was covered with a blue pall bearing the insignia of Columbia University.[65]

A great university thus honored a great teacher, a scholar, and a humanitarian.

[64] "Will of Mary Adelaide Nutting, April 19, 1944," ibid.

[65] Isabel Stewart (New York) to members of the family of Mary Adelaide Nutting, October 7, 1948, ibid. From the George Washington Bridge, high above the Hudson, Adelaide Nutting's ashes were released to the sea.

Afterword

In the years since the death of Adelaide Nutting, phenomenal strides have been made in nursing, nursing education, and nursing administration. Some of these advances she anticipated and labored for; others have gone beyond the range of her vision.

In 1968, 72,348 students graduated from the various nursing programs in the United States: 30,833, or 42 percent from 1,191 practical or vocational nursing programs; 6,213, or 9 percent from the 330 associate-degree or junior-college programs; 28,197, or 39 percent, from the 728 diploma programs open to high-school graduates and largely under the aegis of hospitals; and 7,145 or 10 percent, from the 235 baccalaureate programs under the control of universities and colleges. In 1968–69, in universities offering post-baccalaureate programs, 4,018 students were working toward master's degrees and 258 toward doctorates. In 1968, master's degrees were conferred on 1,615 students and doctorates on 23.[1] In 1958 only two universities had doctoral programs; by 1968 there were six. Over the years an increasing number of nurses with baccalaureate or advanced nursing preparation have entered positions in teaching, administration, and research, but not enough to fill the increasing number of administrative and educational posts created by the expanding health and hospitalization services to meet the needs of a rapidly rising population.

In 1952, after a joint study of structure and function, six national nursing organizations—the NLNE, the NOPHN, the National Association of Colored Graduate Nurses, the Association of Collegiate Schools of Nursing, and the American Association of Industrial Nurses—arrived at a historic decision. They agreed that there should be one organization which offered membership to graduate registered nurses only, and another to serve nurses, non-nurses, schools of nurs-

[1] *Nursing Outlook*, September, 1969, pp. 76–79; *Facts About Nursing, 1965– 66*, p. 7.

ing, and nursing services; they also agreed that membership in the International Council of Nurses should continue to be maintained through the ANA, since the status and usefulness of the council had been enhanced by the establishment of an official relationship with the World Health Organization in 1948. As a result of their deliberations the NLNE, the NOPHN, and the Association of Collegiate Schools of Nursing combined to form the National League of Nursing (NLN); the new league's goals were to foster the improvement of hospital, industrial, public health, and other organized nursing services, as well as nursing education, through the coordinated action of nurses, allied professional groups, citizens agencies, and schools. When the league's final report on structure was presented, the American Association of Industrial Nurses decided to withdraw from the proposed union; the National Association of Colored Graduate Nurses had already been absorbed by the ANA.

Structural changes within the ANA provided "diversity within unity" through seven administrative units: (1) educational administrators, (2) general duty, (3) industrial nursing, (4) institutional nursing service, (5) private duty, (6) public health, and (7) special groups. At the same time, the American Journal of Nursing Company accepted responsibility for two new periodicals—*Nursing Outlook*, which absorbed *Public Health Nursing* and became the official journal of the NLN, and *Nursing Research*, launched in 1952 by the Association of Collegiate Schools of Nursing prior to its merger with the NLN. In 1950, national nursing headquarters were established in New York, with the Journal Company and the nursing organizations occupying adjoining offices. Today the headquarters of the ANA, the NLN, and the Journal Company occupy two floors at 10 Columbus Circle.[2]

Although in the past two decades generous support from private agencies, such as the W. K. Kellogg Foundation, Rockefeller Foundation, Julius Rosenwald Fund, Commonwealth Fund, Russell Sage Foundation, Carnegie Foundation, and Milbank Memorial Fund, has underwritten hundreds of nursing research studies, publications, experimental programs, and institutes, has provided scholarships, and has aided teaching programs in various nursing schools, more is needed if nurses are to keep abreast of the problems created by greater longevity and a rising birth rate.

Federal agencies—especially the U.S. Public Health Service, which acquired a stake in nursing education through the Cadet Nurse Program—have exercised a profound influence on the development of

[2] Mary M. Roberts, *American Nursing: History and Interpretation* (New York: Macmillan, 1954), pp. 575–85.

nursing research and nursing services of all types. The Division of Nursing Resources was set up within the Bureau of Medical Services in 1949 to develop methods of increasing the supply of nurses. With the establishment of the Department of Health, Education, and Welfare in 1953 and the reorganization of the Public Health Service in 1960, the Division of Nursing and the Division of Nursing Resources were brought together within the Bureau of State Services.[3]

In 1961, recognizing that nursing is an essential element in health care and that the major problems confronting the nursing profession could best be solved with the help of constructive public understanding and support, the surgeon general of the Public Health Service appointed a group of consultants to advise him on nursing needs and to identify the appropriate role of the federal government in securing adequate nursing services for the nation.[4] Nursing leaders were well represented in the group and were able to bring to the conferences the weight of careful studies conducted in graduate schools, such as Teachers College, and by the American Nurses Foundation, which had been established by the ANA in 1955 to support research in nursing and to sponsor special projects. Between 1950 and 1955 the ANA alone invested $400,000 in nursing studies.[5] The nursing profession had finally come of age.

The consultants proceeded to develop a blueprint for action based on a population increase of 30,000,000 by 1970. Eight hundred fifty thousand professional nurses would be needed to provide safe, therapeutically effective, and efficient services, but, believing that the acceleration in numbers of nurses had to be safeguarded by sound education if quantitative and qualitative improvements in nursing care were to be attained, the consultants set 680,000 practicing professional nurses as a feasible goal for 1970. To meet this goal, schools of nursing would have to produce 53,000 graduates a year by 1969. The consultants also anticipated the need for 350,000 licensed practical nurses by 1970, but, because the federal support programs for practical-nurse education already in existence offered assurances that this number could be reached, the group concentrated its efforts on programs for expanding schools of nursing and on recruitment programs, both of which would increase the number of nurses prepared to teach, super-

[3] Leo W. Simmons and Virginia Henderson, *Nursing Research: A Survey and Assessment* (New York: Appleton-Century-Crofts, 1964), pp. 105–17.

[4] Surgeon General's Consultant Group on Nursing, *Toward Quality Nursing: Needs and Goals* (Washington, D.C.: U.S. Public Health Service, 1963), p. xiii.

[5] *Ibid.*, p. 54.

vise, and fill other positions of leadership. The consultants urged that federal funds be appropriated to meet these needs.[6]

Subsequently Congress passed the Health Professions Act of 1963 (P.L. 88-129), the Nurse Training Act of 1964 (P.L. 88-581), and the Health Professional Educational Assistance Act Amendment of 1965 (P.L. 89-581), all of which had been actively advanced by the NLN and the ANA. The Nurse Training Act authorized a program of grants to build and renovate schools of nursing; established a program to help collegiate schools of nursing strengthen and improve their training programs, to help diploma schools meet the rising costs of increased enrollment, and to expand the existing facilities for the advanced training of professional nurses; and established a loan system which would enable many talented but needy students to undertake training for a career in nursing. Under the Health Professions Educational Assistance Act Amendment of 1965, the NLN became the nation's approved accrediting agency for all nursing education programs seeking funds under the Nurse Training Act.[7]

The progress made in nursing during the past two decades would have brought Adelaide Nutting satisfaction and joy, especially the inclusion of the behavioral sciences in nursing education; the many nursing studies of care for the newborn, the aged, cardiac patients, the mentally retarded, alcoholics, and rehabilitees; and the remarkable development in nursing literature, both books and periodicals. The new international index of 125 nursing periodicals would have been a special delight.[8]

The nursing profession and nursing education have advanced far from Miss Nutting's student days at Johns Hopkins, when Clara Weeks's *Textbook on Nursing*, Florence Nightingale's *Notes*, and the monthly magazine *Hospital and Trained Nurse* constituted the bulk of nursing literature, and far from the time when nurses reached into their own slender purses to underwrite the hospital economics course at Teachers College.

On September 4, 1964, at the signing of the Nurse Training Act in the Rose Garden of the White House in the presence of members of Congress and leaders of nursing, President Lyndon B. Johnson paid

    [6] *Ibid.*

    [7] Lyndon B. Johnson, "Remarks of the President at Signing of HR 11241—An Act to Amend Public Service Act to Increase the Opportunities for Training Professional Nursing Personnel," September 4, 1964, on file in the Department of Nursing Education Archives, Teachers College.

    [8] The *International Nursing Index* is published quarterly by the American Journal of Nursing Company in cooperation with the National Library of Medicine. The first issue appeared in the spring of 1966.

high tribute to the courageous and dedicated women who had served humanity as nurses throughout the nation's history. "Today's nurse," he said, "must be both humanitarian and scientist. Her great compassion must be matched by much greater competence."[9]

Years before Adelaide Nutting had written, "Compassion may provide the motive but knowledge is our only working power."[10]

[9] Johnson, "Remarks of the President."
[10] M. Adelaide Nutting, "Greeting,' Annual Convention of the New York State Nurses Association, the New York State League for Nursing Education, and the New York State Organization for Public Health Nursing, New York, October 27–28, 1925, MAN Papers.

Bibliography

Writings of Adelaide Nutting

Books

Nutting, M. Adelaide, and Dock, Lavinia L.

1907–
12. *A History of Nursing.* 4 vols. New York: G. P. Putnam's Sons.

1911. Geschiste der Krankenflege. Translated by Agnes Karll. Vol. 1. Berlin: Dietrich Reimer.

Nutting, Adelaide

1912. *Educational Status of Nursing.* U.S. Bureau of Education Bulletin no. 7. Washington, D.C.

1926. *"A Sound Economic Basis for Schools of Nursing" and Other Addresses.* New York: G. P. Putnam's Sons. Cited below as *SEB.*

Articles

Nutting, M. Adelaide

1891. "A Case of Typhoid Fever." *Trained Nurse and Hospital Review,* March, p. 121.

1896. "Statistical Report of Working Hours in the Nurse Training Schools of the United States." *Annual Report,* American Society of Superintendents of Training Schools for Nurses, p. 31. (Also printed in *Trained Nurse,* May, 1896.)

1897. "Address of the President." *Ibid.,* p. 5.

1900. "Studies of Social Conditions." *Ibid.,* p. 68.

"Non-payment System, Johns Hopkins Hospital, Report no. 5." *Ibid.,* p. 24.

1901. "The Preliminary Education of Nurses." *American Journal of Nursing,* March. (Reprinted in *SEB*).

"The Preliminary Course." *The Johns Hopkins Nurses Alumnae Magazine,* December, p. 8.

1902. "Progress in the Hospital." *Ibid.,* March, p. 40.

"Education of Nurses." *American Journal of Nursing,* pp. 799–804. (Also printed in American Society of Superintendents of Training Schools for Nurses, *Annual Report,* 1902, p. 15.)

1903. "Report of the Preparatory Work of Nurses." *American Journal of Nursing,* January, pp. 272–73.

371

"A Word about Training School Libraries, with a Short List of Texts and Reference Books." *Ibid.*, April, pp. 534–36.

"Our Relations to the National Council of Women." *Ibid.*, June, pp. 900–901.

"Work of the Johns Hopkins Alumnae." *Ibid.*, November, p. 104.

"Maryland State Association Organized." *The Johns Hopkins Nurses Alumnae Magazine*, December, pp. 140–43.

1904. "Tuberculosis Exposition, Baltimore." *American Journal of Nursing*, April, pp. 497–98.

"Visiting Nurses in the Homes of Tubercular Patients." *Ibid.*, pp. 500–506.

"State Reciprocity." *Ibid.*, May, pp. 779–85.

"School for Social Workers." *Ibid.*, June, pp. 679–81.

"Report of the Training School." *The Johns Hopkins Nurses Alumnae Magazine*, June, pp. 78–80.

"Suggestions for Educational Standards for State Registration." *Ibid.*, August, pp. 117–32.

"The Home and Its Relation to the Prevention of Disease." *American Journal of Nursing*, September, pp. 913–24.

"Suggestions for Educational Standards for State Registration." *Ibid.*, October, p. 13.

1905. "Some Results of Preparatory Instruction." *Annual Report*, American Society of Superintendents of Training Schools for Nurses, p. 63. (Reprinted in June, 1905, pp. 585–99, and in *SEB*.)

"American Federation of Nurses." *American Journal of Nursing*, July, pp. 653–56.

"Graduating Address." *The Johns Hopkins Nurses Alumnae Magazine*, August, pp. 99–104.

1906. "Visiting Nurses for Tuberculosis." *Charities*, April, pp. 51–55.

"Graduating Address." *The Johns Hopkins Nurses Alumnae Magazine*, August, pp. 121–29.

1907. "Course in Hospital Economics at Teachers College." *American Journal of Nursing*, November, pp. 125–26; January, 1908, p. 279; and October, 1909, pp. 27–30.

1910. Review of *Visiting Nurse in the United States*, by Ysabella Waters. Survey, February 12, pp. 725–26.

"Social Service of the District Nurse." *Household Arts Review*, April, pp. 8–15.

"Nursing and Health." *Public Health Nurses Quarterly*, April, pp. 10–13.

"Address of the President." *Annual Report*, American Society of Superintendents of Training Schools for Nurses, p. 16.

"Brief Account of the Course in Hospital Economics." *Teachers College Record*, May, pp. 1–6.

"The Educational Work of Isabel Hampton Robb." *The Johns Hopkins Nurses Alumnae Magazine*, June, p. 48.

"Nursing Conventions and the Nightingale Anniversary." *Survey*, June 4, pp. 363–64.

"Isabel Hampton Robb: Her Work in Organizations and Education." *American Journal of Nursing*, October, pp. 19–25.

"General Problems in Administrative Work." *Journal of Home Economics*, November, pp. 477–80.

1911. "Address of the President." *Annual Report*, American Society of Superintendents of Training Schools for Nurses, p. 18.

1912. "Nursing and Public Health." *Boston Medical and Surgical Journal*, March 14, pp. 401–5.

"Nursing and Its Opportunities." *Household Arts Review*, May, pp. 1–7.

1913. "Work of the Department of Nursing and Health, Teachers College." *Public Health Nurses Quarterly*, January, pp. 87–91.

"The Nurse as an Educator." *American Journal of Nursing*, September, pp. 927–37.

1914. "How Can We Attract Suitable Applicants to Our Training Schools?" *Ibid.*, May, pp. 601–10.

"Hospital Trustees and the Training School." *Modern Hospital*, July, pp. 57–59. (Also printed in *Annual Report*, American Society of Superintendents of Training Schools for Nurses, 1914, p. 85, and in *SEB*.)

"Responsibility of Trustees." *Public Health Nurses Quarterly*, July, pp. 42–51.

"Training of the Psychopathic Nurse." *Boston Medical and Surgical Journal*, September 24, pp. 473–76.

"The Work of The Johns Hopkins School for Nurses." *The Johns Hopkins Hospital Bulletin*, December, pp. 359–63. (Also printed in *The Johns Hopkins Nurses Alumnae Magazine*, January, 1915, pp. 6–18.)

1915. "The Visiting Housekeeper." *Journal of Home Economics*, April, pp. 167–69.

1916. "A Sounder Economic Basis for Training Schools for Nurses." *American Journal of Nursing*, January, p. 310. (Also printed in *Teachers College Record*, January, 1916, pp. 68–78, and in *SEB*.)

"Education of Nurses for the Home and the Community." *Modern Hospital*, March, pp. 196–200.

"Some Ideas in Training School Work." *Annual Report*, National League of Nursing Education, p. 291. (Reprinted in *SEB*.)

1917. "Obligations of Opportunity." *Teachers College Record*, March, pp. 122–33.

"War and Nursing Education." *Vassar Quarterly*, July, pp. 259–61.

"Statement of Purposes and Plans, Committee on Nursing, General Medical Board, Council of National Defense." *Public Health Nurses Quarterly*, October, pp. 325–26.

1918. "Nursing as It Relates to the War: The Council of Defense." *American Journal of Nursing*, May, pp. 1074–75. (Also printed in *Annual Report*, National League of Nursing Education, 1918, p. 246.)

"How the Nursing Profession is Trying to Meet Problems Arising Out of the War." *Annual Report*, National League of Nursing Education, p. 124.

"Relation of the War Program to Nursing." *Modern Hospital*, October, pp. 338–42.

"Apprenticeship to Duty." *American Journal of Nursing*, December, pp. 159–68. (Reprinted in *SEB*.)

1919. "Relation of the War Program to Nursing in Civil War Hospitals." *Teachers College Record*, January, pp. 66–78.

1920. "Twenty Years of Nursing in Teachers College." *Teachers College Record*, September, pp. 322–36. (Reprinted in *SEB*.)

"Outlook in Nursing." *The Public Health Nurse*, September, pp. 754–65. (Also printed in *Modern Hospital*, September, 1920, pp. 209–13, and in *SEB*.)

1921. "Again the Call to Duty." *American Journal of Nursing*, March, pp. 360–65.

1923. "Thirty Years of Progress in Nursing." *Annual Report*, National League of Nursing Education, June, p. 101. (Also printed in *American Journal of Nursing*, September, 1923, pp. 1027–35 and in *SEB*.)

"Developments in Teaching Since 1873." *Annual Report*, National League of Nursing Education, June, p. 231. (Reprinted in *SEB*.)

"How to Educate the Nurse and at the Same Time Properly Care for the Patient," *Modern Hospital*, September, pp. 305–10.

1927. "Florence Nightingale as a Statistician." *The Public Health Nurse*, May, pp. 207–9.

"The Endowment of Nursing Education." *The ICN*, July, pp. 169–76.

1928. "In Salutation." *Teachers College Nursing Education Bulletin*, January, p. 1.

1929. "The Future of Nursing." *American Journal of Nursing*, p. 903.

"The Future." *The Nursing Journal of India*, November, pp. 278–86.

1930. "The Future in Nursing Education." *World Health*, January–March, pp. 59–65.

1931. "Past, Present, and Future of Nursing." *American Journal of Nursing*, December, pp. 1389–91.

1935. "Thoughts on Our Seventy-fifth Anniversary." *Annual Report*, National League of Nursing Education, June, p. 92.

1936. "Clara Dutton Noyes," *The Johns Hopkins Nurses Alumnae Magazine*, July, pp. 163–66.

Pamphlets and Reprints

Nutting, M. Adelaide

1896. "A Statistical Report of Working Hours in Training Schools." *Annual Report*, American Society of Superintendents of Training Schools.

1907. "Educational and Professional Position of Nurses." Chapter 8 of the *Report of the U.S. Commissioner of Education, 1906*. Washington, D.C.: Government Printing Office.

1910. *Bibliography of Florence Nightingale's Writings*. New York: By the author.

1917. *Relation of Hospital and Training School Organization to the Curriculum*. National League of Nursing Education Bulletin no. 3. Reprinted from National League of Nursing Education, Committee on Education, *Standard Curriculum for Schools of Nursing* (New York: National League of Nursing Education, 1917).

1920. *A Sounder Economic Basis for Training Schools for Nurses*. National League of Nursing Education Bulletin no. 6.

1927. "Some Essential Conditions in the Education of Nurses." Reprinted from National League of Nursing Education, Committee on Education, *A Curriculum for Schools of Nursing* (New York: National League of Nursing Education, 1927).

1929. "Introduction" to *Pioneers of Nursing in Canada*, by History of Nursing Society, School for Graduate Nurses. Montreal: McGill University Press, 1929.

Manuscripts

Nutting, M. Adelaide

n.d. Biographical notes: "Notes on Family History," "Notes on Peasleys and Nuttings," "Notes for Story of Life." MAN Papers.

"How the College Can Help in the Training of Nurses." *Ibid.*

1908. "Opportunity of the Teacher in the Prevention of Tuberculosis." Address delivered at the Anti-Tuberculosis Convention, St. John's, Newfoundland, July. *Ibid.*

1919. "Jane Delano." *Ibid.*

n.d. "Mind of Florence Nightingale." Notes for a projected book. *Ibid.*

"Notes on Mrs. Isabel Hampton Robb." *Ibid.*

1929. "Notes on a Possible International Memorial to Florence Nightingale."

n.d. "Tribute to Anna Maxwell." *Ibid.*

Special Collections

Adelaide Nutting Historical Nursing Collections. Teachers College, Columbia University, New York, N.Y.

Committee on Nursing, General Medical Board, Council of Defense. National Archives, Washington, D.C.: Correspondence, reports, and minutes of meetings.

Department of Nursing Education Archives. Teachers College, Columbia University, New York, N.Y.: historical materials relating to hospital economics course, 1899–1906, 1906–10; Department of Nursing and Health, 1910–22;

Department of Nursing Education, 1922–38; Division of Nursing Education, 1938–42; course announcements, 1899–1965; federal projects; lists of graduates; departmental publications; public health studies; staff meetings; student organizations and activities.

The Johns Hopkins Hospital School of Nursing Archives, The Johns Hopkins Hospital, Baltimore, Md.: applications for admission; "Book of the Teresians," 1906–25; circulars of information; daybooks; code of ethics, 1896; monthly reports to superintendents; records of alumnae; minutes of trustees' meetings; annual reports of superintendents; schedule of lectures, 1889–90 and 1890–91; Dr. Howard Kelly's Nightingale collection; scrapbooks; clippings; Adelaide Nutting's notebooks kept as a student, 1889–91; photographs; Edith Ware's notes for an Isabel Robb biography.

Marshall Papers. Helen Marshall, 960 Tanglewood Dr., Rt. 3, Mountain Home, Arkansas 72653: correspondence relative to Adelaide Nutting and members of her family: letters from former Hopkins and Teachers College students and from friends of Miss Nutting.

Mary Adelaide Nutting Papers (MAN Papers). Teachers College, Columbia University, New York, N.Y.: extensive files of miscellaneous materials; letters to and from nursing students, nursing leaders, physicans, personal friends; class lectures; course outlines, scrapbooks, reports, clippings; 114 letters exchanged between members of the Nutting family, 1882–1946, typed and bound, as well as originals.

Nutting–Stewart Correspondence (MAN–IMS Correspondence). Department of Nursing Education, Teachers College, Columbia University, New York, N.Y.: Letters exchanged between Mary Adelaide Nutting and Isabel Maitland Stewart, 1909–42.

Roberts Papers. Library, American Journal of Nursing Company, 10 Columbus Circle, New York, N.Y.: letters to Mary Roberts from nursing leaders relating to the *American Journal of Nursing*.

Stewart, Isabel M. *Oral History*. 2 vols. New York: Columbia University, Butler Library, 1958.

Stewart Papers (IMS Papers). Department of Nursing Education Archives, Teachers College, Columbia University, New York, N.Y.: letters to and from Isabel Maitland Stewart, 1908–58, lectures, articles, reports, and committee reports.

Wald Papers. New York Public Library, New York, N.Y.: letters to and from Lillian Wald relative to nursing and public health.

Books relating to Canadian Background

Bradley, A. G. *Colonial Americans in Exile*. New York: E. P. Dutton, 1932.

Foster, George C., and Noyes, John P. *Sketches of Some Early Shefford Pioneers*. Waterloo, Quebec: Waterloo Public Library, 1905.

Gosling, Armine Nutting. *William Gilbert Gosling: A Tribute*. New York: Guild Press, 1935.

Grant, George Munro. *Picturesque Canada*. Toronto: Belden Bros., 1882.

Thomas, C. *History of Shefford*. Montreal: Lovell Printing & Publishing Co., 1877.

Works relating to Nurses, Nursing, and Nursing Education

Books

Abdellah, Faye, *et al. Patient-Centered Approach to Nursing.* New York: Macmillan, 1960.

Austin, Anne L. *History of Nursing Source Book.* New York: G. P. Putnam's Sons, 1957.

Billings, John Shaw, and Hurd, Henry M. *Hospitals, Dispensaries, Nursing.* International Conference of Charities, Corrections, and Philanthropy, Chicago, June 12–17, 1893. Baltimore: The Johns Hopkins Press, 1894.

Brainard, Annie M. *The Evolution of Public Health Nursing.* Philadelphia: W. B. Saunders, 1922.

Breay, Margaret, and Fenwick, Ethel Gordon. *History of the International Council of Nurses.* Geneva: International Council of Nurses, 1931.

Breckenridge, Mary. *Wide Neighborhoods: A Study of the Frontier Nursing Service.* New York: Harper & Bros., 1952.

Brown, Esther Lucille. *Nursing for the Future.* New York: Russell Sage Foundation, 1948.

Chayer, Mary Ella. *Nursing in Modern Society.* New York: G. P. Putnam's Sons, 1947.

Chesney, Alan M. *The Johns Hopkins Hospital and The Johns Hopkins University School of Medicine: A Chronicle.* 3 vols. Baltimore: The Johns Hopkins Press, 1943–63.

Cook, Edward Tyas. *Life of Florence Nightingale.* New York: Macmillan, 1942.

Cremin, Lawrence A.; Shannon, David A.; and Townsend, Mary Evelyn. *A History of Teachers College, Columbia University.* New York: Columbia University Press, 1954.

Cullen, Thomas Stephen. *Henry Mills Hurd: First Superintendent of Johns Hopkins Hospital.* Baltimore: The Johns Hopkins Press, 1920.

Cushing, Harvey. *Sir William Osler.* 2 vols. Oxford: Clarendom Press, 1925.

Dock, Lavinia L. *Short Papers on Nursing Subjects.* New York: M. Louise Longeway, 1900.

————. *Hygiene and Morality.* New York: G. P. Putnam's Sons, 1910.

————. *Materia Medica for Nurses.* New York: G. P. Putnam's Sons, 1890.

Dock, Lavinia L., and Stewart, Isabel M. *A Short History of Nursing.* New York: G. P. Putnam's Sons, 1938.

Duffus, R. L. *Lillian Wald: Neighbor and Crusader.* New York: Macmillan, 1938.

Frank, Sister Charles Marie. *Historical Development of Nursing.* Philadelphia: W. B. Saunders, 1953.

French, John C. *A History of the University Founded by Johns Hopkins.* Baltimore: The Johns Hopkins Press, 1946.

Gelinas, Agnes. *Nursing and Nursing Education.* New York: Commonwealth Fund, 1946.

Gibbon, John Murray, and Mathewson, Mary S. *Three Centuries of Canadian Nursing.* New York: Macmillan, 1948.

Giles, Dorothy. *A Candle in Her Hand.* New York: G. P. Putnam's Sons, 1950.

Ginzberg, Eli, et al. *A Program for the Nursing Profession.* New York: Macmillan, 1948.

Goodnow, Minnie. *Nursing History.* Philadelphia: W. B. Saunders, 1953.

Goostray, Stella. *Fifty Years: A History of the School of Nursing, The Children's Hospital, Boston.* Boston: Children's Hospital Alumnae Association, 1940.

Graham, Abbie. *Grace H. Dodge: Merchant of Dreams.* New York: Woman's Press, 1926.

Gray, James. *Education for Nursing: History of the University of Minnesota School.* Minneapolis: University of Minnesota Press, 1960.

Hamley, H. R., and Uprichard, Muriel. *A Study of the Florence Nightingale International Foundation.* London: Grand Council of the International Council of Nurses, 1948.

Hampton, Isabel Adams. *Nursing: Its Principles and Practices.* Philadelphia: W. B. Saunders, 1893.

Hampton, Isabel A., et al. *Nursing of the Sick, 1893.* New York: McGraw-Hill, 1949.

Hurd, Henry. *Institutional Care of the Insane in the United States and Canada.* 4 vols. Baltimore: The Johns Hopkins Press, 1915–17.

Jamiesen, Elizabeth, and Sewell, Mary. *History of Nursing Notebook.* Philadelphia: J. B. Lippincott, 1956.

———. *Trends in Nursing History.* Philadephia: W. B. Saunders, 1934.

Jensen, Deborah MacLurg. *History and Trends of Professional Nursing.* St. Louis: C. V. Mosby, 1955.

Johns, Ethel, and Pfefferkorn, Blanche. *The Johns Hopkins Hospital School of Nursing, 1889–1949.* Baltimore: The Johns Hopkins Press, 1954.

Jordan, Helen Jamiesen. *Cornell University—New York School of Nursing, 1839–1949.* New York: Society of New York Hospitals, 1952.

Kernodle, Portia B., *The Red Cross Nurse in Action, 1882–1948.* New York: Harper & Bros., 1949.

Lambertsen, Eleanor. *Education for Nursing Leadership.* Philadelphia: J. B. Lippincott, 1958.

Lee, Eleanor. *History of the School of Nursing of the Presbyterian Hospital in New York, 1892–1942.* New York: Columbia Presbyterian Hospital, 1942.

Martin, Franklin Henry. *Joy of Living.* New York: Doubleday, 1933.

Munson, Helen W., and Stevens, Katherine. *Story of the National League of Nursing.* Philadelphia: W. B. Saunders, 1934.

Myers, Grace Whiting. *History of the Massachusetts General Hospital, June 1872 to December 1900.* Boston: Griffith-Stellings Press, 1929.

Nightingale, Florence. *Notes on Nursing.* Philadelphia: J. B. Lippincott, 1905.

Osler, William, *"Aequanimitas," with Other Addresses to Medical Students and Nurses.* Philadelphia: Blacton Sons Co., 1905.

Parsons, Sara E. *Nursing Problems and Obligations.* Boston: Whitcomb & Barrows, 1916.

Pavey, Agnes E. *Story of the Growth of Nursing as an Art, a Vocation, and a Profession.* London: Faber & Faber, 1953.

Richards, Linda. *Reminiscences of Linda Richards.* Philadelphia: J. B. Lippincott, 1949.

Riddle, Mary M. *Boston City Hospital Training School for Nurses.* Boston: City Hospital Alumnae Association, 1928.

Roberts, Mary M. *American Nursing: History and Interpretation.* New York: Macmillan, 1954.

Robb, Isabel Hampton. *"Educational Standards for Nurses," with Other Addresses on Nursing Subjects.* Cleveland: E. C. Koeckert, 1907.

———. *Nursing Ethics.* Cleveland: J. B. Savage, 189[?].

———. *Nursing Ethics for Hospital and Private Use.* Cleveland: E. C. Koechert, 1900.

Russell, James Earl. *Founding of Teachers College.* New York: Teachers College Bureau of Publications, 1937.

Sellew, Gladys, and Ebel, Sister M. Ethelreda. *History of Nursing and Its Current Status.* St. Louis: C. V. Mosby, 1956.

Seymer, Lucy Ridgely. *A General History of Nursing.* New York: Macmillan, 1954.

Shyrock, Richard H. *Development of Modern Medicine.* New York: Alfred A. Knopf, 1947.

———. *History of Nursing: An Interpretation of the Social and Medical Factors Involved.* Philadelphia: W. B. Saunders, 1959.

Simmons, Leo W., and Henderson, Virginia. *Nursing Research: A Survey and Assessment.* New York: Appleton-Century-Crofts, 1964.

Spalding, Eugenia Kennedy. *Professional Nursing Trends and Relationships.* Philadelphia: J. B. Lippincott, 1954.

Spalding, Eugenia Kennedy, and Notter, Lucille. *Professional Nursing.* Philadelphia: J. B. Lippincott, 1965.

Stewart, Isabel Maitland. *The Education of Nurses.* New York: Macmillan, 1943.

Stewart, Isabel M., and Austin, Anne L. *A History of Nursing from Ancient to Modern Times: A World View.* New York: G. P. Putnam's Sons, 1926.

Wald, Lillian. *House on Henry Street.* New York: Henry Holt, 1915.

———. *Windows on Henry Street.* Boston: Little, Brown & Co., 1933.

Weeks, Clara S. *Textbook on Nursing.* New York: D. Appleton, 1889.

Werminghaus, Esther A. *Annie W. Goodrich: Her Journey to Yale.* New York: Macmillan, 1950.

Woolsey, Abby Hosland. *A Century of Nursing.* New York: G. P. Putnam's Sons, 1950.

Articles

Banworth, Calista F. "Our Living Memorial: A Brief History of the Florence Nightingale International Foundation." *American Journal of Nursing,* May, 1940, pp. 491–97.

Beard, Richard Olding. "The Making of History in Nursing Education." *American Journal of Nursing*, April, 1922, p. 507.

———. "Report of the Rockefeller Foundation on Nursing Education: A Review and Critique." *American Journal of Nursing*, February, 1923, pp. 358–65; March, 1923, pp. 460–66; and April, 1923, pp. 550–54.

———. "The Social, Economic and Educational Status of the Nurse." *American Journal of Nursing*, August, 1920, pp. 874–962.

Cabot, Richard C. "Suggestions for Improvement of Training Schools for Nurses." *Boston Medical and Surgical Journal*, November, 1921, p. 567.

Carr, Ada M. "Early History of the Hospital and Training School." *The Johns Hopkins Nurses Alumnae Magazine*, June, 1909. Reprint.

Crandall, Ella Phillips. "National Organization for Public Health Nursing." *Modern Hospital*, February, 1917. Reprint.

Cullen, Mary Bartlett Dixon. "Reminiscences." *The Johns Hopkins Nurses Alumnae Magazine*, April, 1949, pp. 50–51.

Cunningham, Elizabeth V. "Education for Leadership, 1899–1959." *Nursing Outlook*, May, 1959. Reprint.

Dines, Alta. "Faithfully Yours, Adelaide Nutting, 1858–1948." *The Johns Hopkins Nurses Alumnae Magazine*, October, 1957, pp. 79–85.

Dock, Lavinia. "Foreign Notes." *Americal Journal of Nursing*, July, 1915, p. 847.

———. "My Recollections of Adelaide Nutting." *The Johns Hopkins Nurses Alumnae Magazine*, April, 1949, p. 49.

Dunbar, Virginia. "The Instructor of History of Nursing." *Nursing Outlook*, May, 1962, pp. 307–10.

Evans, Ernestine, "Adelaide Nutting." *The Woman Citizen*, June 27, 1925, pp. 9–11.

Flexner, Simon. "William Henry Welch." *Science*, November 5, 1920, p. 417.

Goodsell, Willystine. "Mary Adelaide Nutting: Educator and Builder." *Teachers College Record*, January, 1926, pp. 382–83.

Goostray, Stella. "Mary Adelaide Nutting." *American Journal of Nursing*, November, 1958, pp. 1524–29.

"Grading Committee Adopts Official Program." *Modern Hospital*, June, 1927. Reprint.

Gray, Carolyn E. "Yale Honors Miss Nutting." *Modern Hospital*, August, 1922, pp. 128–29.

Hurd, Henry M. "Florence Nightingale: A Force in Medicine." *The Johns Hopkins Nurses Alumnae Magazine*, May, 1910, p. 69.

———. "Relation of the General Hospital to the Training School for Nurses." *Boston Medical and Surgical Journal*, March 5, 1914, pp. 333–47.

———. "Relation of the Hospital to the Community." *Teachers College Record*, May, 1910, pp. 221–33.

"International Committee on Education." *British Journal of Nursing*, October, 1925, pp. 206–8.

"International Florence Nightingale Memorial." *League of Red Cross Societies, Review and Information Bulletin*, June, 1932, pp. 214–15.

"Isabel Robb Memorial Number." *The Johns Hopkins Nurses Alumnae Magazine,* June, 1910.

Jammé, Anna C. "Four Chiefs: A Reminiscence, 1897–1904." *The Johns Hopkins Nurses Alumnae Magazine,* April, 1938, pp. 65–67.

Larimore, Granville. "The Public Health Council: New York's Giant Stride in Public Health." *Health News,* May, 1963.

McGarvak, Eleanor. "Our Changing Attitudes toward Legislation for Nurse Registration." *Trained Nurse and Hospital Review,* April, 1938, pp. 396–403.

McVicar, Jessie Black. "Reminiscences of Mary Adelaide Nutting." *The Johns Hopkins Nurses Alumnae Magazine,* April, 1949, pp. 67–68.

"Mary Adelaide Nutting." *Indiana University Nurses Bulletin,* November 1, 1922, p. 1.

"Mary Adelaide Nutting Award," *American Journal of Nursing,* August, 1943, p. 762.

"Mary Adelaide Nutting Plaque." *American Journal of Nursing,* June, 1944, p. 587.

"Mary Adelaide Nutting as Known by Friends, Students, and Co-Workers." *American Journal of Nursing,* June, 1925, p. 445.

"Medical Women in the Army," *Hospital,* July 27, 1918, p. 658.

Moody, Selma. "Isabel Hampton Robb: Her Contribution to Nursing Education." *American Journal of Nursing,* October, 1938, pp. 1131–39.

Morrison, Jean. "Canadian Girls Nursing Uncle Sam." *The Canada Magazine,* August, 1922, pp. 322–24.

Nevins, Georgia. "My Friend, Mary Adelaide Nutting." *The Johns Hopkins Nurses Alumnae Magazine,* April, 1949, pp. 52–53.

North, Franklin H. "A New Profession for Women." *Century Magazine,* November, 1882, pp. 38–47.

Noyes, Clara D. "Mary Adelaide Nutting: Some Reminiscences." *Red Cross Courier,* June 15, 1925, pp. 13–14.

"One of the Most Useful Women in the World." *Everywoman's World,* September, 1923, p. 3.

"Our Honorable Member, Lavinia Dock, Pickets the White House." *American Journal of Nursing,* November, 1917.

Parsons, Sara E. "Educational Standards for Nursing, State Registration, and Training School Inspection." *Boston Medical and Surgical Journal,* April 9, 1914, pp. 574–75.

————. "Encouraging Signs in Nursing Education." *American Journal of Nursing,* January, 1915, p. 274.

————. "Personal Experience in Training School Organization." *American Journal of Nursing,* June, 1903, pp. 673–77.

"Passing of Florence Nightingale Home, 10 South Street, London." *British Journal of Nursing,* August, 1932.

Pfefferkorn, Blanche. "Nursing Organizations in the United States: Their Origin, Purpose, and Some of Their Results." *Modern Hospital,* February, 1917. Reprint.

"Random Memories of Mary Adelaide Nutting by Former Students." *The Johns Hopkins Nurses Alumnae Magazine*, April, 1958, pp. 38–43.

Robb, Isabel Hampton. "My Association with Illinois Training School." *Quarterly of the Illinois State Association of Graduate Nurses*, May, 1906.

Roberts, Mary M. "Julia Stimson, Col. U.S.A.N.C., 1881–1948." *American Journal of Nursing*, November, 1948, p. 675.

Russell, James Earl. "Thirtieth Anniversary Celebration of the Nursing Education Department, Teachers College." *Nursing Education Bulletin*, Winter, 1929/30, pp. 12–14.

Stewart, Isabel M. "Mary Adelaide Nutting: Educator, Historian, Internationalist." *International Nursing Bulletin*, Winter, 1948, pp. 13–14.

———. "Mary Adelaide Nutting's Philosophy of Nursing and Its Implications for the Future Development of The Johns Hopkins School of Nursing." *The Johns Hopkins Nurses Alumnae Magazine*, April, 1958, pp. 22–23.

———. "An Outline of the History of the Department of Nursing Education." *Teachers College Bulletin*, 17th ser., February, 1920.

———. "Problems in Nursing Education." *Teachers College Record*, May, 1910, pp. 183–202.

Stewart, Isabel M., and Nutting, M. Adelaide. "Educational Value of the Nurse in the Public School." *Ninth Yearbook of the National Society for the Study of Education*. Chicago: University of Chicago Press, 1910.

Taylor, Effie J. "Nursing in Relation to Higher Education." *The Johns Hopkins Nurses Alumnae Magazine*, April, 1958, pp. 28–30.

"Two Early American Schools of Nursing." *American Journal of Nursing*, October, 1948, pp. 611–15.

Van Blarcom, Carolyn C. "Miss Nutting Resigns." *Modern Hospital*, June, 1925, pp. 535–36.

Welch, William H. "Address to Graduates, The Johns Hopkins School of Nursing." *The Johns Hopkins Nurses Alumnae Magazine*, August, 1916, pp. 140–47.

"William Osler," *The Johns Hopkins Hospital Bulletin*, July, 1919, pp. 186–208.

Wolf, Anna D. "Recollections of Miss Nutting," *The Johns Hopkins Nurses Alumnae Magazine*, April, 1958, pp. 24–25.

Reports

American Society of Superintendents of Training Schools for Nurses. *Annual Reports*. Harrisburg, Pa.: Harrisburg Publishing Co., 1894–1949. The Society of Superintendents was known as the National League of Nursing Education from 1912 to 1952 and later became the National League of Nursing.

Burgess, May Ayres. *A Five Year Program for the Committee on the Grading of Nursing Schools*. New York: National League of Nursing Education, 1926.

———. *Nurses, Patients and Pocketbooks*. New York: National League of Nursing Education, 1928.

Committee on Structure of National Nursing Organizations. *New Horizons in Nursing*. New York: Macmillan, 1950.

Flexner, Abraham. *Medical Education in the United States and Canada.* Advancement of Teaching Bulletin no. 4. Boston: Merrymount Press, 1910.

Goldmark, Josephine. *Nursing and Nursing Education in the United States.* New York: Macmillan, 1923.

Martin, Franklin H. *Digest of Proceedings of the Medical Board, Council of National Defense, during World War I.* Washington, D.C.: Government Printing Office, 1934.

National Committee for Improvement of Nursing Services AAIN, ACSN, NACGN, NLNE, and NOPHN. *Nursing Schools at Mid-Century.* New York: The Committee, 1950.

National League of Nursing Education, Committee on Education. *The Case for Shorter Hours in Hospital Schools of Nursing.* National League of Nursing Education Bulletin no. 1. MAN Papers, n.d.

———. *A Curriculum for Schools of Nursing.* New York: The League, 1927.

———. *Curriculum Guide for Schools of Nursing.* New York: The League, 1937.

———. *Standard Curriculum for Schools of Nursing.* New York: The League, 1917.

———. Committee on Grading of Nursing Schools. *Nursing Schools Today and Tomorrow.* New York: The League, 1934.

———. Committee to Secure Rank for Nurses. *Victory.* National League of Nursing Education Bulletin no. 15. August 18, 1920, n.p.

"Organization Meeting of the Association of Collegiate Schools of Nursing, January 20, 21, 1933 [Teachers College, Columbia University]." Mimeographed. MAN Papers.

Palmer, Sophia F. "A Résumé of the Early History of the American Journal of Nursing." *Annual Report,* American Society of Superintendents of Training Schools for Nurses, 1904, pp. 82–84.

Proceedings of the Conference on Nursing Schools Connected with Colleges and Universities, Teachers College, January 21–25, 1928. MAN Papers.

Registered Nurses Association Registry Committee. "Report Submitted to the Board of Directors, September 30, 1927." MAN Papers.

Surgeon General's Consultant Group on Nursing. *Toward Quality Nursing: Needs and Goals.* Washington, D.C.: U.S. Public Health Service, 1963.

Pamphlets

American Journal of Nursing. *Story of the Journal.* New York: The Journal, 1950.

Memorial Meeting in Honor of William Henry Welch, University Club, May 22, 1934. Baltimore: University Club, 1935.

Osler, William. *Doctor and Nurse.* Address to the graduating class of The Johns Hopkins School for Nurses, 1891. Baltimore: Privately reprinted, 1963.

———. *Nurse and Patient.* Address to the graduating class of The Hopkins School for Nurses, 1897. Baltimore: John Murphy, 1897.

Stewart, Isabel Maitland. Introduction to *The Adelaide Nutting History of Nurs-*

ing Collection, Teachers College. New York: Teachers College Bureau of Publications, 1929.

The Training Camp for Nurses at Vassar College. An announcement. 1918.

Manuscripts

"East Harlem Nursing and Health Service: Historical Sketch." September 1, 1930. Department of Nursing Education Archives, Teachers College.

Fisher, Katharine. "Adelaide Nutting and Home Economics." MAN Papers.

Gunther, Emma. "Professor Adelaide Nutting in—Household Administration—Institution Administration." MAN Papers.

Miller, Amy P. "Short History of the Endowment Fund of The Johns Hopkins Nurses Alumnae Association." MAN Papers.

Mitchell, S. Weir. "The Ideal Nurse." Address to the graduating class of the New York Hospital Training School for Nurses, February 28, 1908. MAN Papers.

Specht, Florence. "Biography of Isabel Hampton Robb." MAN Papers.

Stewart, Isabel M. "History and Work of the Department of Nursing and Health, Teachers College." IMS Papers.

———. "I Remember." A notebook of the reminiscences of Adelaide Nutting and other nursing leaders begun a few months before Isabel Stewart's death in October, 1963. IMS Papers.

Newspapers

Baltimore Sun, 1889–1906.

New York Evening Post, 1925.

New York Times, 1900–1942.

The Thermometer, published by the Vassar Campers and Farmerettes, 1918–21.

Waterloo Advertiser, (Quebec, Canada), 1858–1930.

Index

THE JOHNS HOPKINS UNIVERSITY PRESS

This book was composed in Palatino text and Palatino and
Times Roman italic display type by the Monotype Composition Company from a design by Al Madairy. It was printed
by Universal Lithographers, Inc., on S. D. Warren's 60#
Sebago. The book was bound by L. H. Jenkins, Inc., in Hollis-
ton Roxite vellum finish cloth.